Partnerships in community mental health nursing and dementia care

Practice perspectives

Edited by John Keady, Charlotte L. Clarke and Sean Page

Open University Press

Open University Press
McGraw-Hill Education
McGraw-Hill House
Shoppenhangers Road
Maidenhead
Berkshire
England
SL6 2QL

email: enquiries@openup.co.uk
world wide web: www.openup.co.uk

and Two Penn Plaza, New York, NY 10121-2289, USA

First published 2007

A catalogue record of this book is available from the British Library

ISBN-10 0 335 21581 5 (pb) 0 335 21582 3 (hb)
ISBN-13 978 0 335 21581 2 (pb) 978 0 335 21582 3 (hb)

Library of Congress Cataloging-in-Publication Data
CIP data applied for

Typeset by RefineCatch Limited, Bungay, Suffolk
Printed in Poland by OZGraf S.A.
www.polskabook.pl

The *McGraw·Hill* Companies

£24.99

C 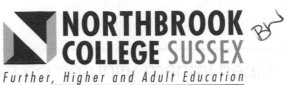 BW

Contents

PART ONE
Models of community support and practice values   5

List of figures

List of tables

Contributors

Trevor Adams teaches dementia care nursing at the European Institute of Health and Medical Sciences, University of Surrey. He has worked alongside people with dementia and their families in hospitals and the community. He has written extensively on dementia care in academic and professional journals and has co-edited three books on dementia care.

Susan Ashcroft-Simpson is Team Leader of the Admiral Nursing Service with the Manchester Mental Health and Social Care Trust. She is an RMN and has spent the majority of her career in dementia care where she has always found new challenges in the field. She has worked in continuing care and day hospital settings, a variety of management posts in which she was able to contribute to the development of new and innovative services and has worked as an Admiral Nurse for the past six years.

Caroline Baker works as a Care Services Director for Four Seasons Health Care and has worked with people with dementia for the past 17 years. Caroline is an RMN and has completed a post-graduate Diploma in Geriatric Medicine. Caroline continues to specialize in the field of Dementia Care and is an Approved DCM Trainer for Bradford Dementia Group. Caroline was Highly Commended in the Rising Star Award (*Nursing Times*) 2003.

Diane Beavis is currently employed as the Specialist Nurse for the Alzheimer's Medication Service in West Dorset (North Dorset Primary Care Trust). She is also actively involved in the Practice Development Unit (PDU) for the Mental Health Service for Older People and was the PDU leader from 2001 until 2004. The Practice Development Unit received full accreditation from Bournemouth University in May 2004.

Catherine Brannan developed her interest in working with people with dementia while supporting a client through the difficult end stage of care. She currently works as a Community Learning Disability Nurse in Edinburgh.

Dawn Brooker is Professor of Dementia Research and Practice at the Bradford Dementia Group, University of Bradford, UK. Dawn is a qualified clinical psychologist who has worked in a variety of clinical, academic and managerial posts in services for older people for the past 20 years.

Shane Burke is a research sociologist in St Patrick's Hospital, Dublin. He has a Master's degree in Applied Social Research from Trinity College, Dublin, and a BA in English and Sociology from University College, Dublin.

Suzanne Cahill is the Director of Dementia Services Information and Development Centre at St James's Hospital, Dublin, and Lecturer in Social Work and Social Policy in Trinity College, Dublin. She is also an Adjunct Associate Professor of Social Work and Social Policy at the University of Queensland.

Caroline Cantley was Professor of Dementia Care, Northumbria University, and Director of Dementia North, the regional dementia services development centre. Her professional background is in social work and she has worked as a manager in health and social services. She is editor of *A Handbook of Dementia Care* (Open University Press 2001).

Peter Caswell has worked in the mental health services for 24 years, during which time he has worked in a diverse range of nursing environments. He has been a community psychiatric nurse for the past 15 years and is currently based with an older adult community mental health team.

Charlotte L. Clarke is Professor of Nursing Practice Development Research, Northumbria University. Her research has covered a range of health and social care issues, with a particular focus on older people and dementia care. At present, she leads the British Academy-funded International Collaborative Research Network on Risk in Ageing Populations, which has projects running in South Africa, India, Australia, the USA and the UK.

Vivienne Davies-Quarrell is Director of Care Services at Kinmel Health Care, founder of Awareness Care and Education (ACE) in dementia services, and Associate Editor of *Signpost* journal of older people and mental health matters. Vivienne has a wealth of experience in service development and the provision of health and social care to older people, people with dementia and their carers in the independent sector. In 2004, she gained an award (highly commended) in the Queen's Nursing Institute Awards for Excellence and Innovation in Dementia Care Nursing; she is a 2005 Florence Nightingale Scholar.

Kenneth Day is an assistant clinical psychologist working for the Learning Disability Service in Lothian, Scotland. He is currently developing a training pack for assisting individuals who have relatives or friends who have dementia.

Kay de Vries' current position is a joint post with the Princess Alice Hospice, Esher, Surrey, and the European Institute of Health and Medical Sciences, University of Surrey, Guildford. These posts involve managing education at the hospice and leading the palliative care pathway for the MSc Advanced Practice at the University of Surrey.

Aine Farrell commenced her psychiatric nurse training in 1988 in St Patrick's Hospital, Dublin, and graduated with honours in 1991. She completed a six-month full-time course in gerontology in James Connolly Memorial Hospital, Blanchardstown, Dublin, in 1996. Since then, Aine has worked with the psychiatry of old age team in St Patrick's Hospital and presently holds the post of community mental health nurse.

Paula Gardiner, at the time of writing, was a community mental health nurse in Essex with a special interest in working with people with dementia and their families. Paula qualified in 1980 and has worked with older people in a variety of general and mental health settings. Paula now works as a mental health nurse practitioner within a general practice.

Sue Gunstone is a nurse lecturer in the School of Nursing and Midwifery at the University of Sheffield. She specializes in mental health nursing with a particular interest in psychosocial interventions in psychosis and older adult dementia care nursing. She teaches both pre-registration and post-basic students and is particularly keen to emphasize the rewards of working with people who experience dementia and their carers.

Philip Hardman gained his mental health nurse registration in 1988 after working as a nursing auxiliary. Currently, Philip works as professional and practice lead for nursing within Older Age Services, Manchester Mental Health and Social Care Trust, and in addition since September 2004, as a Lecturer with Manchester University, School of Nursing, Midwifery and Social Work.

Steve Iliffe has been an inner-city general practitioner since 1979, and is also Reader in General Practice at the Royal Free and UCL Medical School, London. He is co-director of the Centre for Ageing Populations Studies, a research group working on mental health in later life, health promotion and health risk assessment for older people, and service development for an ageing population.

Dee Jones began her early career as a nurse then went on to study and teach law. She is regional manager (North Wales) for Public Service Management Wales (PSMW), Welsh Assembly Government. Previously she was Research Fellow in the Research Institute for Enhancing Learning, University of Wales Bangor; in this post she taught health care law and conducted research in individual and organizational learning.

Gary and Linda Jones met on 17 June 1964, on a Saturday night in Chester and say it was love at first sight. They married in 1967 on 3 April at 2 p.m. in Ellesmere Port. Linda began to have problems with her memory while working as a bank official, a career she had pursued for 30 years. Gary worked for British Steel as a team leader and a couple of years after Linda left work he also took early retirement to look after Linda and he has continued to do so ever since. Linda says, 'He is my rock.' Both Linda and Gary are active in the local branch of the Alzheimer's Society, helping to raise awareness and funds. For the past 15 years they have worked with the MS Society organizing the annual Snowdon Mountain Challenge. Linda and Gary love mountain walking and holidaying in France.

John Keady previously worked as a community psychiatric nurse in a community dementia team in North West Wales before moving into teaching and research at the University of Wales, Bangor, in July 1993. He has maintained an active interest in dementia care and has recently taken up an appointment as Professor of Older People's Mental Health Nursing at the University of Manchester. John is founding and co-editor of *Dementia: The International Journal of Social Research and Practice*.

Cordelia Man-Yuk Kwok is a nurse specialist (psychogeriatric) at Kwai Chung Hospital, the Hong Kong Hospital Authority. Since 1994, she has worked in the first psychogeriatric team in Hong Kong. She has been an Executive Board Member and member of a Training Committee of the Hong Kong Alzheimer's Disease and Brain Failure Association, a Council Member of the Hong Kong College of Mental Health Nursing, and a visiting lecturer at the Hospital Authority Institute of Health Care and the University of Hong Kong.

Jenny Mackenzie is a Senior Lecturer in the Bradford Dementia Group, Division of Dementia Studies at the University of Bradford. She coordinates the MSc Dementia Care and has recently completed research which examined the support needs of family carers of people with dementia from Eastern European and South Asian communities.

Mike Nolan is Professor of Gerontological Nursing at the University of Sheffield and has worked with older people and their carers for over 25 years in a variety of clinical, educational and research roles. Mike has particular interests in promoting partnerships between practitioners, older people and their family carers in both community and care home settings.

Simon T. O'Donovan qualified as an RMN in 1984 and has specialized in the field of mental health services for older people for some 21 years. Simon is an Editor of the prestigious *Signpost to Older People and Mental Health Matters* journal – see www.signpostjournal.co.uk and has recently completed his Doctorate in Nursing, which focused on caregiving burden assessment. Simon is Clinical Director for the Mental Health Services for Older People Directorate and Consultant Nurse Older Vulnerable Adults for Cardiff and Vale NHS Trust.

Sean Page is Clinical Nurse Specialist Team Leader in the Manchester Memory Clinic (Manchester Mental Health and Social Care Trust). He has a pioneering nursing role with an equal focus upon activities related to assessment, diagnosis, non-medical prescribing and the provision of post-diagnostic counselling. In 2004, he won an NHS Innovations award for the introduction of a post-diagnostic counselling service for people with a dementia. Sean is also a Teaching Fellow at the University of Manchester where he lectures on the MSc in Dementia Care.

Emma Pritchard is a Consultant Admiral Nurse with Central and North West London Mental Health NHS Trust. She has specialized in working with older persons with mental health needs, particularly those with dementia, and their supporters and carers, throughout her nursing career. She is also an Associate Fellow with the Royal College of Nursing Practice Development Team.

Jan Reed qualified as a nurse in 1982 and was awarded her doctorate in nursing older people in 1989. She is currently co-editor of the *International Journal of Nursing Older People*, and has authored and edited several books, most recently one on appreciative inquiry as a research method.

Jeannie Robinson is a community mental health nurse working for Sheffield Care Trust (NHS) in an Older Adult Mental Health Team. She has worked with people with dementia and their carers since 1987, and assertive outreach and crisis prevention are an integral part of her work.

David Stanley is Chair in Social Care, a Director of the Centre for Care of Older People (research and practice development) and Head of the Division of Primary and Community Care in the School of Health, Community and Education Studies at Northumbria University, Newcastle upon Tyne, UK. He is immediate past Chair of the Joint Universities

Council for Public Administration, Social Policy and Social Work and is a founding editor of the *Journal of Social Work*.

Fiona Wilkie is currently a community learning disability nurse working for the Learning Disability Service in Edinburgh. She has had a special interest in the links between dementia and Down's syndrome for many years and has contributed to numerous training and educational resources.

Heather Wilkinson is a Senior Research Fellow, directing a programme of work on ageing and dementia, including a number of projects that focus on people with a learning disability. She is based in the Centre for Research on Families and Relationships, University of Edinburgh.

Kevin G. Wood is a Borough Manager/Senior Nurse in the Blaenau Gwent Community Mental Health Team (services for the older adult), Gwent Healthcare NHS Trust. Kevin qualified as a RMN in 1980 and was recently 'highly commended' by the Queen's Nursing Institute Award for Excellence and Innovation in Dementia Care.

Acknowledgements

We would like to acknowledge the contribution of a number of people without whom this book would not have been possible. First, we would like to thank the publisher of the text, especially Rachel Crookes and Rachel Gear, for having faith with the book and helping us, as Editors, to stay on course with its final production. Next, we would like to thank all contributors to the book for their selfless commitment to dementia care and in helping to fulfil the vision for the text. We hope that you will be pleased with the final product. Third, we extend the warmest 'thank you' to Nyree Hulme at the Centre for Health Related Research, School of Healthcare Sciences, University of Wales, Bangor, for her patience, good humour, database and word-processing skills and pivotal role in helping to keep the whole project on track. Finally, 'thank you' to Louise Davies at the School of Nursing, Midwifery and Social Work, University of Manchester, for helping us to pass the finishing post.

Foreword
Mike Nolan

The field of health and social care is constantly evolving and practice must change to reflect both policy initiatives and the new insights into the lives of service users and their family carers that research uncovers. Nowhere is this need more apparent than in dementia care. Practitioners are expected to be 'evidence-based', but with the many competing demands they face, they often struggle to find the latest evidence in a form that is accessible and which highlights for them the practical value of research and theory. Texts which reflect the appropriate balance between research, theory and practice are rare indeed.

One text that did realize this elusive goal was *Community Mental Health Nursing and Dementia Care: Practice Perspectives*, edited by John Keady, Charlotte L. Clarke and Trevor Adams, published in 2003. In the Foreword to that book, I suggested that its publication marked a watershed in the evolution of the CMHN role, and that it provided the impetus for a more inclusive way of working, based on forging creative partnerships between practitioners, people with dementia and their family carers.

It is therefore all the more pleasing to have been asked to write the Foreword for this companion volume, *Partnerships in Community Mental Health Nursing and Dementia Care: Practice Perspectives*. Together, the two texts comprise some 40 chapters addressing the wide-ranging challenges that practitioners face today. Their compass is truly impressive, bringing together contributions from over 50 authors, each recognized authorities in their field. Chapters in this companion volume expand the vision of the first and consider, among other things, such important topics as: legal and ethical issues; the experience of dementia in ethnic minority communities; nurse-prescribing and the CMHN; learning disability and dementia; and palliative care and dementia.

The 2003 book was the first to focus specifically on the role of the CMHN, and this new edition is most welcome. Taken together, the two books constitute a comprehensive and invaluable resource. Moreover, while their focus is on the contribution of the CMHN, there is much that will be of interest not only to practitioners from other disciplines, but also to all those committed to improving the quality of life of people with dementia and their family carers. I would commend them both to you as potentially seminal contributions to advancing practice and understanding in an ever more important and rapidly changing field.

Introduction
John Keady, Charlotte L. Clarke and Sean Page

Welcome to our second book and the companion volume to *Community Mental Health Nursing and Dementia Care: Practice Perspectives* (Keady, Clarke and Adams 2003). Our first book contained 18 chapters and 31 authors and was the first book of its kind to provide a cohesive and discursive account of community mental health nursing practice in dementia care. Moreover, as an editorial team on the first book, we made it an underpinning philosophy to include community mental health nurses (CMHNs) in the dissemination of their own practice and values, as this was the key to unlocking the role, evidence base and ethical/moral standpoint of the profession. As we said in the Introduction to the first book, CMHNs in dementia care must be able to 'define its [own] contribution to the care of people with dementia in a succinct and accessible way if it is to fully understand the contribution that can be made within a multi-disciplinary and inter-agency context' (Adams et al. 2003: xvii). This philosophy continues to drive the production of this second volume. Indeed, we have, arguably, strengthened the practice link in this companion text by including Sean Page, Clinical Nurse Specialist at the Manchester Memory Clinic and Teaching Fellow at the Post Graduate School of Nursing, University of Manchester, as one of the editorial team and main contributors to the book.

So why this second book? Well, primarily, and as we also noted in the Introduction to the first book, the first volume had some significant 'gaps' in its construction that may have inhibited a full appreciation of the CMHN role. These 'gaps', for instance, included the areas of assertive outreach, rural care, activity-based therapies, ethnic minority practice, the learning disability interface, health promotion/education, younger person services, care home working, assessing vulnerabily, engaging in end-stage care, legal implications of practice, and listening to user perspectives on the CMHN role. We also failed to accommodate views and experiences from other parts of the world, such as Ireland and Hong Kong, where CMHNs' work in dementia care remains integral to community-based provision for people with dementia and their families. As editors of this second volume, we are pleased to say that we have located contributors for each of these 'gaps' and have included discussion where more marginalized people with dementia may be located (such as in prison, homeless or seeking asylum), but where a literature base remains scarce and a CMHN role is still in its genesis, if anywhere at all.

In the four years since our first book appeared, the pace of change in the United Kingdom's (UK) health and social care policy has been breathtaking. To take but two examples, the publication of *Everybody's Business: Integrating Mental Health Services for Older Adults* (Department of Health 2005) provided telling insights into the need for inter-agency services and collaboration with service development underpinned by the following core values: to provide a person-centred approach; to improve people's quality of life; to meet patients' complex needs in a coordinated way; and to promote age equality. These values need to be integral to the vision of practice adopted by CMHNs. Similarly, opportunities to apply national benchmarking standards, such as those outlined in the *Essence of Care* document (NHS Modernisation Agency 2001) and its accompanying benchmarking tool (NHS Modernisation Agency 2003), have emerged to provide a context for CMHN work and a way of applying the vision to practice.

Additionally, in 2006, two reviews of mental health nursing have been published. In Scotland, this has taken the form of the Scottish Executive's (2006) review *Rights, Relationships and Recovery: The Report of the National Review of Mental Health Nursing in Scotland*, while the Department of Health (2006) has published the Chief Nursing Officers' review of Mental Health Nursing entitled *From Values to Action*. In Northern Ireland, at the time of writing (September 2006), the Bamford Review of Mental Health and Learning Disability is taking place and one of the interlinked reviews deals with 'Dementia and mental health conditions of older people' (www.rmhldni.gov.uk/ – accessed 28 September 2006). The implications of these reviews will have a significant influence upon the future direction and scope of practice for CMHNs in dementia care. It is important to point out, however, that mental health nursing, certainly in Scotland and England, is attempting to unify its approach to practice through the application of a 'recovery model' (Anthony 1993), an approach that is yet to be fully considered within dementia care nursing. We will return to this discussion in the final chapter to the book.

The structure of the book

This book is divided into three Parts, as follows:

1   Models of community support and practice values
2   Professional role and clinical work
3   Moving forward: changing and developing CMHN practice.

Part 1, 'Models of community support and practice values', contains seven chapters and places the work of CMHNs within a multi-professional and service context while looking to identify its unique contribution to both nursing and team working. The opening chapter is written by the three editors, led by Sean Page, and roughly uses a ten-year time-frame (1996–2006) to trace policy and practice development in health and social care and highlight the CMHN's role at each point in time. Chapter 2 is written by Steve Iliffe and presents a (practising) general practitioner's viewpoint on the role of the CMHN, focusing mainly upon the value and efficacy of the 'wrap-around' model as a tailored process of care. Within the service philosophy developed by Vivienne Davies-Quarrell as part of the ACE club in North Wales, Chapter 3 includes the contributions of Linda and Gary Jones, who, as service users, outline the importance of CMHNs working in collaboration in order to build a sense of purpose and well-being in their lives. Continuing this 'user' theme, in Chapter 4 Sue Gunstone and Jeannie Robinson draw upon their practice and local experience in Sheffield to outline steps for service user involvement in care pathways. Chapter 5 is written by Dee Jones and explores legal and ethical boundaries for CMHN practice; case study examples and expert commentary are integral to this chapter. In the penultimate chapter in Part 1, Jenny Mackenzie provides an authoritative commentary upon culture and identity in order to enlighten, and develop, a user–provider relationship that informs CMHN practice. The final chapter in this Part, Chapter 7, is written by Trevor Adams and Paula Gardiner and highlights the importance of relationships to the work of the CMHN and the need to develop negotiated plans of care with people with dementia and their families.

Similar to the structure of the first book, the 'hands-on' nature of Part 2 is deliberately designed to be its largest component. In this Part, entitled 'Professional role and clinical work', the editors have sought the contribution of practising CMHNs (and academics with strong practice links) in the UK, Eire and Hong Kong to help illustrate the richness, diversity and depth of CMHN activity. Each of the 12 chapters in Part 2 either confronts areas of CMHN practice in dementia care that were not featured in the first volume, or augments role dimensions that were addressed there. Chapter 8, written by Diane Beavis, reviews holistic practice in an early intervention rural community service – the Alzheimer's Medication Service, West Dorset, UK – while also exploring the CMHN's role in health education. Sean Page, in Chapter 9, develops his focus on memory clinic work from the first book and outlines the role of the CMHN in nurse prescribing; in so doing, Sean draws upon his own work as part of the Dementia Treatment Clinic in South Manchester to provide the theory–practice bridge. In Chapter 10, Aine Farrell, Suzanne Cahill and Shane Burke trace the history and development of the role of CMHN in Ireland from the 1960s and present the results of a survey of CMHNs in Ireland (N = 19) on their role and patterns of rural working. Chapter 11 changes direction a little and presents evaluative work undertaken by Jan Reed, Charlotte L. Clarke, Caroline Cantley and David Stanley in the North-east of England that focuses upon services for younger people with dementia delivered within a multi-disciplinary context. In their chapter, Jan Reed and her colleagues tease out the role of the CMHN within this team and spell out lessons for practice and service development. Drawing on an extensive literature and knowledge base, Simon T. O'Donovan, in Chapter 12, develops the notion of risk from the first book and applies concepts of vulnerable adults and effective risk management strategies to the abuse of people with dementia and the role of the multi-disciplinary team/CMHN. Next, in Chapter 13, Fiona Wilkie, Catherine Brannan, Kenneth Day and Heather Wilkinson address a much overlooked area of practice, the Community Learning Disability Nurse and a specialist focus on learning disabilities and dementia; in this chapter, the authors also discuss the process of diagnosing dementia in a person with a learning disability. Chapter 14 then draws upon the inspirational work of Kevin Wood in South Wales to highlight opportunities for CMHNs to augment cognitive models of intervention with people with dementia and their families with creative art approaches. In Chapter 15, Caroline Baker and Dawn Brooker demonstrate the power of Dementia Care Mapping as a tool for CMHNs to use in their interface with the care home sector and potential referrals of people with dementia labelled as 'challenging'. Chapter 16, by Caroline Cantley and Peter Caswell, describes an innovative pilot project undertaken in the Hull and East Riding Community Health NHS Trust to evaluate the role of the CMHN in an assertive outreach service for people with dementia. Here, the focus on time-limited, intensive interventions with those living with the most complex needs certainly chimes with current policy and practice rhetoric. In the next chapter, Chapter 17, Cordelia Man-Yuk Kwok and Philip Hardman take an international comparative approach to dementia care and illustrate CMHN practice from Manchester, UK, and Hong Kong, China. The penultimate chapter in Part 2, Chapter 18, is written by Kay de Vries and draws on data from her PhD study to describe the palliative care experience of people with Creutzfeldt-Jakob disease; the role of the CMHN in specifically addressed within this context of practice. Chapter 19, written by Sean Page and Philip Hardman, explores marginalized groups within the dementia care community, focusing on people with dementia in the prison service, who are homeless or who may find themselves as asylum seekers.

The third Part is entitled 'Moving forward: changing and developing CMHN practice' and consists of three chapters. Chapter 20, written by Emma Pritchard and Sue Ashcroft-Simpson, reviews the educational options that are ahead of CMHNs as they attempt to develop their specific area of professional interest; an example of portfolio development from the Admiral Nurse service is shared as a 'good practice' exemplar. The next chapter, Chapter 21, is written by one of the editors of the book, Charlotte L. Clarke, and explores the complex relationships and inter-relationships between practice communities (of which CMHNs are one) and people with dementia and their families. The final, brief, chapter of the book is written by the combined editors of the two volumes and presents a series of statements that pinpoint some of the challenges and opportunities facing CMHNs in dementia care as we move into the twenty-first century.

We hope that you will enjoy the book.

References

Adams, T., Keady, J. and Clarke, C. (2003) Introduction, in J. Keady, T. Adams and C. Clarke (eds) *Community Mental Health Nursing and Dementia Care: Practice Perspectives*. Maidenhead: Open University Press, pp. xvii–xxvii.

Anthony, W.A. (1993) Recovery from mental illness: the guiding vision of the mental health service system in the 1990's, *Psychosocial Rehabilitation Journal*, 16: 11–23.

Bamford Review of Mental Health and Learning Disability (2006) *Dementia and Mental Health Conditions of Older People*, www.rmhldni.gov.uk/ (accessed 28 September 2006).

Department of Health (2005) *Everybody's Business: Integrating Mental Health Services for Older Adults*. London: Department of Health.

Department of Health (2006) *From Values to Action: The Chief Nursing Officer's Review of Mental Health Nursing*. London: Department of Health.

Keady, J., Clarke, C.L. and Adams, T. (eds) (2003) *Community Mental Health Nursing and Dementia Care: Practice Perspectives*. Maidenhead: Open University Press.

NHS Modernisation Agency (2001) *Essence of Care*. London: NHS Modernisation Agency.

NHS Modernisation Agency (2003) *Essence of Care Guidance*. London: NHS Modernisation Agency.

Scottish Executive (2006) *Rights, Relationships and Recovery: The Report of the National Review of Mental Health Nursing in Scotland*. Edinburgh: Scottish Executive.

PART ONE

Models of community support and practice values

1

Models of community support for people with dementia

Where does the CMHN fit in?

Sean Page, John Keady and Charlotte L. Clarke

Introduction

> Most people with dementia live at home, this is where they want to live, this is where their families want them to live, and this is where the government wants them to live.
>
> (Graham 2003)

Community care has, in all meanings of the word, become big business. However, lengthening the time that people with dementia spend at home is not necessarily the most appropriate indicator of success or quality of life for all concerned. As an outcome, it fails to appreciate whether or not the person with dementia finds life organized around a 'care package' a satisfying experience, and sight may be lost of the fact that for many people with dementia, admission into a care home can be a positive choice and a rewarding experience. Despite these concerns, community care is 'here to stay' and this chapter explores some of the tension, issues and opportunities around its socio-political rise in importance in the health and social care field, its current provision and future profile. Allied to this exploration is an analysis of the role that the community mental health nurse (CMHN) can actively play in promoting quality of life for people with dementia, and their family networks as they make use of the available support services.

Community care: the changing landscape

The development of traditional asylums has its roots within the successful economic boom of the Victorian era, coupled with a desire to fund what was for the time an enlightened and humane approach towards the 'mentally ill'. This asylum tradition has meant that for the greater part of the twentieth century the provision of mental health care was dominated by institutionalization and institutional caring practice (Nolan 2003). From the 1960s onwards, this landscape began to change with less political enthusiasm to financially maintain the institutions and a growing perception that less expensive and more individualized options were available (Turner 2004). Plans were outlined in the early 1960s to restrict hospital services to providing only acute psychiatric care, while responsibility for continuing care (within a community model) would pass to the local authority (Ministry of Health 1963).

Supporting this process of change were evolving criticisms about the stigma of mental illness, the negative impact of 'institutional neurosis' and the neglect, abuse and inadequate care practices commonly associated with the mental hospital (Jones 1993). In coining the term, the 'old culture of dementia care', Kitwood (1997) later described and condemned the impact of such practices upon the very personhood of people with dementia living within these environments. Notwithstanding the impetus, and need, for services to be provided outside of the closed world of the asylum, it is clear that community care options have never been adequately funded. In alluding to this, the Griffiths Report (Department of Health 1988) offered the illuminating analogy that community care was 'Everyone's distant relative but nobody's baby.'

Following hot on the heels of this report, the *Caring for People* White Paper (Department of Health 1989) called for no further hospital closures until 'a funded community-based alternative was in place'. Paradoxically, there was no central provision of funding established to develop community services while asylums were sold and redeveloped. Through the mid to late 1980s market forces influenced the provision of community care and the private sector offered services at a lower cost than institutional care. The steep decline in National Health Service psychiatric bed numbers in the decade from 1982 was mirrored, and possibly exceeded, by an increase in provision within the private residential and nursing homes sector (Davidge et al. 1993).

Now, virtually all the 'traditional' mental hospitals have now closed with the long-stay residents having died, drifted into homelessness or more typically been absorbed into community-based care facilities. With this change the previous dominance of the institution has disappeared and been replaced by an overwhelming belief in the value of community care and support. Concerns are, however, being expressed that although this has largely been a positive and bloodless coup, vestiges of the old regime remain very much at the heart of care provision. For instance, Holloway (2004) collectively describes all community care provision as simply forming a 'virtual asylum' reflecting concerns that realizing the potential of person-centred care with the ideals of autonomy and empowerment is restrained by an old cultural resistance to, and fear of, change from those who deliver the care (Edwards 2004).

By clinging on to the ethos of the 'old' regime, it can be seen how the traditional model of community support (see Figure 1.1) influences the current landscape and prevents change from occurring. At the apex of the support pyramid are the two domains, *acute care* (crisis management) and the *frail older people* (dependency management), that attract the greater proportion of available resources.

While these are, indeed, deserving of attention, their dominance suffocates any attempt to intervene at an earlier stage to either prevent crisis or to improve the (mental) health and well-being of older people more generally. What emerges is the maintenance of stereotypes that in turn maintain an ageist agenda towards service provision. As an example, cost ceilings on care packages are so much lower in comparison to adults of working age, that older people receive only 'safety net' services and are forced into residential care earlier than should be the case (Joseph Rowntree Foundation 2003).

It must also be acknowledged that this change agenda has had an overall impact on the practice of the CMHN. Banerjee and Chan (2005) have rehearsed these arguments and began by reflecting that the deinstitutionalization process has led to the number of

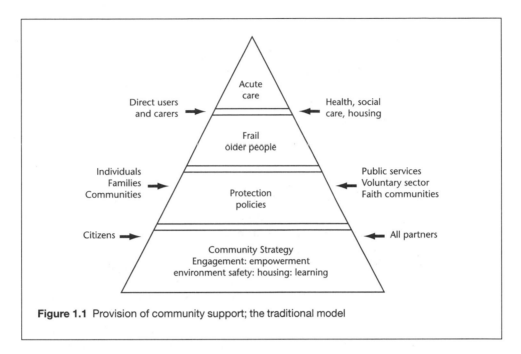

Figure 1.1 Provision of community support; the traditional model

continuing care beds in a hospital setting being 'tiny' in comparison to numbers available in the past; an outcome that has implications for people with dementia requiring general nursing care. In equally small numbers are the acute admissions beds available to older people with mental health problems. Consequently, the threshold for severity of illness, which triggers admission, has significantly risen, and usually only those people who present with the 'highest levels of risk' may be admitted into hospital.

This reduced provision has a number of implications that, unless solutions can be found, will potentially prevent change from occurring. For example, people with dementia are now experiencing rationing of services on the basis of severity of illness or risk, with the bulk of community support provision going to those at the apex of the support pyramid (Figure 1.1). The opportunities to engage with people at an earlier stage of their condition become fewer and the traditional model of support is therefore perpetuated. This is despite a policy agenda that is aimed at early intervention (DOH 2001). There is potential for the resources of the CMHN to be increasingly targeted towards those people with dementia who present with high levels of risk and disturbance, yet are below the threshold for receiving hospital care. Only in the most 'severe' cases will specialist mental health services be involved, and far greater community support will be provided by primary care, social services or other agencies. It is with these issues and concerns in mind that we will now consider the current provision of community support services in the UK.

Models of community support provision: a contemporary appraisal

Over time, the experience of living with a dementia leads to a high level of dependency and a reliance on care services (family and/or service-based) to maintain personal integrity and esteem. In acknowledging this, it may be considered that the move towards community-based services is not an alien concept to most old age psychiatric services. For instance, Arie (1970) set out the fundamental principles that have subsequently come to influence the development of such services across the UK for more than three decades; high on the list is the importance of assessing, treating and maintaining people in their own homes. We now explore some of the models of community support that are currently available to/for people with dementia and uncover areas where the CMHN is making an active contribution.

The family

It is one of the paradoxes of dementia care that the family carer is at one and the same time the greater provider and user of community support services. By far the greatest contribution to maintaining people with dementia in their own homes comes from the family of the person and the move towards deinstitutionalization, as outlined earlier, has increased this responsibility. It is estimated that the value of services provided by unpaid family carers, about £57 billion, equates to the same amount of total healthcare funding for the UK over a 12-month period (Alzheimer's Society 2004), and that some two million carers devote at least 50 hours per week to this voluntary activity (Office for National Statistics 1995). While services provided by the family may be played down as simply a natural or normal extension of the family relationship, they have become essential to maintaining people with dementia in the community and are highly influential in terms of outcomes. It is recognized, for example, that those people with spouse or daughter, acting as carer, are significantly less likely to enter institutional care than those with other or no carers (Melzer et al. 1997).

It is also well established that the caring role can be arduous with frequently documented stress, increased psychological morbidity, diminished social life, reduced employment prospects, exhaustion and ill-health. The family carer becomes as much 'at risk' of social isolation as the person with dementia and while there are limits, particularly increasing behavioural disturbance, for example, much of the research draws attention to the increased commitment and sense of obligation found among spouse and daughter carers (Levin et al. 1989). It is also important to balance this rather negative construction of the caring experience with the rewards of caring that are seen and reported by carers of people with dementia, particularly in the areas of maintaining the dignity of the person with dementia, sustaining their general sense of 'happiness', tending to their needs and ability to give the 'best' care possible (Nolan and Keady 2001: 167).

If carers are adequately supported within their role, then people with dementia may live at home for much longer. On the other hand, support means that a range of services to meet family needs and expectations has to be in place and that an emphasis on promoting family empowerment and adaptive coping moves beyond the rhetorical and into the practical. The challenge often comes when resources are patchy, ineffective or non-existent (Graham 2003). Accessing support for family carers is fraught with potential difficulties. The GP may often be the first port of call but may well not fully perceive, or accurately estimate, the extent of difficulties, may not be convinced of the value of community support provision or may not adequately know what kind of support is available (Pollitt et al. 1991). If referral by the GP is problematic, then self-referral by the carer is seen as being potentially 'hazardous' (Bruce and Patterson 2000) as many will be easily discouraged, or confused, when presented with inadequate information or inappropriate signposting.

Timing of a referral to social services to allow carers to access an array of community support has to be correctly judged. The whole issue of involving outside care providers of any kind signals a watershed in the caring experience. If it is presented too early, it can be damaging to the morale of the carer, especially when allied to concerns about how the person with dementia will react. Similarly, delaying referral may mean that the support on offer is simply 'too little, too late' to impact upon the severity of problems and challenges. As Alison Soliman (2003) demonstrated in our previous book, CMHN support geared explicitly to the needs of family carers can have a positive impact upon the quality of life of the person with dementia and benefits the family system.

Early intervention services

Increased social awareness of dementia, improved diagnostic services and the arrival of potential drug therapies have meant that increased numbers of people are receiving a diagnosis of dementia at a much earlier stage than at any other time. While such a move reflects what people with dementia have said they want (Pratt and Wilkinson 2001), it raises needs and expectations that the traditional model of support cannot realistically meet. Alzheimer's Scotland – Action on Dementia (2003) has previously articulated these needs as including the provision of relevant and accurate information, the meeting of emotional needs and the provision of appropriate social support. These needs are probably universal to all people with long-term conditions, but if we consider that the profile of people known to have dementia and their supporters is changing, then it follows that their needs may best be met well before a crisis point is reached. Greater emphasis is therefore being placed upon the early introduction of support to promote adjustment and coping with the diagnosis, and emerging symptoms. Box 1.1 outlines a range of interventions that may be used to provide this support.

The early introduction of appropriate medical treatments alongside psychosocial interventions not only improves the well-being of people with dementia, but also potentially reduces carer stress to an extent that the need for residential care may be postponed. Early intervention services are therefore specifically designed to support people through the early stages of a dementia and are rooted in the move towards crisis prevention (Department of Health 2001).

Box 1.1 Early interventions for people with dementia and their supporters

- Diagnosis.
- Pharmacological therapies.
- Accurate information provision.
- Counselling and emotional support.
- Support groups.
- Rehabilitation programmes.
- Advocacy services.
- Support or befriending.
- Aids, technologies and adaptations.

One of the best examples has been the Dementia Advice and Support Service (DASS). Established in 1998 by the Mental Health Foundation, DASS operates across the UK through a small number of pilot schemes. Each scheme provides a domiciliary-based service to people who have received a diagnosis of dementia. The minimum ranges of services are: the provision of information, advice, support, signposting and befriending. Additionally, some schemes offer complementary services such as respite, advocacy or counselling and their overall aims are presented in Box 1.2.

Services aimed at post-diagnostic counselling form one area of early intervention that is growing in prominence and, as this (see Chapters 8 and 9) and the previous CMHN dementia care text revealed (Page 2003), can be undertaken by the CMHN working in specialist settings such as in the memory clinic. As an intervention, post-diagnostic counselling is drawn, almost exclusively, from the work of Yale (1999) and aims to promote the notion that people with dementia are able to use strategies that allow them to 'take on their diagnosis' and 'work it through', emphasizing the aspiration of reaching a point, and life, beyond diagnosis. The intention of support would therefore appear to be inherently prophylactic, utilizing educational and psychological mechanisms to enhance coping strategies. Clear comparison can be made with the nature and psychological processes of palliative care support services and in this respect the promotion of problem-focused solutions, rather than emotion-based ones, is the desirable outcome. Arguably, post-diagnostic counselling may therefore represent a vital element in the early introduction and development of a palliative care approach towards the experience of living with dementia.

There appears to be agreement that meeting in groups affords the opportunity for meaningful discussion and aligns with the goals outlined above. What needs to be reinforced, though, is that not everyone is comfortable with the group format (Yale 1999) and therefore the CMHN, as an experienced and confident practitioner, can use a post-diagnostic counselling process with an individual person or family. Where they are used, group sessions may be structured, unstructured or a combination of both and most programmes use some component of education alongside the opportunity for participant-led dialogue.

As to the efficacy of the group approach, Bender and Constance (2005) argue that

---

Box 1.2 DASS project aims

- Improve the availability of information, advice and support to people in the early stages of dementia and their families.

- Extend the period of community-based living for people with dementia.

- Promote user and carer well-being and help users and carers 'manage' dementia more effectively.

- Develop a range of practical, replicable models of service delivery.

- Increase the involvement of GPs in diagnosing and treating dementia in its early stages.

- Act as a catalyst for extending the network of services available.

- Develop a body of knowledge about the role and effectiveness of early intervention for older people with dementia, including ethnic minority elders.

- Demonstrate the potential for using volunteers alongside paid staff.

benefits of participation can be viewed from the perspective of the leaders, the relatives and (most importantly) the participants. They found that group participation was for some the only regular social contact, reinforcing findings from Mason et al. (2005) that the most significant benefit, for participants, was framed in terms of the social network that group participation facilitated. This was in direct contrast to the multiple social losses being experienced in the participant's everyday lives, and the role of the group in the maintenance of a sense of self was seen as crucial.

Social care

While overall social care provision encompasses a broad array of activities from home helps to nursing home placement, this section considers those services that are collectively referred to as 'home care' – essentially, the provision of assistance with domestic tasks or personal care provided through social services or a care agency. The focus is upon those tasks and activities that are central to the older person being maintained at home and the intensity of the service is measured by virtue of the amount of time the service is required by an individual and calculated through 'contact hours'. A little help to many people in need is of enormous significance to people with dementia who live alone and to family carers who are encountering difficulty of some description. Currently, more intensive home support is quantified as the requirement to provide more than five contact hours per week and six or more visits per week.

A review of demands placed upon community support services by people with dementia (Alzheimer Scotland – Action on Dementia 2003) estimated that there are 1,100 people with dementia within a population of 100,000. Of these, 60 per cent live at home and almost all are in receipt of some kind of community support. The largest group (63 per cent) required only a standard service that includes some help with personal care or the use of day centres, whereas the smallest group (6 per cent) required more intensive packages of care. It is this 6 per cent of people with dementia who are struggling to remain at home and who may require almost constant supervision, who have personal needs which will need to be met day and night, and whose main carer will need the support of planned respite or input from specialist CMHN. Because the traditional model of service coordination places significant demands upon the family carer, it is unlikely that people with dementia living alone could be effectively maintained at home even with this high degree of support, and it would not be uncommon for them to experience earlier admission into a continuing care home. Additionally, the reality of home support is often poor. The independent provision of domestic care services has proliferated over the past decade and this may have been at the expense of quality and training (Godber and Rosenvinge 1998). A vital role for the CMHN emerges in terms of vigilance for indicators of abuse, whether intentional or otherwise, advocating on behalf of people with dementia and advising domestic carers about appropriate behaviour, communication approaches, daily living skills, and so on.

In responding to problems in service delivery, some non-statutory agencies, predominantly housing associations, have recently started to turn their attention to increasing the amount of support they can offer to their tenants who may have particular needs. An integrated in-house model of support 'Extra Care' is offered by the Anchor Housing Association (Tench 2003) and views a single provider of both housing and care working in partnership with external providers, such as GPs and pharmacists. The key principle of

'Extra Care' is to provide people with dementia (among others) with housing specifically designed to promote social inclusion and maximize independent living. Instrumental to this philosophy is the availability of a 24-hour domiciliary care team with the ability to respond to an individual tenant's changing needs. Overall, the 'Extra Care' model is influenced by interdependence, particularly in relation to decision-making regarding tenancy offers or managing relationships with neighbours. Interdependence also emphasizes the importance of commitment from all stakeholders, thereby ensuring that people with dementia are appropriately placed and supported in the community setting.

In adding a mental health dimension to home support, Murphy (1997) has differentiated between two different types of care needs which she terms 'ordinary' and 'special'. Ordinary needs are those required by every citizen and include such things as: a place to live, companionship, protection from harm, meaningful occupation, meals, etc., and this would fall within the remit of the social care provider. Special needs are those that are generated directly by a mental illness, they are those things that specialist mental health services would provide and include: medical treatment, psychological treatment and rehabilitation.

Placing these in the context of home support, Lawley and Inasu (2003) describe an intensive home support service for older people with mental illness which aims to address these special needs and by so doing prevent hospital admission. Audit of the service provided mixed and interesting results. People with a dementia and severe psychiatric symptoms associated with increased risk could be effectively maintained within the community when they would otherwise have been compulsorily detained in hospital. The negative effect of this was that again the severity threshold for admission was raised and consequently expectations were placed upon other community support providers to participate in managing more seriously ill people. A proportion of the intensive support team's time was therefore reallocated to training and supporting these other providers.

A further finding was that some patients who needed admission had this delayed until a greater crisis was reached. Previously, Richman et al. (2003) found that where preventing admission is used as a successful outcome measure, then the act of admitting a person to an assessment ward, or similar environment, becomes seen as a failure. Consequently, the CMHN may start to adopt a stance that is more about preserving his or her own self-esteem than it is about the best interest of the patient, and the finding underlines the importance of clinical supervision for the CMHN when taking on new and challenging roles.

Rehabilitation and intermediate care

It is suggested that much rehabilitation work associated with Old Age Psychiatry occurs not in the community but in the few remaining hospital beds that psychiatrists have access to (Bullock 2002). In the short term, this is related to time-limited admissions into acute admissions beds for people who develop another coexisting mental health problem, such as severe depression. The emphasis is upon regaining stability over illness symptoms, with achievable goals for dictating discharge back into the community being identified on admission (Bullock 2002). Long-term rehabilitation in this context is used to describe admissions into NHS 'continuing care' beds for a period of time longer than 12 weeks, while the patient is subject to a goal-focused intervention rather than being the recipient of continuing care.

Introducing a concept of rehabilitation to dementia care has a number of advantages. First, it redefines the use of the NHS continuing care beds as rehabilitation beds. Accordingly, it challenges the acute sector to cease perceiving them as the appropriate place to move on the 'bed blockers', a pejorative term used to describe older people, some with dementia, who, while fit for discharge, have no community or residential provision available. Second, and more fitting for the context of this chapter, it shows that rehabilitation is possible for people with dementia and raises their profile as being equal recipients of intermediate care. In placing people with dementia into the context of intermediate care, we naturally return to the theme of community support.

The Nuffield Institute (2002) claim that people with dementia who have been admitted to general hospital care are too easily moved on to the residential home sector instead of being assisted to return home. At the heart of this is the poor care that many receive in acute hospital wards. These are frequently cited as over-medication, dehydration and communication failure, leading to deteriorating physical health and consequently to deterioration in mental health. Associated with this are the attitudes towards dementia, which are found in the traditional model, that is, people with dementia are vulnerable, burdensome, problematic, draining of resources and incapable of rehabilitation (Godfrey et al. 2004).

Moreover, there are deficiencies with the current ethos of intermediate care with few rehabilitation opportunities being offered to people with dementia, despite the concept of intermediate care being enthusiastically supported in political terms (Department of Health 2001) and receiving an annual budget in the region of £900 million. This disparity is claimed to be due to intermediate care staff having limited experience of mental health problems and inadequate assessment skills which may lead them to conclude that those with dementia cannot benefit from rehabilitation (Nuffield Institute 2002).

This negative stance is rejected by Gilliard (2003) who advocates that there are many skills and abilities which can be relearned and not only can people with dementia return home but also their vulnerability to further transition can be prevented. In further promoting this viewpoint, Dementia Voice (2002), the Dementia Services Development Centre for the South West, have developed a framework for developing intermediate care services around the needs of people with dementia. They begin by stating the aim as being:

> To enable people with dementia to retain or regain abilities where the loss of these abilities would lead to significant change in their quality of life, and/or living arrangements, and such change would not be consistent with their understood wishes.
> (Dementia Voice 2002)

Intermediate care for people with dementia is therefore no different than it is for any other older person. Interventions are targeted at times of transition when existing living and support arrangements are breaking down and when it is indicated that intervention can prevent such breakdown. It may, however, be different in that a specialist mental health practitioner should manage its coordination. This is an acknowledgement of the extra dimension that dementia brings to the situation and the essential requirement for both risk assessment and decision-making to be influenced by holistic, person-centred practice.

Clearly this creates a role for the CMHN to be attached to existing intermediate care teams and to coordinate or case manage rehabilitation for people with dementia. By doing so, it may be that not only do people with dementia achieve a greater equity of access to rehabilitation leading to greater opportunities to return and remain home, but also that their participation in decision-making is enhanced. One concept that might be useful in building a bridge between practice reality and academic thinking is that provided by McCormack (2003) who introduces the concept of 'authentic consciousness' as a method for assisting older people to reach decisions that are their own rather than influenced by external pressures, such as worries of family members or demands from acute care staff. Achieving authenticity in decision-making is rooted in values, of a right to self-determination, and activities, focused on the therapeutic relationship, which are to be found at the core of the professional practice of mental health nursing and as such may come easier to the experienced CMHN.

It may also be argued that while the CMHN has become active in supporting the residential care and nursing home sector to better understand and respond to the needs of residents with dementia (Furniaux and Mitchell 2004), there is little in the way of complementary provision to hospital wards. This liaison role is a clear and present opportunity for service development and an augmentation to the CMHN role.

Day care

The aim of day care is to provide a service that offers some relief to home care providers and an alternative means of respite for carers of people with dementia. In addition to this, it is strongly advocated that day care should be designed to offer something of significance to the person with dementia, whether this be to relieve distress, disability exclusion or isolation (Murphy 1997). Traditionally, these services have been provided by both the health service (day hospitals) and social services (day centres) and both have been not too dissimilar. However, as we have argued, times have changed and the two types of service provision are now much more distinct.

The day centre has a clear focus on the provision of long-term community care and offering people with dementia some structure to life and opportunities to engage in meaningful and purposeful activity, while also providing carers with vital time apart. The day hospital remit has changed and become more associated with aiding the assessment process and treating acute mental health problems which would otherwise warrant institutional admission. The day hospital also provides psychotherapy, behavioural intervention and monitoring of pharmacological therapy regimes and its long-term support provision is targeted towards those who are 'at risk' of relapse (due to a coexisting functional illness), or those whose needs may not be fully met by the day centre.

While both services offer much to people with dementia, one of the commonest challenges faced to their use is that of the person's refusal to attend. Frequently, this is described as being a consequence of loss of insight due to dementia (Fairburn 1997) that culminates in rejection, or restriction, in the care package being delivered, increased caregiver burden and potentially earlier admission to care. Alternatives have been proposed to the 'insight assumption' that may act as a further element of blame and stigma. Keady and Nolan (1994) proposed the adjustment stage of 'suffering in silence' whereby people with dementia, although acutely aware of changing abilities, are not psychologically prepared to be open with others about this and consequently appear to be in denial. Moreover, it can be that people with dementia, or their families, make an informed decision that they simply do not want this type of service in their lives.

Recognizing that refusing the offer of day care is not simply an 'insightless act' but, perhaps, a more determined strategy aimed at self-preservation requires an understanding and empathy that are best found in an experienced practitioner. Here, there is a valid role for the CMHN to work towards a meaningful therapeutic relationship, based on principles of interdependence, through which the person with dementia can be supported to make a decision on the place, and meaning, of day care in their lives.

Discussion

People with dementia are entitled to live as 'normal a life as possible' for as long as is possible and one of the primary aims of health and social care services should be to provide the means to make this happen. Sadly, over the past decade, the services afforded by either health or social care providers have become unbalanced (Department of Health 2001). Health aspects have become fairly well developed in respect of assessment, diagnosis and medical treatment, while social care support aimed at promoting satisfactory community living has been overwhelmed, in some cases reduced to the rudimentary, and in some cases, such as intermediate care, may be almost lacking.

The current situation represents a struggle for people with dementia to live productively in a place of their choosing within the community, and the reality is that they have frequently been disadvantaged by the lack of specific and dedicated support.

As mentioned earlier, just a little help to many people in need is of enormous significance to either people with dementia who live alone, or to family carers who are encountering difficulty of some description. Unfortunately, the 'little help' is disappearing as a service option as the eligibility thresholds for social care are constantly raised due to resource pressures (Godfrey et al. 2004). Many people remain isolated, and living at home, alone, with no support may be as disempowering and unstimulating as admission into the most depressing of care facilities.

However, a new paradigm may be emerging. Its roots are encapsulated within the 'From welfare to well-being' report (Joseph Rowntree Foundation 2003) which is published with one eye on the future demographic challenges facing the UK, while seizing an opportunity to promote 'positive ideals' for community support provision. The report makes a number of key recommendations (see Box 1.3) raising philosophical themes that are as applicable to people with dementia as they are to older people generally. There is a reflection of the value placed on the individual and an acknowledgement of the aspirations older people have to retain independence, choice and control. Throughout there is a theme that making efforts to engage more effectively with older people, or those who use support services, has been the most significant catalyst in changing policy.

Change in policy is evidenced by a growing desire being placed upon the movement away from a traditional focus upon ill-health and the frail elderly towards preventive strategies. In the context of dementia care, this move is therefore away from a focus predominantly upon services that respond to those people with severe symptoms or carers in crisis. This is to be welcomed as an opportunity to see a real departure from the traditional, often nihilistic, model that has promoted late referral and response and is at odds with the ethos of the National Service Framework for Older People (Department of Health 2001), as it applies to England.

We seem to be on the verge of a new and positive policy agenda which is influenced by quality of life, well-being, anti-ageism, equality, social inclusion, empowerment and valuing the individual. It represents a seismic change that has led to a debate about how best to

> **Box 1.3** Key recommendations of the Joseph Rowntree Foundation report, 'From welfare to well-being'
>
> - *Vision and culture:* a new vision and culture are required to celebrate old age and recognize the value of older people in society, both individually and as a whole.
>
> - *Ageism and discrimination:* a stronger legal framework is required, based on age equality and a rights-based approach.
>
> - *Poverty and income in retirement:* a comprehensive review and reform are needed both legally and financially to address income in retirement and poverty.
>
> - *Information and resources for choice and control:* improvements are needed to enable older people to have greater choice and control particularly at times of transition.
>
> - *Meeting the market needs of older people as consumers:* need to address the failure of the market to meet demands for products and services that older people want to retain independence, choice and control.
>
> - *Quality of life and well-being:* action is needed to promote a quality of life and well-being approach.
>
> - *Housing and support options:* a broader set of options is required to support independence in old age.
>
> - *Strategy, resourcing and commissioning:* a stronger and more comprehensive framework is required.

commission, provide and deliver services, which not only reflect these ideals, but also identify and address barriers to change. The Association of Directors of Social Services and Local Government Association (ADSS and LGA 2003) suggest that preventive strategies are the key to realizing a new landscape of community care provision. They are critical of the traditional model and propose an alternative (Figure 1.2), and argue that:

> Future services need to reverse the trend by inverting the triangle so that the community strategy and promotion of well-being is at the top of the triangle and the extension of universal services for all older people is seen as crucial to all agencies.
>
> (ADSS and LGA 2003)

The recent White Paper, *Our Health, Our Care, Our Say* (DH 2006) has begun to articulate how we might realistically invert the triangle of care. Through the Partnerships for Older People Projects (POPPS) (Care Services Improvement Partnership 2006), local authorities are starting to test mechanisms that will act to shift resources across whole systems, thereby encouraging preventive strategies to flourish. The aim is to move away from the current 'patchwork', characterized by inconsistent, incoherent and uncoordinated services with unstable resources, towards a 'network' of services with consistency in commissioning and funding. Under POPPS, many services, including those aimed at low-level need and prevention, will be commissioned and evaluated and there appears to be a built-in preparedness to learn from mistakes.

Overall, while investing in the prevention of illness and crisis is suggested as cost neutral, the philosophy involves a better use of resources and public services working together more effectively (ADSS and LGA 2003), it is also suggested that in judging value the emphasis moves away from quantifiable reductions in expenditure towards improve-

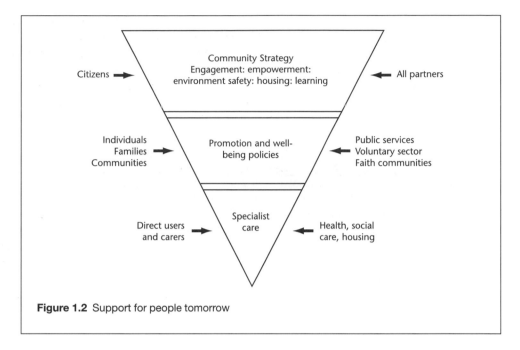

Figure 1.2 Support for people tomorrow

ments in quality of life and independent living, as perceived by older people themselves. If these are to be the new standards by which we measure services, then it becomes evident that preventive strategies should aim to promote quality of life and not simply focus upon the prevention of admission to hospital or institution. At the local level the involvement of the CMHN may be fundamental to the overall success of this strategy.

The Chief Nursing Officer for England and Wales recognizes the valuable contribution that all community nurses play in supporting people with long-term conditions (Department of Health 2005a). In doing so, she draws attention to concerns about those with complex needs who experience uncoordinated care and frequent unplanned crisis interventions or admissions. We have earlier identified such problems as being characteristic of the traditional model of community support provision and agree with her statement that these people are not effectively supported and their ability to remain at home is compromised. They receive care that is intermittent, ad hoc, and reactive to crisis and has little relation to preventive strategies. Although many professionals and specialists may be involved, no one assumes overall responsibility for ensuring that all health and social care needs are met.

A framework for impacting upon this is offered (Department of Health 2005b), and while its emphasis upon the 20–30 per cent of people in greatest need continues to reflect the traditional model, it does also focus much upon the value of preventive interventions. The apex of the model is concerned with two groups; those who have complex needs (level three) and those who are highly at risk of developing complex needs (level two). Considering this model a little further allows us an opportunity to reflect on the role of the CMHN as a specialist involved in community support and preventive intervention.

Those people with dementia falling into the level two category (at risk of developing complex needs) will be those who require better disease management to promote their wellbeing and reduce their risk of deterioration. The CMHN probably works most frequently at this level of specialist intervention and both editions of this book are a testament to the diverse array of possibilities that exist for the CMHN to preserve the integrity of people with dementia and their families and promote optimum levels of health. In addition, level two is characterized by nurses from different backgrounds working closely together to meet needs by implementing protocols to protect vulnerable adults from abuse (see Chapter 12 by Simon T. O'Donovan) or for non-medical prescribing of medications to people with dementia (see Chapter 9 by Sean Page). Overall, there is an emphasis at level two on developing a comprehensive care plan with the active involvement of both the person with dementia and their family networks, or supporters. This places us squarely within a triadic approach to CMHN practice, an ideal in which all three parties (person with dementia, their family/support network and the CMHN) act as a partnership with equality in communication and decision-making, assuring that none of the parties becomes marginalized (Fortinsky 2001). See also Chapter 7 in this book by Trevor Adams and Paula Gardiner.

In moving into level three (those with complex needs), the situation changes considerably, as does the degree of complexity and risk; here we may well see more people with dementia falling into this category as demographic changes (more females in the workforce, more lone parents, more single people choosing to live alone, increased family mobility and less traditional marital relationships, allied to a reluctance to take on (future) caring responsibilities) impact upon society's dependence upon the family to provide the bulk of community care. Indeed, those at level three present with more severe illness, polypharmacy, limitations to activities of daily living and several coexisting medical conditions. As an example, it is not uncommon for a person with Alzheimer's disease to also have other medical complaints, such as cardiovascular disease, diabetes, and so on. This emphasis moves towards effective case management within which all care needs (health and social) are identified and met in an integrated way by skilled and knowledgeable practitioners.

For some time now in the United Kingdom case management has been regarded as central to government policy for the management of people with long-term conditions who, with specialist and intensive support, are able to remain at home longer and have increased choice on health and social care options (Department of Health 2005a). The case manager is seen as being both the provider and procurer of care and assumes responsibility for ensuring that all needs are identified and met. The underpinning principles of case management are set out in Box 1.4 and a number of advantages have been identified.

Box 1.4 Principles of case management

- Provide least invasive care in least invasive setting.
- Support effective primary care.
- Focus on patients in the community carrying the highest burdens of disease.
- Build partnerships with hospital care clinicians and social services.
- Identify patients who are at high risk of unplanned hospital admission.
- Enable each patient to have a personalized care plan based on his or her needs, preferences and choices.
- Integrate the patient journey throughout all parts of the health and social care system.

Among these advantages are: the identification of those people in the community who have complex needs; the development of a multi-faceted care plan to meet those needs, an overall emphasis on preventive strategies; and an opportunity for patients and carers to make future plans and to exercise choice over the range of possibilities.

The role of 'Community Matron' is proposed as a means of delivering effective case management and is defined as being very much a nursing role for those with high-level skills in assessment, medicines management, negotiation, decision-making, resource allocation and enabling or empowerment of patients (DOH 2005a). While nurses with a district nursing background will fill the majority of roles, there is no barrier on mental health nurses also doing so, indeed, it is even suggested as a means of developing the Care Programme Approach for older people (DOH 2005a). It is, however, a requirement that all Community Matrons are sited within primary care and, although this does raise questions about the efficacy of primary care involvement with dementia care, it opens up a new possibility for the CMHN to be more closely aligned to GP practices and, additionally, to become more involved in early and ongoing intervention work.

Summary

If, as intimated earlier, community care has become 'big business', then it is a business that struggles with the reality that demand will always exceed supply; consequently, the traditional model of community support often fails to meet the needs and expectations of its customers. Available resources are targeted towards the most vulnerable while preventive strategies for those in less need are inadequately provided for. What this achieves is a perpetuation of an inherently flawed model as the risk of vulnerability is neither addressed nor reduced, and we are forced to conclude that many people with dementia are condemned to move towards a point of crisis and, ultimately, into continuing care without access to the choice, equality and autonomy of will that are becoming central to public policy and legislation (see Department of Health 2005a, 2005b).

Despite the laudable efforts of many who provide community care and support services, we have to acknowledge that the traditional system is inadequate. We are also minded to acknowledge that there are early signs of a new paradigm, focused on recovery, crisis prevention and the promotion of well-being, which is offered for discussion. The concern has to be that changing community care is such a mammoth task that any debate finds itself stuck at a stage of evangelical rhetoric with no movement occurring. To counter this, change must be evolutionary, rather than revolutionary, and we are seeing this pragmatic approach emerging from the Department of Health with an emphasis being placed on preventive strategies (Department of Health 2005b) and on the contribution that nurses and nursing can make to meet the needs of the most vulnerable while reducing future crisis for others (Department of Health 2005a).

Whatever the future may hold, it seems evident that the CMHN is conceptually and practically well placed to play a significant role in the provision of community care and support, whether this be under the traditional model or a radically different inverted pyramid model or perhaps, more realistically, in the transition between the two.

Lessons for CMHN practice

- People with dementia are entitled to live as 'normal a life as possible' for as long as is possible and a fundamental aim of health, social care and voluntary systems should be to provide the mechanisms to make this happen.

- People with dementia and their families are currently disadvantaged by a lack of dedicated and specific support.

- Implementing preventative strategies in the community to 'ward off' crisis points is a positive and necessary re-orientation of service values and support.

- The CMHN has an active and positive role to play in promoting quality of life for all people with dementia who are living in the community.

References

Alzheimer Scotland (2003) *Making the Journey Brighter: Early Diagnosis and Support for People with Dementia and their Carers*, policy report. Edinburgh: Alzheimer Scotland – Action on Dementia.

Alzheimer's Society (2004) *Policy Position: Carer Support*, available at: www.alzheimers.org.uk

Arie, T. (1970) The first year of the Goodmayes psychiatric service for old people, *Lancet*, ii: 1175–82.

Association of Directors of Social Services and Local Government Association (ADSS and LGA) (2003) *All Our Tomorrows: Inverting the Triangle of Care*. London: ADSS and LGA.

Banerjee, S. and Chan, J. (2005) Organisation of old age psychiatry services, *Psychiatry*, 4(2): 73–6.

Bender, M. and Constance, G. (2005) Wadebridge Memory Bank: a psychoeducation group, *Journal of Dementia Care*, 13: 28–30.

Bruce, D.G. and Paterson, A. (2000) Barriers to community support for the dementia carer: a qualitative study, *International Journal of Geriatric Psychiatry*, 15(5): 451–7.

Bullock, R. (2002) *Building a Modern Dementia Service*. Middlesex: Altman.

Care Services Improvement Partnership (2006) Partnerships for Older People Projects (POPPS), available at: www.cat.csip.org.uk

Davidge, M., Elias, S., Jayes, B., Wood, K. and Yates, J. (1993) *Survey of English Mental Illness Hospitals*. Birmingham: Inter-Authority Comparisons and Consultancy, University of Birmingham.

Dementia Voice (2002) Template for intermediate care for people with dementia, available at: www.dementia-voice.org.uk/consultancy/intermediate_care2

Department of Health (1988) *Community Care: Agenda for Action*. London: Department of Health.

Department of Health (1989) *Caring for People: Community Care in the Next Decade and Beyond: Caring for the 1990s*. London: Department of Health.

Department of Health (2001) *National Service Framework for Older People*. London: Department of Health.

Department of Health (2005a) *Supporting People with Long Term Conditions: Liberating the Talents of Nurses who Care for People with Long Term Conditions*. London: Department of Health.

Department of Health (2005b) *Supporting People with Long Term Conditions: An NHS and Social Care Model to Support Local Innovation and Integration*. London: Department of Health.

Department of Health (2006) *Our Health, Our Care, Our Say: A New Direction for Community Services*. London: Department of Health.

Edwards, P. (2004) Is it time for a bit of tough love? *Journal of Dementia Care*, September–October: 17.

Fairburn, A. (1997) Insight and dementia, in M. Marshall (ed.) *State of the Art in Dementia Care*. London: Centre for Policy on Ageing.

Fortinsky, R.H. (2001) Health care triads and dementia care: framework and future directions, *Aging and Mental Health*, 5 (Suppl. 1): 35–8.

Furniaux, J. and Mitchell, T. (2004) Community Mental Health Nursing Liaison Project, *Mental Health Nursing*, 24: 4–8.

Gilliard, J. (2003) Intermediate care and people with dementia, paper presented at the Intermediate Care and Dementia LIN Conference, London, November.

Godber, C. and Rosenvinge, H. (1998) 'Services', in R. Butler and B. Pitt (eds) *Seminars in Old Age Psychiatry*. London: Royal College of Psychiatrists.

Godfrey, M., Townsend, J. and Denby, T. (2004) *Building a Good Life for Older People in Local Communities: The Experience of Ageing in Time and Place*. York: The Joseph Rowntree Foundation.

Graham, N. (2003) Editorial: Dementia and family care: the current international state of affairs, *Dementia* 2: 147–9.

Holloway, F. (2004) Reprovision of the long stay patient, *Psychiatry*, 3(9): 5–7.

Jones, K. (1993) *Asylums and After: A Revised History of the Mental Health Services: From the Early 18th Century to the 1990s*. London: Athlone Press.

Joseph Rowntree Foundation (2003) From welfare to well-being: summary conclusions of the JRF task group on housing, money and care for older people, avialable at: www.jrf.org.uk

Keady, J. (1996) The experience of dementia: a review of the literature and implications for nursing practice, *Journal of Clinical Nursing*, 5(5): 275–88.

Keady, J. and Nolan, M.R. (1994) Younger onset dementia: developing a longitudinal model as the basis for a research agenda and as a guide to interventions with sufferers and carers, *Journal of Advanced Nursing*, 19: 659–69.

Kitwood, T. (1997) *Dementia Reconsidered: The Person Comes First*. Buckingham: Open University Press.

Lawley, D. and Inasu, P. (2003) Dementia, decision-making and domicile. *Old Age Psychiatrist*. Winter: 8–9.

Levin, E., Sinclair, I. and Gorbach, P. (1989) *Families, Services and Confusion in Old Age*. Aldershot: Avebury.

McCormack, B. (2003) A conceptual framework for person-centred practice with older people, *International Journal of Nursing Practice*, 9: 202–9.

Mason, E., Clare, L. and Pistrang, N. (2005) Processes and experiences of mutual support in professionally led support groups for people with early stage dementia, *Dementia*, 4(1): 79–112.

Melzer, D. et al. (1997) Cognitive impairment in elderly people: population based estimate of the future in England, Scotland and Wales, *British Medical Journal*, 1(315): 462.

Ministry of Health (1963) *Health and Welfare: The Development of Community Care*. London: HMSO.

Murphy, E. (1997) Dementia care in the UK: looking towards the millennium, in C. Holmes and R. Howard (eds) *Advances in Old Age Psychiatry: Chromosomes to Community Care*. Wrightson Biomedical Publishing Ltd.

Nolan, M. and Keady, J. (2001) Working with carers, in C. Cantley (ed.) *A Handbook of Dementia Care*. Maidenhead: Open University Press, pp. 160–72.

Nolan, P. (2003) Voices from the past: the historical alignment of dementia care to nursing, in J. Keady, C. Clarke and T. Adams (eds) *Community Mental Health Nursing and Dementia Care: Practice Perspectives*. Maidenhead: Open University Press.

Nuffield Institute for Health (2002) *Exclusivity or Exclusion? Meeting Mental Health Needs in Intermediate Care*. London: Nuffield Institute.

Office for National Statistics (1995) *General Household Survey*. London: Office for National Statistics.

Page, S. (2003) From screening to intervention: the community mental health nurse in a memory clinic setting, in J. Keady, C. Clarke and T. Adams (eds) *Community Mental Health Nursing and Dementia Care: Practice Perspectives*. Maidenhead: Open University Press.

Pollitt, P.A. et al. (1991) For better or worse: the experience of caring for an elderly dementing spouse, *Ageing and Society*, 11: 443–69.

Pratt, R. and Wilkinson, H. (2001) Tell me the truth: The effect of being told the diagnosis of dementia, *Mental Health Foundation Updates*, 3(1):

Richman, A., Wilson, K. and Scally, L. (2003) Service intervention: an outreach support team for older people with mental illness, *Psychiatric Bulletin*, 27(99): 348–51.

Soliman, A. (2003) Admiral Nurses: a model of family assessment and intervention, in J. Keady, C. Clarke and T. Adams (eds) *Community Mental Health Nursing and Dementia Care: Practice Perspective*. Maidenhead: Open University Press.

Tench, T. (2003) *Extra Care Housing: Living with Dementia*. Kidlington, Oxon: Anchor Housing.

Turner, T. (2004) The history of deinstitutionalisation and reinstitutionalisation, *Psychiatry*, 3(9): 1–4.

Yale, R. (1999) *Developing Support Groups for Individuals with Early Stage Alzheimer's Disease*. Baltimore, MD: Health Professions Press.

2

How others see us

General practitioner reflections on the role and value of the community mental health nurse in dementia care

Steve Iliffe

Introduction

The diagnosis of dementia involves a series of transactions between medical personnel, often with general practitioners (GPs), and the person with dementia or their families (Downs et al. 2002). At first sight there is little role for the community mental health nurse (CMHN) in the diagnostic process, and even in the disclosure of the diagnosis to the individuals and families concerned. Responses to problems that arise during the course of the dementia process, and educational and health promotion tasks aimed at both people with dementia and their carers are very different activities, and arguably belong more in the realm of specialist nurses than in the GP domain, or in that of the practice nurse. From this perspective, the role of the CMHN is a clear one in which the longer-term support for the person with dementia lies in the community mental health nurse's domain once the diagnosis has been made. This Fordist model of illness and care is one that we have learned during our training, but it is now a problem for both disciplines. It sees the person with dementia being delivered to one end of a conveyor belt (the diagnostic step) and then acted upon (the care pathway) as she moves along the production line (the disease trajectory). Reality is more complicated, professional roles are more blurred, and the model both objectifies the person with dementia and omits important figures, such as spouses and family members.

This Fordist approach starts from the professional boundaries and historically formed job descriptions of different disciplines, not from the viewpoint of the person with dementia, nor that of their carers. In this chapter I will argue that the Fordist model is inappropriate, at least in the sense of professionals having highly differentiated roles at different positions in the diagnostic and care process, and that we can envisage an approach to dementia care that is more person-centred, perhaps to the extent that it is so tailored to individuals that it could be called 'wrap-around' (Longley and Warner 2002). In such a tailored process of care CMHNs will have a role to play (if often an indirect one) in the diagnostic process, while contributing in the domains of health promotion and problem-solving to the professional development of other medical and nursing disciplines. This alternative model will replace the Fordist production line not simply because we wish it to do so, but because the demand for services from an ageing but also increasingly critical population makes the production line model obsolete and unworkable.

There are two reasons for this alternative view. The first is that recognition of dementia is intrinsically difficult, obstructed by professional and lay anxieties about the diagnosis, and a source of clinical difficulty or even anxiety to many general practitioners. The second is that CMHNs are relatively scarce workers who unaided will be unable to staff a production line carrying an increasing number of people with dementia. On the other hand, as skilled professionals, often with years of experience in working with people with dementia, they have the potential to transfer some of their skills to others, including GPs. Given the historical differences between medicine and nursing, and the different work cultures of GPs and CMHNs, this skills transfer may not be easy. This chapter will discuss how it may come about, first by reviewing the scale of the problem of dementia care, then by considering the empirical evidence supporting different approaches to inter-professional working, and, finally, by examining the skills needed in dementia care, albeit seen from a general practice perspective.

The scale of the problem

The problem is due to three factors:

1   the skills deficit
2   the changing prevalence of dementia
3   the workforce deficit.

The skills deficit

The National Service Framework for Older People (NSFOP) (DOH 2001), emphasizes the need for early detection and diagnosis of dementia in primary care, to allow access to treatment and planning of future care, and to help individuals and their families come to terms with the prognosis. Similarly, the Audit Commission report, *Forget Me Not 2002* (2002) recommends that general practitioners make increased efforts to diagnose dementia early. This report points out that the cost of failing to diagnose early is often a crisis situation for the person with dementia and his or her family, with specialist services being called in at too late a stage to establish supportive care packages.

In the Audit Commission's survey of 8051 general practitioners in 73 areas in England, 60 per cent agreed that an early diagnosis of dementia was important (Renshaw et al. 2001). This figure is essentially the same as that from the Audit Commission's pilot data from 12 areas, collected in 1999, suggesting that a significant minority of general practitioners remain unconvinced (Audit Commission 2000). It is known that general practitioners may not recognize patients with early dementia for multiple and complex reasons. A range of factors are likely to be important in impeding the recognition of and response to dementia in primary care, which have been summarized in reviews by De Lepeleire and Heyrman (1999), Iliffe et al. (2000) and van Hout et al. (2000), but there is little doubt that we have a problem of under-recognition and under-response to dementia in primary care (Camicioli et al. 2000; Valcour et al. 2000). This under-recognition and under-response may be due in part to failure to recognize signs of a complex and slowly evolving disorder, and in part to negative attitudes towards the diagnosis and assessment of dementia (Boise et al. 1999). General practitioners may be embarrassed or anxious about carrying out cognitive function tests (van Hout 2000), and do not benefit from using standard diagnostic criteria presented as clinical guidelines (Downs et al. 2000). Practitioners who have most difficulty in making the diagnosis of dementia also have more problems in disclosing the diagnosis, particularly to the person with dementia (Cody et al. 2002).

Practitioners may be sceptical about the benefits of anti-dementia drug treatment, inhibited in making early diagnoses by the limited availability of local resources to support the person with dementia (Olafsdottir et al. 2001), uncertain about the clinical management of people with dementia (Freyne 2001), or have difficult relationships with patients and carers (Fortinsky 2001). A willingness to accept a family's reluctance to disclose the diagnosis may clash with a desire to communicate honestly and directly with a patient (Gordon and Goldstein 2001), creating dilemmas for long-term relationships. Practitioners are being encouraged to undertake activities that they find particularly difficult, but are urgently needed (Marriott 2003), such as providing education, offering psychological support for carers and mobilizing carer social support (Cohen et al. 2001). The medical response to co-morbidity in patients with dementia, where effective communication with patients and with carers is essential, is similarly problematic when the professionals lack skill or confidence (Brauner et al. 2000). It is hardly surprising, then, that general practitioners consistently say that they feel inadequately trained to respond to the needs of people with dementia and their families (Alzheimer's Disease Society 1995; Audit Commission 2000; Downs et al. 2000).

What should such training include? A recent qualitative study using nominal group techniques with 144 general practitioners in three purposively selected settings identified six key themes that explain the complexity of dementia diagnosis and management: (1) the pre-eminence of problem-solving over differential diagnosis as a working style; (2) the existence of gaps in support services; (3) problems of confidentiality; (4) rules governing disclosure of diagnoses; and (5) heuristics (rules of thumb) for distinguishing dementia from normal ageing or other pathologies. In addition, the practitioners identified principles governing medication use, issues around carers' needs and implications for professional education (Iliffe and Wilcock 2005). Community mental health nurses may identify common themes in that list that pose problems for them in their professional activity and development, suggesting that both disciplines could benefit from an exchange of experiences.

The changing prevalence of dementia

Dementia is one of the most pressing problems facing health and social care. Approximately 5 per cent of those over 65 years and 20 per cent of those 85 years old have some kind of dementia, prevalence rates that appear similar across Europe (Hoffman et al. 1991). A recent review of dementia prevalence studies in the EU estimated that 3.8 million people (6.4 per cent of this age group) had dementia (Lobo et al. 2000). Given the ageing of the European population (Launer and Hoffman 1992; Ott et al. 1998), the incidence of dementia is likely to be 10 new cases per 1000 people per year, or 600,000 per year across the European Union. In 1998, it was estimated that there were nearly half a million people with dementia in the UK, and this figure was predicted to rise to 650,000 by 2021 (Bosanquet et al. 1998). A general practice in the United Kingdom with a demographically typical list size should expect a current case-load of 10 to 12 people with dementia and an incidence of 1.6 new patients with dementia per GP per year (Iliffe et al. 2002). A practice serving a young population (for example, in the inner city areas) may not notice much change as out-migration of retired people changes the population profile further, but in retirement areas general practitioners may already have 20 or so people with dementia registered with them, and this will rise to nearer 25. In such a locality, a group practice of five full-time equivalent GPs may be managing a caseload of 100 individuals with dementia, and should anticipate adding another 25 in the next few years. Given the increased awareness of the public about dementia, and an increasingly consumerist attitude among younger generations towards the care of their parents, we should prepare for an expanding workload, without necessarily being able to enlarge the workforce proportionately.

The workforce deficit

The existing workforce in health and social care is too small to implement all the changes required by the National Service Frameworks for older people (Department of Health 2001) and for mental health. Early estimates from the Department of Health's Older People Care Group Workforce team suggest that we will need 9 per cent more general practitioners, 29 per cent more old age psychiatrists, 15 per cent more community mental health nurses, 14 per cent more clinical psychologists, 35 per cent more health care assistants and 39 per cent more social workers by 2010 to deliver service to the NSFOP's 'gold standard'. These are large increases in staffing which may not be achieved, even if the resources are available to train and pay all these new workers. Recruitment and retention of staff are particularly problematic in nursing and social work, and this problem is emerging in some areas even in high status and high income medical disciplines. How then can we achieve desirable objectives like optimal care for people with dementia in such a context? The temptation is either to seek organizational solutions that proffer apparent efficiencies by promoting closer collaboration, or to invest in joint training programmes that are intended to enhance and share knowledge. Both these approaches have much merit, and need exploring further.

| Solutions

The solutions suggested to the problems are:

1   practice attachment of CMHNs
2   outreach and education
3   adult learning.

Practice attachment of CMHNs

General practitioners have a positive view of what CMHNs can offer their patients (Stansfield et al. 1992; Monkley-Poole 1995), although in early surveys practitioners commonly noted a lack of communication about patients and limited feedback on treatment outcomes (Briscoe and Wilkinson 1989). A decade ago GPs reported that they wanted to be able to refer directly to CMHNs rather than to psychiatrists, and also wanted CMHNs to be based in general practice (Stansfield et al. 1992). The latter arrangement – practice attachment – seemed to become increasingly popular with general practitioners during the 1990s (Boardman 1997).This desire for location of CMHNs in general practice was not specific to CMHN attachment, but reflected a wider view that all community services should orientate themselves around practice populations rather than localities.

The logic behind practice attachment for CMHNs seems to be supported by evidence that such arrangements improve the quality of care given to older people. The relationship between GPs and CMHNs seems to affect the number and appropriateness of referrals, with accessibility and the GPs' familiarity with the CMHN role being important factors (Thomas and Corney 1993). In seeking co-location with CMHNs, GPs want to gain diagnostic clarity plus clinical guidance in the care of people with dementia, and support for family carers with rapid access to services (Williams 2000).

A recent survey of GPs' perceptions of CMHN roles in dementia care (Blunden and Long, 2002) found that two-thirds of respondents thought they had a good understanding of the role of CMHNs, which included investigation and medical diagnosis, provision of emotional and practical support for carers as opposed to the person with dementia, and training for primary care professionals. Blunden and Long (2002) were surprised by the diversity of expectations that GPs had about what CMHNs could offer older people with dementia, and their families, commenting that this diversity was incongruent with the NSFOP's aim to reduce variations in service access and referral patterns. They also described the GP view that CMHNs would offer medical diagnoses as a 'fundamental misunderstanding', although other commentators see CMHNs as offering support to their colleagues in primary and social care services as an alternative to medical assessment (Rolfe and Phillips 1995), which takes the nursing role close to the diagnostic function of medicine.

Certainly the expectations documented by Williams (2000) and reinforced by Blunden and Long (2002) appear to be an odd mixture of diagnosis (a medical role) and care-giving tasks that might more realistically lie with social services or voluntary organizations. While many CMHNs see carer or family support as a key activity, this is not always evident to families (Clarke et al. 1993; Pickard and Glendinning 2001) and more precise tasks, such as the use of scales and assessments tools, are not standard features of pre- or post-qualifying nurse training (Keady and Adams 2001). Such a mismatch in expectations and actual role could be problematic for a policy of practice attachment, although, as we have seen, the presence of a CMHN within a practice may alter the behaviour of clinicians in beneficial ways, essentially by rapidly altering expectations and understanding of roles. The issue for mental health services, however, may be whether the service has the resources available for such a professional development project, on top of current caseloads.

Outreach and education

The solution to problems of CMHN caseloads and mental health service staffing levels may be to use CMHN expertise in a more overt educational role (Keady and Adams 2001), without necessarily adopting the practice attachment model. The NSFOP requires mental health services for older people to offer outreach and support, acting as a bridge between primary care and mental health services (Barnes 1997), and to develop care protocols for referral and continuity of care (Department of Health 2001). These approaches may constitute a more efficient model of working across the boundary between specialist and generalist services than co-location of professionals.

The value of CMHNs working with older people with dementia has been recognized (Audit Commission 2000) and, despite variation in their roles and numbers, they have been seen as potential specialists in dementia care (Dewing 2000) or advanced nurse practitioners in this area (Rolfe and Phillips 1995; Hawkins and Eagger 2002). Analysing these roles, the Royal College of Nursing (Traynor and Dewing 2002) concluded that the eight core competencies for Admiral Nurses specializing in community dementia care are:

1   therapeutic work

2   sharing information about dementia and carer issues

3   advanced assessment skills

4   prioritizing work

5   preventative work and health promotion

6   ethical and person-centred care

7   balancing the needs of the carer and the person with dementia

8   promoting best practice.

There is, of course, a difference between the ambitions of professional leaders (or the hopes of NHS managers) for a professional group such as community mental health nursing and the, perhaps, more realistic perceptions of practitioners in the field, and we need to be aware of that in making any plans for CMHN outreach work. There is, though, some evidence from CMHNs that supports the idea of an expanded role for CMHNs within primary care, albeit with some qualifications. Manthorpe et al. (2003) report a survey on dementia care involving 79 CMHNs, in which self-reported skills, knowledge and attitudes were compared across different disciplines within nursing (mainly practice and community nursing). Three findings from this study are particularly important for this discussion. First, CMHNs were more likely than other community nurses to over-estimate the prevalence of dementia, perhaps because of their more frequent contact with people with dementia. This has implications for services because over-estimating prevalence may under-estimate the capacity of existing teams to meet demand, and create a pessimistic rather than realistic mood among professionals, particularly if ageist attitudes and the pessimistic environments of long-stay institutions influence the nursing culture (Keady and Adams 2001).

Second, CMHNs were more confident than other nurses in their diagnostic skills in dementia, but (like everyone else including old age psychiatrists) experienced early dementia as very difficult to recognize. This suggests that the task of timely recognition will not easily be delegated to CMHNs, however much general practitioners would like this. Finally, CMHNs found some tasks in working with people with dementia relatively easy, compared to their community and practice nurse colleagues, especially recognition, advice on behavioural and psychological problems and providing information. There is nothing surprising about this finding, but it does support the argument that CMHNs are a potential source of experience that could contribute to the professional education of other disciplines, particularly when experiential approaches to adult learning are used (see below).

Manthorpe et al. (2003) concluded that CMHNs could develop the skills and confidence of their nursing peers while learning from them about their abilities to provide instrumental support as well as the management of care. While this conclusion is consistent with the evidence from this survey, and from other studies, there is also evidence that CMHN skills themselves need enhancing, particularly given the apparent tendency to over-estimate the burden of dementia in the population. It appears that experience can have both a positive and a negative effect on awareness of dementia, leading to understanding and misunderstanding of the problems. The question for those developing dementia services is how to reinforce the positive effects of experience while countering the negative. In my opinion, the answer lies in the methods of adult learning.

Adult learning

The principles of professional development are well understood, and give pointers to how community-based practitioners can enhance their skills in recognizing and responding to the onset of dementia in a timely way (Iliffe et al. 2002). As adult learners, practitioners of all disciplines must identify their own learning needs, formulate their own objectives, identify resources, evaluate their learning (Knowles 1980), and take the first step towards seeking knowledge (Grant et al. 1998). Such awareness of learning needs and of motivation to update skills and knowledge is linked to expected benefit (Willis and Dubbin 1990), which itself depends on recognition of under-performance or lack of knowledge. Learning occurs most easily when concrete practice is related to conceptual models in order to solve problems (Brookfield 1986) and explicit recognition of complexities, uncertainties and conflicting values seems essential to this process (Cervero 1988). Learners prefer a mixture of formal (didactic) and informal (experiential) styles corresponding to a mix of propositional (factual) and experiential knowledge (Eraut 2000). Peers and colleagues can be effective educators (Nowlem 1988), but this must be qualified by the apparent reluctance of general practitioners to learn *with* other professionals, even when they are often willing to learn *from* them (Grant et al. 1998).

We do not know to what extent community-based practitioners dealing with heavy caseloads, multiple requirements to meet new service standards set by National Service Frameworks, obligations to satisfy new forms of appraisal and revalidation, and major anxieties about future funding, can and do identify their learning needs, recognize under-performance, and find and use educational resources to enhance dementia care. However, we do know that some of the widely used educational approaches to enhancing and extending professional knowledge and competence – like joint training – have their limitations, so before time and resources are committed to joint training, these limitations need exploring.

Inter-professional and inter-agency educational events do seem to provide opportunities to consider professional role changes and their impact on others, and to debate the impact that delegation may have on a service system. A recent overview of studies of inter-professional education (Freeth et al. 2002) found general evidence of positive change in knowledge/skills and attitudes, and also the potential to influence organizational behaviour, although evidence of benefit to patients is lacking. On the other hand, in practice, joint training is no more popular than joint working, perhaps for the good reason that it does not necessarily improve performance (Thompson 2002) but it is often presented uncritically as a solution to service difficulties where the fundamental problem is service capacity and connectedness, not dementia awareness. A focus on joint working may even have a negative dimension, representing avoidance behaviour among professionals, through delegation of tasks to others (e.g. nurses need to use screening instruments) or diffusion of responsibility (e.g. the whole team needs to be more aware) (Iliffe and Manthorpe 2004).

Nevertheless the Audit Commission has recommended that local mental health practitioners should provide training and support for the whole primary care team (Audit Commission 2002), noting an association between receipt of training for GPs and the perceived value of early diagnosis of dementia for their patients (Renshaw et al. 2001). It is not clear how these educational relationships will evolve. Evidence suggests that busy practitioners dislike the lecture format and want professional education to relate to practice. In contrast, specialists such as consultants prefer to deliver formal teaching and consider that teaching conducted around practice, such as referrals, is too time-consuming and variable (Marshall 1998). Different types of educational input also seem relevant with medical consultants reporting being more influenced by medical journals and conferences, and GPs by medical newspapers and meetings (Allery et al. 1997). Given such contradictory expectations, what role can the CMHN have in promoting multi-disciplinary working? If the answer is anywhere, it is in helping to identify the range of skills needed for dementia care, and mapping their availability on each locality. Taking this approach means that we can reframe the tasks of professional learning in a person-centred way rather than in terms of traditional professional roles, without losing the insights, techniques and benefits of organizational modes like attachment or liaison, or of joint training. Such a task is not one that can fall on CMHNs alone, and in fact must be led by old age psychiatrists and local service managers, who need to be aware of the educational and organizational complexities of professional development, but CMHNs can contribute a great deal of information about local services and also counter naive enthusiasm for 'quick fixes'.

Enhancing skills

The implications for the labour-intensive work of dementia care are clear. If the job categories cannot expand as fast as needed, the tasks of dementia care will have to be redistributed, which means that skills will have to be shared and transferred between different disciplines. This need for skills transfer will be particularly acute where economic factors like housing costs deter new entrants to health and social care disciplines. The alternative to this smarter working is no improvement in the quality of care, at least in the short to medium term.

A series of nominal groups with general practitioners, interviews with specialists in old age psychiatry and community mental health nursing, participant observation studies of multi-disciplinary training events about dementia care, and consultations with those engaged in dementia collaboratives, have all provided insights into the skills issues in dementia care. From this we have developed a model of the generic skills that could be shared across disciplines, as core competencies usable by doctors, nurses and social workers (Iliffe et al. 2004a). Our focus has been on dementia care in the community, and not the special skills needed in care homes, and it may reflect the general practitioner perspective more than that of the CMHN. Nevertheless, we offer it as a contribution to the educational debate.

We have identified 12 competencies needed on the dementia care pathway. We all possess them to greater or lesser extent, all can be enhanced by experience, and all can be taught. They are summarized in Figure 2.1.

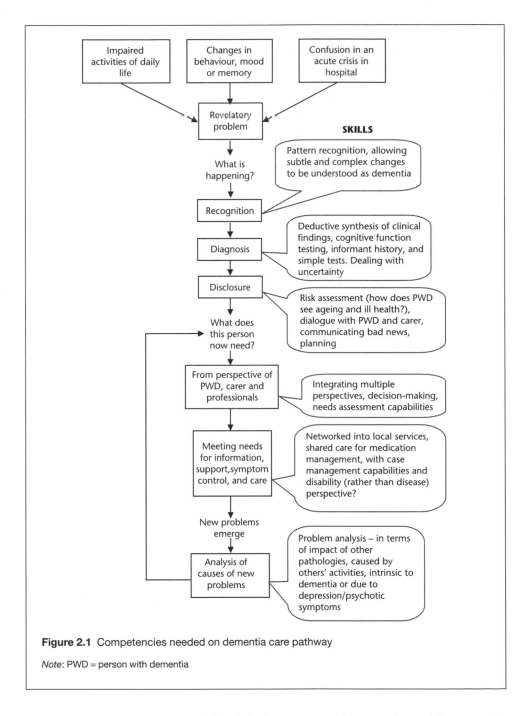

Figure 2.1 Competencies needed on dementia care pathway

Note: PWD = person with dementia

1   *Pattern recognition.* Dementia is relatively uncommon for general practitioners and is hard to recognize, especially in its early stages, but all professionals need to do to enlarge their experience is to listen to those with plenty of it – people with dementia, their family members, or experienced community nursing staff. The educational

resource for recognition of dementia is readily available, but under-used, particularly in undergraduate and post-graduate medical training.

2 *Deductive synthesis*. This involves interpreting clues about how different bits of evidence fit together. When the pattern of symptoms is not immediately obvious, the diagnostic task involves fitting together and making sense of the accounts given by individuals, the descriptions given by family members or friends, and the results of interviews and tests. This may seem a very professional task, but we have some evidence that no professional group has a monopoly of expertise; the experienced social worker will do it as well as the general practitioner, and the same is likely to be true of CMHNs.

3 *Dealing with uncertainty*. What do you do if are not sure whether your suspicions about the early signs of dementia are correct, or when there are disagreements between people with different points of view, or when there are anxieties about the risks run by someone with early dementia? Handling uncertainty by seeking advice, networking with experts and planning a strategy is teachable and learnable, but it is not the same as referral. Liaison activity by CMHNs can meet this need.

4 *Risk assessment*. General practitioners and other professionals can come into conflict over the significance of risks, the former being more likely to emphasize risks and encourage moves into institutional care than the latter. Explicit discussion about how judgements about risk are made may be necessary but uncommon, suggesting that this is a focus for joint training across disciplines.

5 *Dialogue*. Assumptions about the superiority of expert knowledge on the one hand, and the absence of knowledge in the person with dementia on the other, can get in the way of sensible conversations. Promoting a problem-solving approach that starts with an open discussion of the problem will foster dialogues rather than monologues.

6 *Communicating bad news*. Nobody likes this task, and some are better at it than others. There is much to be learned from fields like cancer care and learning disability on how to communicate the bad news about a diagnosis of Alzheimer's disease. This may be another theme where joint training may have more benefits than risks.

7 *Integrating different perspectives*. This is more than fitting together jigsaw pieces, but a more complicated task of mixing different viewpoints into a workable plan that all can implement. It entails compromise, and is a measure of collaborative working.

8 *Networking*. Medical practice is founded on hierarchical relationships or referral upwards and delegation downwards, while social care tends towards horizontal relationships – networking. Knowing what resources are available locally is key to dementia care in the community, and CMHNs may be an important source of enlightenment for general practitioners.

9 *Shared care*. At the moment this tends to mean joint responsibility between general practitioners and specialists for monitoring medication use, but working to a shared plan could also apply to psychosocial interventions for dementia, and may be very relevant to the growing number of memory clinics.

10 *Case management*. Not to be confused with care management in social work, but not so different from it, case management means the systematic monitoring of and response to dementia over time, with organized follow-up, a sharp eye for change and

the capacity to act and intervene. Nursing training emphasizes it, and medicine is weaker at it, so CMHNs may function as role models for primary care.

11 *Disability perspectives.* Is dementia a disease or a disability? Emphasize the former and you are likely to underline the degenerative neurological processes and the lack of any disease-modifying treatment. Emphasize the latter and you are more likely to identify remaining capabilities and strengths, and find ways to offset losses. Doctors tend to learn their craft in disease terms, although general practitioners are aware of the disability perspective; nurses seem to orient their thinking and action towards a disability model.

12 *Problem analysis.* Without stepping back for a longer view of behaviour problems in dementia it is easy to reach for the prescription pad. Problem analysis means at least thinking about behaviour change in terms of pain experienced but not expressed directly, activities of others that are provocative to the person with dementia, behaviours like stroking or wandering that are intrinsic to dementia, and depression. Problem analysis is easy to teach and learn, and all disciplines will benefit from it.

Each of us can assess our strengths and weaknesses in these 12 competencies, and no doubt in aggregate CMHNs and general practitioners would differ in the balance of abilities. But the individual variation would be great, and we may well find that the experienced CMHN performs better than the novice or even competent general practitioners in some domains, while the experienced GP could teach the novice CMHN a thing or two. The challenge for professionals in every locality is to map their own and others' competencies and match their efforts to the skill mix available; Chapter 20 in this text by Emma Pritchard and Sue Ashcroft-Simpson provides an example of how this has been approached by the Admiral Nurse Service. The leadership of mental health services will play a crucial role in orchestrating this process. With 12 competencies this may seem a huge task, even with inspired leadership, but there is a way into the mapping process through the one competency that is built into the National Service Framework for older people, shared care.

Shared care

The NSFOP focuses on the potential value of shared care in the management of anti-dementia medication, and required all Primary Care Trusts (and all general practices) to have a shared-care protocol in place by 1 April 2004. In a study of different perspectives on dementia care in general practice, old age psychiatry and community mental health nursing we found that the idea of shared care – and, to a lesser extent, the practice – extended well beyond the use of medication (Iliffe et al. 2004b). It proved possible to partition the tasks of dementia care roughly into generalist and specialist fields, the former including practice nurses as well as general practitioners, the latter including CMHNs as well as old age psychiatrists, psychologists and social workers. This bipartite division is shown in Table 2.1.

A service development plan that consciously addressed the generalist and specialist tasks, according to the distribution of local skills would, if implemented, cover most if not all of the 12 competencies. It could be done at a level of principle – training in how to establish shared care for medication use initially, when to use cognitive screening tests, how to break the news of the diagnosis, where to seek information, support and help – and in

Table 2.1 Roles in developing shared care

Generalists' tasks	Specialists' tasks
informing primary care staff about key issues in dementia;	enabling memory clinics to cope with rising referral rates;
carry out simple cognitive function test;	providing training in cognitive function testing;
awareness of local specialist services and their roles;	informing primary care about services and resources available;
telling the patient there is a problem needing investigation;	providing a reliable diagnostic process;
playing an agreed role in breaking bad news;	playing an agreed role in breaking bad news;
contributing to changes in shared care programmes;	formulating and communicating a treatment plan Initiating Acetylcholinesterase Inhibitor (ACEI) therapy where appropriate;
participating in follow-up and monitoring medication effects and adverse effects;	participating in follow-up and making decisions about cessation of medication;
responding to needs and problems in dementia course;	responding to needs and problems over time;
providing continuity until death.	supporting all, including other professionals.

practice, through case discussions in the surgery, the home of the person with dementia, or over the phone. Community mental health nurses may then be surprised at how much they contribute to diagnostic processes, how much they learn about disclosure, how supportive they are (without at first realizing it) to colleagues in general practice and nursing, how their perspective on the accumulative burden of dementia care changes, and how their skills diffuse into a wider workforce.

Summary

The desire to enhance and standardize the quality of dementia care written into the NSFOP is a worthy one, but it will be brought about by diversification of efforts to achieve change, unified by a common framework of understanding. Community mental health nurses can play a catalytic role in these processes, which will develop differently in different localities, precisely because they have transferable skills enriched by wide experience. Organizational issues, like attachment and liaison, will matter less than an awareness of the matrix of skills (and skill deficits) within which they work. The creation of a local learning environment that includes generalists and specialists, nurses and doctors, will allow the expertise held by CMHNs to be deployed well beyond their current caseload.

Lessons for CMHN practice

- CMHNs are a potential source of experience and expertise that could contribute to the professional education of other disciplines.

- Joint training is often presented uncritically as a solution to service difficulties, but it does not necessarily improve performance.

- CMHNs can contribute a great deal of information about how local services actually work to the task of service re-configuration, and also counter naive enthusiasm for 'quick fixes'.

- The tasks of dementia care will have to be redistributed, which means that skills will have to be shared and transferred between different disciplines.

- The challenge for professionals in every locality is to map their own and others' competencies and match their efforts to the skill mix available.

References

Allery, L.A., Owen, P.A. and Robling, M.R. (1997) Why general practitioners and consultants change their clinical practice: a critical incident study, *British Medical Journal*, 314: 870.

Alzheimer's Disease Society (1995) *Managing Dementia in the Community*. London: Alzheimer's Disease Society.

Audit Commission (2000) *Forget Me Not*. London: The Audit Commission.

Audit Commission (2002) *Forget Me Not 2002: Developing Mental Health Services for Older People in England*. London: Audit Commission.

Barnes, D. (1997) *Older People with Mental Health Problems Living Alone: Anybody's Priority?* London: HMSO.

Blunden, P. and Long, R. (2002) Dementia and GP referrals to CPNs, *Mental Health Nursing*, 22(4): 8–12.

Boardman, J. (1997) Community Psychiatric Nursing occasional paper 40, London: Royal College of Psychiatrists.

Boise, L., Camicioli, R., Morgan, D., Rose, J. and Congleton, L. (1999) Diagnosing dementia: perspectives of primary care physicians, *Gerontologist*, 39(4): 457–64.

Bosanquet, N., May, J. and Johnson, N. (1998) Alzheimer's Disease in the United Kingdom: burden of disease and future care. Health Policy Review paper 12, London: Imperial College School of Medicine.

Brauner, D., Muir, J. and Sachs, G. (2000) Treating nondementia illnesses in patients with dementia, *JAMA*, 283(24): 3230–5.

Briscoe, M. and Wilkinson, G. (1989) General practitioners' use of community psychiatric nursing services: a preliminary survey, *J Royal Coll General Practitioners*, 39(327): 412–14.

Brookfield, S.D. (1986) *Understanding and Facilitating Adult Learning*. Maidenhead: Open University Press.

Camicioli, R., Willert, P., Lear, J., Grossmann, S., Kaye, J. and Butterfield, P. (2000) Dementia in rural primary care practices in Lake County, Oregon, *J Geriatr Psychiat and Neurology*, 13(2): 87–92.

Cervero, R.M. (1988) *Effective Continuing Education for Professionals*. San Francisco: Jossey-Bass.

Clarke, C., Heyman, R., Pearson, P. and Watson, D. (1993) Formal carers: attitudes to working with the dementing elderly and their informal carers, *Health and Social Care in the Community*, 1: 227–38.

Cody, M., Beck, C., Shue, V.M. and Pope, S. (2002) Reported practices of primary care physicians in the diagnosis and management of dementia, *Aging and Mental Health*, 6(1): 72–6.

Cohen, C.A., Pringle, D. and LeDuc, L. (2001) Dementia caregiving: the role of the primary care physician, *Can J Neurolog Sciences*, 28: S72–S76.

Department of Health (2001) *National Service Framework for Older People*. London: HMSO.

De Lepeleire, J. and Heyrman, J. (1999) Diagnosis and management of dementia in primary care at an early stage: the need for a new concept and an adapted structure, *Theoretical Medicine and Bioethics*, 20: 215–28.

Dewing, J. (2000) Developing a specialist role for nurses in dementia care, *Journal of Dementia Care*, 8: 22–4.

Downs, M., Clibbens, R., Rae, C., Cook, A. and Woods, R.T. (2002) What do general practitioners tell people with dementia and their families about the condition? A survey of experiences in Scotland, *Dementia*, 1: 47–58.

Downs, M., Cook, I., Rae, C. and Collins, K.E. (2000) Caring for patients with dementia: the GP perspective, *Aging and Mental Health*, 4: 301–4.

Eraut, M. (2000) *Developing Professional Knowledge and Competence*. London: Falmer Press.

Fortinsky, R.H. (2001) Health care triads and dementia care: integrative framework and future directions, *Aging and Mental Health*, 5: S35–S48.

Freeth, D., Hammick, M., Koppel, I., Reeves, S. and Barr, H. (2002) *A Critical Review of Evaluations of Interprofessional Education*. London: LTSN Centre for Health Sciences and Practice.

Freyne, A. (2001) Screening for dementia in primary care – a viable proposition? *Irish J Psychological Medicine*, 18(2): 75–7.

Gordon, M. and Goldstein, D. (2001) Alzheimer's disease – to tell or not to tell, *Canadian Family Physician*, 47: 1803–8.

Grant, J., Stanton, E., Flood, S., Mack, J. and Waring, C. (1998) *An Evaluation of Educational Needs and Provision for Doctors within Three Years of Completion of Training*. London: Joint Centre for Education in Medicine.

Hawkins, D. and Eagger, S. (2002) Group therapy: sharing the pain of diagnosis, in S. Benson (ed.) *Dementia Topics for the Millennium and Beyond*. London: Hawker Publications, pp. 73–5.

Hoffman, R., Rocca, W., Brayne, C., et al. (1991) The prevalence of dementia in Europe: a collaborative study of 1980–1990 findings, *Int J Epidem*, 20: 736–48.

Iliffe, S. and Manthorpe, J. (2004) The recognition of and response to dementia in primary care: lessons for professional development, *Learning in Health and Social Care*, 3(1): 5–16.

Iliffe, S., Walters, K. and Rait, G. (2000) Shortcomings in the diagnosis and management of dementia in primary care: towards an educational strategy, *Aging and Mental Health*, 4(4): 286–91.

Iliffe, S. and Wilcock, J. (2005) The identification of barriers to the recognition of and response to dementia in primary care using a modified focus group approach, *Dementia*, 4: 12–23.

Iliffe, S., Wilcock, J., Austin, T., Walters, K., Rait, G., Turner, S., Bryans, M. and Downs, M. (2002) Dementia diagnosis and management in primary care: developing and testing educational models, *Dementia*, 1(1): 11–23.

Iliffe, S., Wilcock, J. and Haworth, D. (2004a) A toolbox of skills to share across dementia care, *Journal of Dementia Care*, 12(4): 15–17.

Iliffe, S., Wilcock, J. and Haworth, D. (2004b) Shared care for people with dementia, *Journal of Dementia Care*, 12(3): 16–18.

Keady, J. and Adams, T. (2001) Community mental health nurses in dementia care: their role and future, *Journal of Dementia Care*, 9(2): 33–7.

Knowles, M.S. (1980) *The Modern Practice of Adult Education from Pedagogy to Androgogy*, 2nd edn. New York: Cambridge Books.

Launer, L.J. and Hofman, A. (1992) Studies on the incidence of dementia: the European perspective, *Neuroepidemiology*, 11: 127–34.

Lobo, A., Launer, L.J., Fratiglioni, L., Andersen, K., Di Carlo, A., Breteler, M.M., Copeland, J.R., Dartigues, J.F., Jagger, C., Martinez-Lage, J., Soininen, H. and Hofman, A. (2000) Prevalence of dementia and major subtypes in Europe: a collaborative study of population-based cohorts, *Neurology*, 54: 11 (Suppl. 5): S4–9.

Longley, M. and Warner, M. (2002) Alzheimer's disease: an introduction to the issues, in M. Warner,

S. Furnish, M. Longley and B. Lawlor (eds) *Alzheimer's Disease: Policy and Practice across Europe*. Oxford: Radcliffe Medical Press.

Manthorpe, J., Iliffe, S. and Eden, A. (2003) Nurses' knowledge, experience and confidence in the early recognition of dementia, *J Advanced Nursing*, 44(2): 183–91.

Marriott, A. (2003) Helping families cope with dementia, in T. Adams and J. Manthorpe (eds) *Dementia Care*. London: Arnold, pp. 187–201.

Marshall, M.N. (1998) Qualitative study of educational interaction between general practitioners and specialists, *British Medical Journal*, 316: 442–5.

Monkley-Poole, S. (1995) The attitudes of British fundholding general practitioners to community psychiatric nursing services, *J Adv Nursing*, 21(2): 238–47.

Nowlem, P.M. (1988) *A New Approach to Continuing Education for Business and the Professions*. New York: Macmillan.

Olafsdottir, M., Foldevi, M. and Marcusson, J. (2001) Dementia in primary care: why the low detection rate? *Scand. J Primary Health Care*, 19(3): 194–8.

Ott, A., Breteler, M.M., van Harskamp, F., Stijnen, T. and Hofman, A. (1998) Incidence and risk of dementia: the Rotterdam Study, *American Journal of Epidemiology*, 147: 574–80.

Pickard, S. and Glendinning, C. (2001) Caring for a relative with dementia: the perceptions of carers and CPNs, *Quality in Ageing*, 2: 3–11.

Renshaw, J., Scurfield, P., Cloke, L., and Orrell, M. (2001) General practitioners' views on the early diagnosis of dementia, *Br J of Gen Practice*, 51: 37–8.

Rolfe, G. and Phillips, L.-M. (1995) An action research project to develop and evaluate the role of an advanced nurse practitioner in dementia, *Journal of Clinical Nursing*, 4: 289–93.

Stansfield, S., Leek, C., Travers, W. and Turner, T. (1992) Attitudes to community psychiatry among urban and rural general practitioners, *BJGP*, 42: 322–5.

Thomas, R. and Corney, R. (1993) Working with community mental health professionals: a survey among general practitioners, *BJGP*, 43(375): 417–21

Thompson, R. (2002) Are two heads better than one? *The Psychologist*, 15(12): 616–19.

Traynor, V. and Dewing, J. (2002) *Admiral Nurses Competency Project: Final Report*. London: RCN Institute.

Valcour, V., Masaki, K., Curb, J. and Blanchette, P. (2000) The detection of dementia in the primary care setting, *Arch Int Medicine*, 160(19): 2964–8.

van Hout, H., Vernooij-Dassen, M., Bakker, K., Blom, M. and Grol, R. (2000) General practitioners on dementia: tasks, practices and obstacles, *Patient Education and Counselling*, 39: 219–25.

Williams, I. (2000) What help do GPs want from specialist services in managing patients with dementia? *Int J Geriatr Psychiatr*, 15(8): 758–61.

Willis, S.L. and Dubin, S.S. (eds) (1990) *Maintaining Professional Competence*. San Francisco: Jossey-Bass.

3

Beyond respite

Working in collaboration with younger people with dementia and their families in designing support services that 'enhance life'

Vivienne Davies-Quarrell, Linda Jones and Gary Jones

Introduction

Life certainly has its twists and turns and can rarely be as predictable as our plans and dreams perhaps would aspire to, but this surely is the fabric of life itself. Consider for a moment your own plans and aspirations for the future. What is it that you expect or expected to be doing in your forties and fifties? Perhaps diligently progressing with your career or enjoying the benefits of the role and status you have already achieved. Maybe even riding the crest of a wave, feeling comfortable and content with life – its purpose and progress.

Many people at this stage in their lives are actively planning for the future, considering it as the culmination or reward for the path taken thus far. Imagine then receiving a diagnosis of dementia at this stage of one's life. What would happen now to those plans and aspirations? The previously held vision for the future seemingly snatched away; life begins to pass by, memories seem to just ebb away into a mist, and with them go those dreams. What direction would one have now?

How do people faced with this scenario find the ability to recapture and rebuild their lives to a different plan? Do they, in your experience, have people around who can help, or are they floundering too, focused on their own losses and the impact that this condition has on their life and the vision of their shared future lives together?

Are younger people with dementia facing a future where other people lead and they follow? A future where they are the ones in receipt of care instead of providing it? A future where they are regarded as incapable and where well-intentioned people seem to want to keep them safe at all costs, thinking that they surely must be a risk to themselves – after all, they do have dementia.

Are they offered a choice of a range of flexible support and respite services that provide accessible appropriate information and opportunities to enable them to successfully adjust and adapt? Maybe they are in some areas but more often than not, it is a different story. The only services available are home care or weekly attendance at a day centre with 80- and 90-year-olds who also have a dementia. Or respite for a week at the local care home for older people, if there is a bed available and always assuming that the registration allows for people under the age of 65. Maybe the only real option is regular booked respite on a psycho-geriatric assessment ward, where they have to go even if their family doesn't need the break, because it has been booked and the family are afraid of losing that place when they may well need it in the future.

In these all too common circumstances younger people with dementia and their families feel that the course of their life suddenly becomes predictable, they feel powerless in its progression and assume that the final chapters of their life have already been written by someone else.

Age-appropriate flexible local services that will work in collaboration in an endeavour to find ways to support younger people with dementia and their families as they come to terms with the diagnosis, review their lives, their relationships and their future, are needed in order that these people can begin to address living in the present and successfully manage their daily lives; and community mental health nurses have a valuable role to play in this process.

This chapter shares the experience of younger people with dementia and their marital partners who have found support and enjoyment in an inclusive and collaborative approach, pioneered by the writer, an independent mental health nurse in the community. It is an approach that aims to help those people with a diagnosis of dementia and their families to face the future and to continue to love and live life in all its guises. This approach is best described by Gary and Linda themselves.

Gary

Before Linda was diagnosed with Alzheimer's disease, she was a very independent woman; she had a good job working in a bank. One of her favourite hobbies was cooking and I would often find her in the kitchen, knee-deep in ingredients.

When things started to go wrong and I noticed changes within Linda, I had to take the decision to put Linda's cooking onto the back boiler, so to speak. This was heartbreaking for both of us and Linda's confidence was shattered.

Unbeknown to Linda, her colleagues at work had also noticed problems, and this was when we began to look for the cause. It was a long and difficult time in our lives. Linda was diagnosed and treated for depression but that didn't make any sense to us, she had always been such a sociable, confident and capable person, there didn't seem to be any reasons for her to be depressed.

The antidepressants didn't help, so eventually the doctors looked at other possibilities. It was some time before we were given the diagnosis of Alzheimer's disease, years in fact, but after everything we had been through it was a relief to find out what it was. Linda was relieved that it was a recognized condition and not simply just 'her'.

Linda

Life had changed so much during the time it had taken to get a diagnosis. I had given up my job and was spending more and more time in the house. I stopped going on nights out with my former work colleagues because I was afraid that I would get lost on the way to or from the loo! I felt anxious and embarrassed that maybe I couldn't keep pace with the conversation; I know now that those anxieties probably made matters worse than they really were. Shopping was also so difficult; I had just lost so much of my confidence and my will. The fun had gone, I was withdrawing from nearly everyone and everything that had been important in my life.

After the diagnosis I was told about a new service that had started for younger people who had dementia and so Gary and I went along to the Alzheimer's Society branch meeting to meet with the nurse who had set up this up.

Gary

We didn't know to expect, we thought it might be like a 'day care' service that older people attend and we wouldn't have wanted that. We thought we would go along to the branch meeting and find out more. We were reassured after meeting with Vivienne that the new service was far from what we feared; it was a group of active younger people and so we thought it was worth a visit to this 'club' to see for ourselves.

Once Linda started attending the ACE Club, she began to rebuild her confidence. Gradually she was encouraged to take the risk and to start cooking again at the Club venue. I fully supported this as I wanted my wife to feel useful again.

Family members also attend the Club and so it really didn't take long for me to see Linda's confidence come back; she was soon cooking homemade soups and dishes for all the club members. I could see Linda was still very 'capable' and was enjoying cooking again. Reassured, I began to see how I could find ways of supporting this at home. We decided to look for a more suitable cooker so she could start cooking at home again. The cooker we eventually found was great for Linda; all the dials for the left and right are on the same side as the rings and not in a line across the front, making it much easier to use, even for me! I also put up a fire blanket, like the one in place at the Club, close to the cooker in case of an emergency.

Cooking is not the only thing that Linda steadily regained her confidence and skills in. For a long time she was scared of lighting the coal fire, now I only need to prompt her, she is capable and safe. Linda now has more confidence to go out with her former work colleagues, where previously she would not leave the house.

Linda

Washing the clothes and bedding was always a disaster. I would put clothes in the machine and not turn it on and later take out a load of unwashed clothes, or I would turn on the machine and leave the clothes in it for days. Either way, the clothes all had to be washed again. Now Gary has marked the dials to make it easier for me. He still worries about me doing the ironing; he is afraid I will pick up the iron the wrong way round and burn my hands but I tell him 'anyone could do that'.

I want my independence and I enjoy time on my own at home doing the usual day-to-day activities. Gary was anxious to leave me at first but I feel so much more confident now that I reassure him! If I become anxious I will phone a friend and he is happy with this.

Everyone should be encouraged to decide in their own right what risks they want to take in life. It is hard to be told by someone else that you can't do this or you can't do that until the paperwork is completed and then a decision will be made! This is my life and I have learnt how to live it even in the face of dementia.

Gary

The thoughts of Linda and I had regarding the Club cannot be put into words but without the vision of Vivienne (the nurse) seeing an unmet need for people in Linda's predicament, I would not know what sort of a future we would have. The help and support we receive from all those involved in the ACE have made coping with our situation easier.

If Vivienne had not seen the need to allow people to continue being in charge of their lives and encouraging them to take control and of their need to belong, then life would be a very unhappy experience. She knew that the traditional day care available was not appropriate to the needs of younger people with dementia and that, if offered, this type of service would have a detrimental effect on the lives of younger people with dementia.

Linda wants to live for today, to try new experiences and to *make* the choice to say no. ACE is appropriate for her needs, and for me it helps to support the changing needs that affect us; it has given me new relationships and new friends.

Linda

ACE has shown me that I can look forward to life. It has given me laughter and unconditional friendship. I can be myself.

Vivienne (CMHN)

It is human nature to aspire to a life that is full and blessed with such riches as love and friendship, challenge and achievement, happiness and contentment. There are many facets to achieving a full life and the values of these differ between individuals, and at times can even be elusive to ourselves. Continuing, however, to live a full and rich life in the face of a diagnosis of early onset dementia, either for oneself or for someone one cares deeply for, is a challenge indeed.

It is a challenge not only for the person with the diagnosis and members of their immediate family and extended social network, but also a real challenge to us as nurses, to find creative and effective ways to provide and facilitate appropriate support for individuals and families, who are facing the daily challenges that living with dementia brings, particularly when younger people with dementia appear to have no clearly defined place within our diverse healthcare landscape.

I was presented with just this challenge when I was contracted by the local branch of the Alzheimer's Society to design and provide a dedicated service for younger people with dementia that would afford a period of respite to the family carer. Being presented with a 'blank sheet' was a real opportunity to harness all my nursing experience and skills to positively influence the experiences of younger people with dementia and their families in the local community.

On reflection, I also drew on family values to inform this developmental work. As a

43-year-old at the time (only two years younger than the first member of the ACE Club and coincidently the same age as his wife, also a registered nurse), I contemplated my own life and that of my husband, children and friends. I considered the potential impact that a diagnosis of early onset dementia would have within my own family and wider circle. This led me to look more closely at the issues that younger people with a diagnosis of dementia and their families faced on a daily basis, and from this period of contemplation, I began to identify what may be helpful, and as importantly, what would not. I was able to empathize with those individuals who were experiencing dementia for real.

It was my observation that younger people with a diagnosis of a dementia together with their partners and families, far too often fell between two stools when it came to service design and provision, and more often than not, they were tagged onto existing support services for older people, where they became passive recipients of a model of care that was inappropriate to their real needs.

It became evident that the clinical assessment and diagnosis of a dementia in a younger person can often be protracted and that subsequent care pathways were at worst non-existent, and at best, fraught with bureaucratic difficulties. I met with many individuals who over several years had experienced such difficulties compounded by their receiving various diagnoses before eventually being referred to a memory clinic, neurologist or psychiatrist for a specialist in-depth assessment.

This had often been a demoralizing and disempowering journey, during which time a range of losses were experienced. Many individuals commented that over the years, they found out who their real friends were, poignantly illustrating a shrinking social circle, often including the loss of their job, an inability to maintain their career progression, and a withdrawal from a previously active and fulfilling social life. I witnessed the changing family dynamics and the toll this took on close relationships and the resultant negative impact on the individual's and family's sense of well-being and quality of life.

I formed the opinion that younger people who have a diagnosis of dementia were at risk of being disempowered both by circumstance and the very nature of the diagnosis; by the social stigma and the common misconception that dementia only affects 'old people'. The reality of malignant social psychology was all too evident and they were often victims of an unwitting prejudice, born out of ignorance and active disablement, fuelled through a paucity of accessible appropriate information and proactive support services.

It appeared to me, that the individuals I met who were enduring these circumstances, felt that their lives of were out of balance and in many respects had become increasingly out of their control, both at home and in the wider community.

The persons with the dementia had lost their self-esteem and their confidence in a whole range of daily living activities and they had experienced heightened anxieties in the course of normal social interactions. As individuals, even within a family, they often felt isolated and alone. Interestingly, these feelings were also commonly experienced by the marital partner who more often than not had assumed the role of supporter and carer. They also expressed their feelings of guilt, because out of fear for the safety of their partner and out of a lack of understanding of the symptoms and presentation of dementia, they had too easily lost confidence in their partner's remaining skills and abilities.

I didn't need to conduct extensive cognitive assessments to form the opinion that much of the withdrawal and the decline in activity and abilities was more due to a combination of a lack of confidence, a decrease in self-esteem and increased anxiety, than to the effects of dementia. I was hopeful that if these areas could be addressed by means of appropriate support for both the person with the dementia and for the partner/family carer, then learning and strategies would follow to compensate for any actual decline in abilities due to memory difficulties. Additionally, by bringing people together who were in similar situations, we were reducing the sense of isolation and providing an environment where new relationships and friendships could flourish without the usual anxieties that so many people had experienced. This was to be the focus of my work.

ACE was established with the aim of restoring the homeostasis and is grounded in an underlying philosophy of facilitation and empowerment for its members. ACE embraces the involvement of family and friends. It encourages and supports inclusive activities and provides opportunities for couples and families to share everyday experiences, as well as some more adventurous antics as diverse as belly dancing and falconry.

One of the many benefits of such an inclusive approach is that family members can see for themselves how much enjoyment their partner is having and the subtle progress being made, they can exchange and learn strategies for coping and enabling, and they can share experiences with fellow members. As a result, some strong and enduring friendships have developed that are sustained outside of the normal meeting times of the Club. Information gleaned and strategies employed inform the care and support that the family continue to provide at home. 'The Club has helped me in maintaining a normal life within the home. We have gained some freedom from the constraints of the illness' (Joan and Alan, ACE members).

ACE has evolved into a collaborative of younger people with dementia who are enabled to be Autonomous, Confident and Empowered, not words one would normally hear associated with people with dementia. However, the recognition that behind every individual lie the achievements and challenges they have conquered, and that before them lie new horizons and endless possibilities has enabled members to develop and sustain their own philosophy for living, 'Loving Life and Daring to Live it!'

Actively engaging with our members as equals, has restored their self-esteem and self-determination. We are all members of ACE and traditional nurse–patient roles have been redefined. We do not have an over-reliance on formal assessments and care plans; it is rather a process of acting on what we hear. By actively listening to the personal stories of their achievements and challenges, and by facilitating open expression of their aspirations, we can identify personal goals and within a culture of saying 'Yes', we encourage and support individuals to achieve their aspirations as and when they emerge, to re-hone faltering skills and to recognize the potential for supporting and developing new abilities. This has assisted people to come to terms with their condition and regain a sense of purpose and a measure of control over their own lives and over the lives of those they care about. 'Our Club, for that is how I now think about it, has proved to me that life does not need to stop with such a diagnosis; it gives you that little push in the right direction to help you think for yourself' (Mo, ACE member).

This level of empowerment took many months to achieve. There was a great deal of work to be done, people were used to being passive in the unfolding chapters of their own lives, their expectations of themselves, of each other and somewhat sadly, of dementia support services in general, were incredibly low. Here lay the real challenge, not only for myself and our 'enablers' but crucially for those younger people with dementia and their families.

In many respects we all felt we were treading virgin ground but we found truth in the saying, *safety in numbers*. None of us was doing this alone, there was constancy in sharing the journey and learning together. As the pioneer of this approach, I learnt to appreciate the uncertainty it brought, as this indicated to me that we were indeed effectively facilitating by empowering others.

As professionals, we are constantly exposed to service policies and procedures that extol the virtues of person-centred care and empowerment. The paradox is that the more a service strives towards empowerment through policy and procedure, the more unlikely it is to succeed. To achieve person-centred care, empowerment needs to come first. Empowerment, like person-centred care, is a philosophy that should be nurtured; it is not prescriptive, it is a dynamic and creative process that constantly evolves and goes with the natural flow of people's lives, changing abilities and aspirations and it happens at ground level, at that all-important interface between one human being and another.

One cannot achieve empowerment with people who have dementia without also empowering the individuals who are providing the day-to-day support, be this family members or professionals. The role of community nurses in this respect is paramount. Just ask yourself why you came into this profession in the first place. What did you, and what do you, want to achieve? What difference do you want to make to people's lives and how are you to achieve this?

Mental health nurses are skilled in rehabilitation and proactive approaches and these can and should be used with people with dementia and their families. People with dementia and their carers are the experts in living with dementia and they have a great deal of expertise to contribute. Combined knowledge and skills are resources that can be shared and disseminated across allied professions and cascaded through the family and support networks of people with dementia within the community. As nurses, we have a responsibility to ensure that our interventions are sustainable even in our absence, otherwise the imbalance of power and reliance becomes disabling.

Community nurses have a vital role in equipping people with the knowledge and the skills, empowering people with the confidence and enabling people to thrive and to achieve a state of well-being, irrespective of age, disability or changing circumstances.

This may sound like a tall order and a challenge indeed, but it can achieved through collaboration and partnership, through passion directed at solutions, through a willingness to be flexible and creative, through values and attitudes and through commitment and loyalty.

There are hidden potentials to identify and opportunities for community nurses to make a substantial impact on the philosophies and design of support and services that meet local need and impact positively on the quality of life that their clients and their families experience. We should act as leaders of change and advocates for those in our care and not always just accept the status quo. As our ACE belly dancers would say, 'We should all be movers and shakers!'

My journey began alongside those younger people with dementia and their families who were once alone, withdrawn and isolated. Encouraging active participation and valuing and respecting the contribution that they and others have made, and continue to make, to the design and ongoing development of ACE, has opened up new horizons for all of those involved.

Enabling our members to follow their own path and to rewrite their earlier perception of the final chapters of their own life has been a humbling and inspirational experience.

I cannot overstate the importance of the focus on facilitation and empowerment that enables people to 'Love Life and Dare to Live it.' The experience of every day *is* what counts and community mental health nurses in collaboration with others can positively influence this experience for many people.

Dementia pays no respect to race, creed, sexuality or age. Community nurses are guests in people's lives and in their homes and, as such, should have an appreciation of how such differences relate to the services that are provided. People with dementia are not a homogenous group, and in dementia care services, one size does not fit all.

'As individuals we can contribute, as a group we have a voice and as ACE we can and do make a difference to our lives and to the lives of others' (Members of ACE 2004).

4

The right route

Service user involvement in care pathways

Sue Gunstone and Jeannie Robinson

Introduction

Service user involvement in the planning and delivery of care is a much talked about topic. Participants at a King's Fund seminar (Easterbrook 1999) talked about their experience of working with older people, and in particular what they themselves would want should they ever need assistance. The message coming from those present was clear: there is a real need to retain a sense of dignity and to be able to exercise real choices and have autonomy in one's life, Easterbrook noted, 'People want a life, not a care plan' (1999: 3). Being dependent on another person can make your sense of self-esteem and dignity fragile and may lead to mental health problems.

Over the past 10 to 15 years, a major theme of UK government health and social care policy has been to encourage services to change the way they relate to the people who use them (Department of Health (DOH) 1989a, 1989b, 2000, 2001c, 2003). These papers advocated that service users should be involved in the design and evaluation of services and in individual care planning. This is slowly changing the way service users and carers are being perceived by health and social services. This change, in part, can be attributed to lobbying by pressure groups, and the change in healthcare philosophy to a belief in person-centred care. Nursing has attempted to move from seeing the patient as a passive recipient of care, to a responsible and active partner in care (Page 2003).

Alongside this move towards service user and carer involvement, the government recognized the need to address the problems of the 'postcode lottery of care' that exacerbates health inequalities. The drive to introduce effective and equitable care delivery to older adults with mental health problems has gained momentum in the past five years. Policy documents such as the National Service Framework (NSF) for Older Adults (DOH 2001a) and both *Forget Me Not* reports (Audit Commission 2000 and 2002) identified the wide variations in identified standards, practice and resources available. There is also an expectation that managers will provide a service that is open to scrutiny in relation to efficiency and effectiveness (DOH 1997). Care pathways enable services to address these issues as they provide a clear framework for service users, carers and professionals that ensures that the care being given and received is efficient, effective and equitable.

Care pathways also provide a means of negotiating care decisions with clients and in this way they encourage the need for service user involvement. Naleppa (1996) found that people who are involved in decision-making are more satisfied with and more likely to comply with their care plan and they benefit both psychologically and physically. This is due to both the empowerment that effective service user involvement brings and the increased communication between the service user and clinician, which is a natural part of service user involvement in care pathways. This, in turn, leads to increased job satisfaction for the clinician, as the care plan is a shared document, which both the service user and clinician work through collaboratively. Both parties are clear about the process and its goals and therefore the responsibility for its implementation and success is shared.

Service user involvement

The term 'service user' has many interpretations. Usually it would be the recipient of care who would be termed the service user. In dementia care, the carer may also be described as a user of services. The role of carers has been acknowledged alongside the recognition that they need to be supported and involved in decision-making, not only in direct care, but also in policy-making and the delivery of care. However, it needs to be remembered that carers' views when used in their own right are valuable but when used as a proxy do not always coincide with the views of the person with dementia (Moriarty 1999). The public as potential service users also have a role in service user involvement in care provision; they have their own perspectives about people with mental health problems – views that may well change if they become actual service users. For the purpose of this chapter and bearing in mind Moriarty's caution, the term 'service user' includes carers as they have a large contribution to make in developing care pathways for people with dementia. We will touch only briefly on the public's role in service user involvement.

The term 'involvement' can also be interpreted in many ways. Recently there has been a move from consultation, which stems from the early 1990s (DOH 1990), to participation, reflecting a shift in the balance of power towards service users and carers (DOH 2001b).

The driving forces

There has been diversification and strengthening of the service user movement (Bowl 1996) and, following on from this, increased government advice that service users should be involved in the planning and management of services (DOH 1989a, 1990, 2001b, 2001c, 2003). Although service user involvement is an issue that has been around for over 20 years, care pathways are a relatively new concept in government documents (DOH 2001a) and there appears to be a strong political will to ensure their use. This sits well with service user involvement as both the development of, and use of, care pathways lend themselves to effective service user involvement both on a local and personal level.

The document, *Patients and Public Involvement in Health: The Evidence for Policy Implementation* (DOH 2004) has provided scientific evidence to support the benefits of public and patient involvement in developing and delivering health care. Harry Cayton (Director for Patients and the Public, DOH) states that prior to these papers 'there had been a nagging sense that patient and public involvement is a nice idea with little real justification' (DOH 2004: 1). The evidence base is now there.

The way forward – national, local, personal

Service users and carers need to feel genuinely valued to avoid tokenism (International Alliance of Patients Organizations (IAPO) 2006). In Dodds' (2003) investigation of service user involvement in education, it was clear that there is a need to ensure that service users feel included rather than exploited. The transfer of power to service users and carers is crucial for any meaningful exchange to take place (Bowl 1996). Service users have to be involved from the beginning; they need to be part of a continuous process. They need to be included in setting the agenda, and involvement should be at national, local and individual level. See Box 4.1 for examples of how service users and carers can be involved in their care.

From a national perspective, service users need to be involved in policy decision-making at government level. Organizations such as the Alzheimer's Society, Age Concern, Help the Aged and carer pressure groups, such as The Princess Royal Trust, have a valuable contribution to make in representing the views of people with dementia and their carers at national level.

The success of national policy implementation depends on local implementation plans and initiatives. Patients' Councils, Patient Advice and Liaison Service and Independent Complaints Advocacy Service go some way in influencing the way care is delivered to an individual. At our local level, Sheffield Care Trust (NHS) Mental Health and Wellbeing has established 'The Council' for service users and carers, which is an independent body.

Box 4.1 Examples of user and carer involvement

- Commission for Patient and Public Involvement in Health (CCPPIH)
- Independent Complaints Advocacy Service (ICAS)
- Patient Advice and Liaison Service (PALS)
- Patient and Public Involvement Forums (PPIF)
- Overview and Scrutiny Committee (OSC)
- Patient and Public Involvement Forums (User and Carer Councils)
- Expert Patient programme
- Satisfaction questionnaires
- Comments boxes
- Links with voluntary agencies who represent carers and users
- Workshops
- Focus groups
- Representation at meetings on specific topics
- Involvement in research and education
- Involvement in interviews for staff posts
- Day-to-day contact with service users and carers – non-verbal and verbal communication
- Support groups
- Copies of letters written between professionals about the person's care.

The aim of this body is to ensure that the voice of service users and carers is heard at the highest level. The Chairperson is a co-opted member of the Sheffield Care Trust Executive Board. Also on the board are two non-executive positions, one for a service user and one for a carer. 'The Council' has three sub-groups, Mental Health, Older Adults Mental Health and Learning Disabilities. Council members sit on a range of sub-committees such as Clinical Governance and Finance. The Chief Executive of Sheffield Care Trust and other senior staff attend 'The Council' meetings and this high-level commitment to service user and carer involvement has clearly had an impact on the success of the organization (Sheffield Care Trust Council 2004).

Council members are involved in the following activities:

- working directly with services to make improvements now and in the future;
- holding the Trust to account for things it says it will do;
- providing the Trust with information about service users and carers' experiences;
- working with those in the city who have influence in planning and shaping services;
- making sure there is good coordination of service user involvement in a way that values diversity and avoids duplication;
- developing networks and links with other relevant service user groups in the city;
- influencing the development of service quality through involvement in staff training service, evaluation and audit;
- working to emphasize the importance of well coordinated and joined-up services.

A strong and genuine commitment is obviously essential to enable service users and carers to influence policy and practice development. There is a recognized need to give training and support. This can take the form of:

- training in assertiveness and confidence building;
- group work and committee skills;
- knowledge of budgeting, planning systems and the function and structures of local services;
- reimbursement for their time, effort and expertise;
- inclusion in the decision-making process;
- availability of a contact person throughout the process.

(Sheffield Care Trust 2004; Bowl 1996)

In considering service user involvement at a personal level, it is necessary to acknowledge that dementia is a very complex illness, requiring different approaches at different stages. There may be an assumption that if a person has dementia they are unable to participate in the development of their own care pathway. However, people in the early stages can be articulate and readily communicate their needs and wishes and can give advanced directives about how they would wish to be treated in the future. Those in the later stages of the illness will require different skills and care settings. It is the responsibility of the professionals, of the advocates and of the carers to enable the person with dementia to communicate their views and needs. Traditionally, proxies have been used because of the view that people with dementia are unable to express their opinions. However, there is evidence from education, research and practice in the dementia field of service users' views being successfully obtained to the benefit of everybody (Goldsmith 1996; Allan 2000, 2001a, b; Rose 2001; Killick 2003, 2004; Cantley et al. 2005; McAndrew and Taylor 2006).

Communication with someone with dementia requires particular attention, and may have to be flexible, spontaneous and intuitive. Thought needs to be given to the pacing and timing of communication, and there needs to be an awareness of the impact of the environment (Cantley et al. 2005; McAndrew 2006). Goldsmith (1996) identified the need to be opportunistic in order to gain service user involvement with people with dementia. It was when people were engaged in activities that staff were able to communicate in a more meaningful way. Bruce (2000) advocates for a better use of interpreting non-verbal communication and using this to inform practice. Nurses tend to be very good at noting non-verbal communication but there is not necessarily a culture of interpreting and acting on that information. For example, a client's challenging behaviour should be explored for its meaning rather than being seen just as behaviour to be managed (Allan 2001a). Dementia Care Mapping (Bradford Dementia Group 1997) which looks at well-being and ill-being is an ideal tool for examining the client's subjective experience of care.

Pritchard (1999), Allan (2001b) and Dodds (2003) demonstrated that once professionals set aside conventional thinking, the service user and professional relationship blossomed, creating satisfaction for all. An attitudinal shift is required to enable staff to listen actively to service users' views and preferences, both for their individual care and for service development (Fryer 1999). In-service training can be used to increase the staff's ability to use a wide range of skills to engage in the process. No one is suggesting that this process is easy (Allan 2001b; McAndrew and Taylor 2006). Allan (2001b: 27) recognized:

> staff need to be able to switch from doing one thing to another as the need arises, when this is done well, it looks easy, but in fact I am sure it is rather difficult, the demands on their attention and energy are multiple and complex and the work is so tiring that to change gear in the way that communication work often requires is problematic.

It is reassuring that Allan (2001b) was able to demonstrate that even in a busy clinical area it was possible to involve service users in their own care. This had the additional effect of improving staff morale.

Bringing people together in small group settings also has benefits. In Sheffield, regular 'Coping with Forgetting' and 'Caring and Coping with Loss in Dementia' groups are available. These groups enable the clients and carers respectively, to explore the experience of dementia and the impact it has on their lives. The information gleaned from these groups enables services to be planned in a sensitive person-centred way.

Information gained from all the above approaches should work on two levels, first, on the immediate care for a person, and second, by feeding into the development of care pathways at local level.

Barriers to service user and carer involvement

There is a range of issues that form barriers to service user involvement, including attitudes to mental health, diagnosis sharing, identification with being a service user, and ethical dilemmas of practice. Where the public are seen as part of the user consultation process, it needs to be recognized that they come with their own agenda. Bowl (1996: 167) believed that the public were concerned with 'issues of safety and segregation and as tax payers who fund service provision'. The public may have fears about people with mental health problems guiding their own destiny and this may act as a barrier to service user involvement in consultation and participation. Hopefully, the situation will slowly change as political will supports patient and public involvement in health (DOH 2004). There has also been a drive to educate the public about mental illness in an effort to reduce stigma, for example, Alzheimer's Awareness Week and World Mental Health Day.

In the early 1990s, Ramon and Sayce (1993) and Stevenson and Parsloe (1993) found that staff were reluctant to consider service user involvement, but there is more recent evidence that the situation is changing (Allan 2000; Thorp 2004). With appropriate support and training, Allan (2000) found that health and social care staff both enjoyed and benefited from the experience of seeking service users' views, but they acknowledged that the experience was not without its challenges.

One consequence of ageism in our society and the stigma associated with a diagnosis of dementia is a reticence to diagnose dementia and then share that diagnosis with the individual. Milne et al. (2000) found 20 per cent of general practitioners (GPs) were very reluctant to give a diagnosis of dementia. Indeed, Brooke and Greaves (2004) identified that only one in ten patients with dementia receive a diagnosis. Service users cannot be expected to make informed choices about their care if they are not given a diagnosis. Iliffe et al. (2004) stated that GPs are not trained to identify the illness during opportunistic consultation as they see so few people with dementia, the estimate being two new patients with dementia per year. Brooke and Greaves (2004) challenge this view, believing this number to be an underestimate. While acknowledging that they are GPs with a special interest in dementia care, they find that they regularly refer one to two patients a month to the specialist services. There appears to be a culture that denies the fact that there are significant numbers of people living with dementia in the community under the care of the primary care team. This culture allows GPs to dismiss their need for training, as it is not seen as a priority issue.

A precurser to being involved in care decisions and service developments is that the individual has to recognize that they may be unwell and present to the appropriate service, usually the GP. Brooke and Greaves (2004) found that service users and carers were not presenting early while Ndoro and Marimirofa (2004) and Godfrey (1997) found that service users and carers don't always recognize their condition as an illness. They noted that families thought the deterioration in their relatives' abilities was a normal part of the ageing process. Furthermore, carers do not always recognize themselves as carers, seeing what they do as part of their responsibilities within a relationship (Rogers 2000). Therefore, service users and carers did not always present early to access services.

Once this hurdle of diagnosis has been overcome, another important issue to be considered is people's reluctance to express critical views. Bowl (1996) found mental health service users in the younger age group were reluctant and fearful of expressing critical views, as they were frightened of either personal sanctions or that their service might itself be threatened. This applies equally, if not more so, to the older adult age group as the balance of power shifts incrementally the older one becomes (Rudge 2002). When someone has the added difficulty of mental health problems, the situation is further compounded (Breeze 2002).

When service users and carers feel able to become involved in service development, the issue of whose views they are representing – their own or the wider service user and carer population – was sometimes confused (Bowl 1996). Good support and training are required to tackle this problem.

There are ethical and moral issues for professional staff should service users and carers choose a course for their own care that differs from the one staff would recommend. Having gathered and documented the views of service users, carers and professionals, a care plan can be developed. Staff need to ensure that both the person with dementia and the carer have been enabled to make an informed choice about the care they wish to receive. If a member of staff feels that the choice made constitutes a risk for either the carer or service user, then the Care Programme Approach can be used to manage the situation, ensuring that all members of the multi-disciplinary team and the service user and carer are involved in the decision-making process. Staff will need support and training to be able to deal with issues of ability and competence of the person with dementia and carers' subjectivity. Good clinical supervision is an essential component that supports the decision-making process.

The barriers related to service user involvement are by no means insurmountable but they are present and obvious. Not least, there needs to be a commitment from the statutory agencies to support this process. For example, there is a need for funding to provide for expenses such as travel, sitting services and reimbursement for time given. In truth, there is the need for a cultural change in the mind-set of the statutory services and the general public. That said, it is achievable, as the policy set out in *Patients and Public Involvement in Health* (DOH 2004) has demonstrated.

Care pathways

Before discussing the term 'care pathways', it is necessary to highlight the confusion that surrounds the subject. This confusion is caused by the abundance of terms used to describe care pathways. See Table 4.1 for a list of alternative terms.

De Luc (2000: 80) defines care pathways as 'multi-faceted tools comprising a number of different elements that have the primary purpose of supporting clinical processes'. The National Health Service Modernisation Agency/National Institute for Clinical Excellence (NICE) (2002: 1), discussing protocol-based care, stated they are 'the detailed descriptions of the steps taken to deliver care or treatment to a patient and are sometimes called Integrated Care Pathways'. Shuttleworth (2003: 6) provides a more comprehensive definition:

Table 4.1 Alternative terms for care pathways

Anticipated recovery pathway/path	Care map	Care profile
Care protocol	Care track	Case management (micro level)
Clinical algorithm	Clinical pathway	Collaborative care plan
Collaborative care track	Critical care method	Critical pathway/path
Expected recovery pathway	Integrated care pathway	Multi-disciplinary action plan
Multi-disciplinary pathways of care	Patient pathways	Personalized care pathway
Protocols	Shared care protocols	

Care protocols set out the treatment to be given to patients with specific conditions. They can be relatively simple covering a single procedure or more complex and multidisciplinary. Protocols that involve MDTs and cover a whole episode of patient care are usually known as Integrated Care Pathways (ICPs).

Care pathway is also a term used in a general way, meaning the various ways patients and carers move into and through the system (Johnson 1997). As such, there have always been care pathways, for example, a GP would pick up the phone to make a referral to the consultant psychiatrist or ring the community mental health team for a chat with the community mental health nurse (CMHN).

In an attempt to standardize care, the NSF for Older Adults (DOH 2001a) stated that Primary Care Trusts will ensure that every general practice is using a local protocol agreed with specialist services to treat and care for patients with depression or dementia. The process of developing the dementia referral and assessment pathway in Sheffield included the views of service users and carers. This pathway provides clear guidance on the process and structure of referral to a community mental health team and dictates the quality of information given to the multi-disciplinary team (MDT). For example, if a person presents at a GP surgery complaining of memory problems, under the current pathway we would expect the GP to do relevant blood tests to identify any physical cause of the confusion. They would also use the Abbreviated Mental Test Score (Hodkinson 1972), and when making the referral to community mental health team, they would state present and past medical history and any medication being taken. It is hoped that in time service users and carers will become more aware of these protocols. It will become routine for service users and carers to receive a copy of their relevant care pathway. Should clinicians deviate from the pathway, service users and carers will be able to challenge the decision.

As a team at local level we can choose to monitor if GPs are adhering to the referral/ assessment pathway but this is not an in-built part of the process, unlike an integrated care pathway. It is inherent in an integrated care pathway that variations of care are be identified, recorded and acted upon. This is known as variance tracking (de Luc 2000). Integrated care pathways are not common in mental health and they are particularly scarce in dementia care.

Barriers to using care pathways

We work in a culture of constant change and this can be a barrier to the implementation of care pathways, particularly integrated care pathways. For example, the ability to carry out the audit or upgrade an integrated care pathway in the light of new guidelines may get lost, in the attempt to keep up to date with other changes. If the original champion of the integrated care pathway moves on without somebody else taking up the mantle, an integrated care pathway can quickly become an outdated document. This would be worse than no document at all because we would be moving away from evidence-based practice. This applies equally to local protocols.

Multi-agency and multi-organization working creates difficulties in putting care pathways into practice as everyone comes with their own agenda (Atwal 2002). If any professional group belonging to the multi-disciplinary team is not committed to service user involvement or care pathways, it will have a major impact on pathway development.

However, if the process is managed properly, everyone's concerns can be taken into account and their views heard.

There can be dissonance between managerial and clinical expectations (Atwal 2002). For example, clinicians may recommend permanent care in a particular instance but it is not available because of a cost analysis by managers. The political drives towards care pathways, which are evidence-based and agreed by all, will hopefully facilitate managerial and clinical expectations to merge.

There are concerns that integrated care pathways limit the scope for professional development (Atwal 2002). However, if implemented properly, integrated care pathways actually improve professional and clinical development through variance tracking. It is not expected that clinicians will carry out procedures or tasks that they feel are inappropriate, but they will be expected to document why they deviated from the proposed plan, thus allowing everyone to learn from the process.

Benefits of care pathways

At the present time there is limited evidence of the use of care pathways to improve patient care. This is due to the newness of the strategies and the fact that research in this area is limited. However, benefits have been identified, with de Luc (2000) and Atwal (2002) finding that it increased collaboration between disciplines as they worked closer together following the joint development of the pathway. Care pathways also reduce duplication and improve communication, as all professionals work with the same set of notes.

The use of care pathways may also improve professional decision-making. Staff who are novices in the clinical area will tend to adhere to the care pathway and benefit from the guidance it provides. However, experienced staff may deviate from the pathway justifiably, where appropriate. In the case of an integrated care pathway, their course of action will be monitored by the analysis of the variance tracking. As the pathways are developed from an evidence base, it ensures all patients are given appropriate care, leading to more effective clinical care. With the current drive to service user and carer involvement, they will increasingly play a vital part in the development and review of all new care pathways.

User involvement, care pathways and the CMHN

From the perspective of the CMHNs, service user involvement at a personal level is the area they encounter on a daily basis. It is widely recognized that CMHNs work in a triadic partnership between themselves, the person with dementia and the carer (Adams et al. 2003). The need to work in partnership has recently been highlighted in the Chief Nursing Officer's review of mental health nursing (DOH 2006). Page (2003) recognized that service users and carers are no longer passive partners – it is a relationship where we learn from each other (Peplau 1988). For some older adults, health professionals are held in awe and therefore it is difficult for them to voice their preferences. This can be further complicated when there is a close therapeutic relationship, as the person with dementia or carer may wish to please the member of staff and will not challenge the care plan. The role of the CMHN is to facilitate the empowerment of service users and carers to enable them to make informed choices. For example, it is now established practice to share correspondence between professionals, with the service user and, where appropriate, their carers; however, the CMHN needs to make sure the correspondence is understood.

An issue that CMHNs are regularly confronted with is the issue of confidentiality. Carers are recognized as an essential part of the caring team and therefore they require information to carry out their responsibilities. This situation needs to be addressed on an individual basis. Carers cannot be shut out of the loop under the guise of confidentiality. Likewise, the person with dementia should not be disempowered by staff ignoring their wishes. When somebody is being cared for by a member of the family or friend, the dynamics of the relationship changes and this can cause difficulties of adjustment for both the person being cared for and the care giver. The fluidity of confidentiality is just one aspect of the changing relationship. The skills of the CMHN are essential in resolving these issues.

The sometimes diverse views of service users, carers and staff need to be managed. It is not always possible to please everyone, but CMHNs need to work with service users and carers to enable them to reach an informed decision, which is 'the best fit' for all concerned. For example, they might encourage the carer to accept extra home care rather than respite, to enable the person with dementia to stay at home, while they have a holiday. Likewise, they may encourage the person with dementia to accept respite to enable the carer to have a break. It is the nurse's responsibility to ensure that service users and carers understand the consequences of any decisions they make regarding the care pathway. For example, it is not professionally acceptable to offer a service and then unquestioningly accept its refusal without examining the consequences of the decision with the person with dementia and carer.

A care pathway is a guide to a person's needs and should be dynamic. Where there is variance between the care needs and the care pathway, professionals need to make informed decisions about the most appropriate way forward. It is important that variance in care is documented and used to inform future practice and further development of the care pathway and resources, ensuring that evidence-based equitable care is provided to all service users and carers. CMHNs need to become involved in service development, ensuring their views and those of people with dementia and their carers are heard. They also need to provide the opportunity for service users and carers to become involved in decision-making at a local level, for example, patient forums.

CMHNs must ensure they have access to supervision and staff development to ensure they have the confidence to practise in this turbulent and constantly changing world (Carradice et al. 2003). Moreover, it needs to be recognized by organizations that working to empower service users and carers results in nurses moving away from their traditional power base, and this creates vulnerability, which requires support.

Summary

When we embrace service user involvement we are providing truly person-centred care. It is an exciting and challenging prospect, which requires nurturing and commitment to enable it to develop. CMHNs are in a prime position to facilitate this process, however, they require support from their organization to do this.

As nurses, we live in an ever-changing world where innovations come and go, and people could be pardoned for not getting excited about the latest trend. Service user involvement is different; it is about you and me; it is what we would want for ourselves; and that is a strong motivator to ensure we provide it for our client group. It now has a 20-year history and is growing in strength all the time.

Care pathways have a shorter history, but there is a strong political will to ensure their use. Recently the Care Services Improvement Partnership/National Institute for Mental Health England (2006) identified 10 high impact changes for mental health services, one of which includes the need for ICPs. The lines between primary and secondary care services have blurred over the last few years and there needs to be a framework to facilitate the transfer of care back and forth. Care pathways provide this framework. Development of shared pathways between primary and secondary services has improved communication between professionals, and has clarified roles. However, there is still some way to go before service users and carers are automatically informed of the pathways relevant to them and nurses need to ensure that this happens.

Integrated care pathways have been shown to improve communication, collaboration, and care delivery within CMHTs. However, dementia is a complex illness, which makes developing an integrated care pathway a daunting task, but every journey starts with the first step. The multi-disciplinary team, including service users and carers, need to be involved from the beginning to ensure success. Service user involvement and care pathways need to be embedded in the culture of service provision to allow them to hold firm while everything around them changes.

Lessons for CMHN practice

- Service user involvement improves the care experience.
- Care pathways provide an evidence-based equitable service to all.
- CMHNs are in a prime position to facilitate these developments.
- CMHNs require support to undertake these actions.
- 'People want a life, not a care plan'. (Easterbrook 1999: 3)

References

Adams, T., Keady, J. and Clarke, C. (2003) Introduction, in J. Keady, C. Clarke and T. Adams (eds) *Community Mental Health Nursing and Dementia Care: Practice Perspectives*. Maidenhead: Open University Press.

Allan, K. (2000) Drawing out views on services: a new staff-based approach, *Journal of Dementia Care*, Nov/Dec: 16–19.

Allan, K. (2001a) Drawing out views on services: ways of getting started, *Journal of Dementia Care*, Jan/Feb: 23–5.

Allan, K. (2001b) Drawing out views on services: meeting the many challenges, *Journal of Dementia Care*, March/April: 26–9.

Atwal, A. (2002) Do multidisciplinary integrated pathways improve inter-professional collaboration? *Scandinavian Journal of Caring Science*, 16: 360–7.

Audit Commission (2000) *Forget Me Not: Mental Health Services for Older People*. London: Audit Commission.

Audit Commission (2002) *Forget Me Not 2002: Developing Mental Health Services for Older People in England*. London: Audit Commission.

Bowl, R. (1996) Legislating for user involvement in the United Kingdom: Mental Health Services and the National Health Services Act, *International Journal of Social Psychiatry*, 42(3): 165–80.

Bradford Dementia Group (1997) *Evaluating Dementia Care: The DCM Method*, 7th edn. Bradford: University of Bradford.

Breeze, J. (2002) User participation and empowerment in community mental health nursing practice, in J. Dooher and R. Byrt (eds) *Empowerment and Participation: Power, Influence and Control in Contemporary Health Care*. Wiltshire: Mark Allen Publication Limited.

Brooke, P. and Greaves, I. (2004) Screening tools in primary care, *Dementia Bulletin*, May: 1–4.

Bruce, E. (2000) Looking after well-being: a tool for evaluation, *Journal of Mental Health Care*, Nov/Dec: 25–7.

Cantley, C., Woodhouse, J. and Smith, M. (2005) *Listen to Us: Involving People with Dementia in Planning and Developing Services*. Newcastle upon Tyne: Dementia North/Northumbria University.

Care Services Improvement Partnership/National Institute for Mental Health England (2006) *10 High Impact Changes for Mental Health Services*. London: DOH.

Carradice, A., Keady, J. and Hahn, S. (2003) Clinical supervision and dementia care: Issues for community mental health nursing, in J. Keady, C. Clarke and T. Adams (eds) *Community Mental Health Nursing and Dementia Care: Practice Perspectives*. Maidenhead: Open University Press.

de Luc, K. (2000) Care pathways: an evaluation of their effectiveness, *Journal of Advanced Nursing*, 32(2): 485–96.

Department of Health (1989a) *Caring for Patients*. London: HMSO.

Department of Health (1989b) *Working with Carers*. London: HMSO.

Department of Health (1990) *National Health Service (NHS) and Community Care Act*. London: HMSO.

Department of Health (1997) *The New NHS: Modern, Dependable*. London. HMSO.

Department of Health (2000) *The NHS Plan: A Plan for Investment, a Plan for Reform*. London: The Stationery Office.

Department of Health (2001a) *National Service Framework for Older People*. London: The Stationery Office.

Department of Health (2001b) *Shifting the Balance of Power*. London: The Stationery Office.

Department of Health (2001c) *Health and Social Care Act, Section 11*. London: The Stationery Office.

Department of Health (2003) *Building on the Best: Choice, Responsiveness and Equity in the NHS*. London: The Stationery Office.

Department of Health (2004) *Patients and Public Involvement in Health: The Evidence for Policy Implementation*. London: The Stationery Office.

Department of Health (2006) *From Values to Action: The Chief Nursing Officer's Review of Mental Health Nursing*. London: Department of Health.

Dodds, P. (2003) Involving the recipients of dementia care in training for staff, *Mental Health Practice*, 6(10): 34–6.

Easterbrook, L. (1999) *When We Are Very Old: Reflections on Treatment, Care and Support of Older People*. London: King's Fund Publishing.

Fryer, D. (1999) Commentary, *International Journal of Geriatric Psychiatry*, 14: 133–4.

Godfrey, M. (1997) The user perspective on managing for health outcomes: the case of mental health, *Health and Social Care in the Community*, 5(5): 325–32.

Goldsmith, M. (1996) *Hearing the Voices of People with Dementia: Opportunities and Obstacles*. London: Jessica Kingsley Publishers.

Hodkinson, M. (1972) Evaluation of a mental test score for assessment of mental impairment in the elderly, *Age and Ageing*, 1: 233–8.

Iliffe, S., Wilcock, J. and Haworth, D. (2004) A 'shared care' model for people with dementia, *Journal of Dementia Care*, May/June: 16–18.

International Alliance of Patients' Organizations (2006) http://www.patientsorganizations.org/showarticle.pl?id=590&n–962 (accessed 14/07/06).

Johnson. S. (1997) *Pathways of Care*, Oxford: Blackwell Science.

Killick. J. (2003) Dementia described from the inside, *The Journal of Dementia Care*, 11(6): 28–30.

Killick. J. (2004) Charts for sailing alongside voyagers with dementia, *The Journal of Dementia Care*, 12(1): 24–5.

McAndrew, F. and Taylor, R. (2006) How all voices are heard for strategic planning, *Journal of Dementia Care*, May/June: 22–4.

Milne, A., Woolford, H., Mason, J. and Hatzidimitriadou, E. (2000) Early diagnosis of dementia by GPs: an exploratory study of attitudes, *Aging and Mental Health*, 4(4): 292–300.

Moriarty, J. (1999) Use of community and long-term care by people with dementia in the UK: a review of some issues in service provision and carer and user preferences, *Aging and Mental Health*, 3(4): 311–19.

Naleppa, M.J. (1996) Families and the institutionalised elderly: a review, *Journal of Gerontological Social Work* I, 27(1–2): 87–111.

Ndoro, R. and Marimirofa, M. (2004) West African older people in the UK with dementia, *Mental Health Practice*, 7(9): 31–2.

NHS Modernisation Agency, National Institute for Clinical Excellence (2002) *What is Protocol-Based Care?* London: The Stationery Office.

Page, S. (2003) From screening to intervention: the CMHN in a memory clinic setting, in J. Keady, C. Clarke and T. Adams (eds) *Community Mental Health Nursing and Dementia Care: Practice Perspectives*. Maidenhead: Open University Press.

Peplau, H. (1988) *Interpersonal Relation in Nursing*. Basingstoke: Macmillan Education Ltd.

Pritchard, E. (1999) Involving older users in education and evaluation, *Elderly Care*, 11(8): 16–17.

Ramon, S. and Sayce, L. (1993) Collective user participation in mental health: implications for social work education and training, *Issues in Social Work Education, and Training*, 13(2): 53–70.

Rogers, H. (2000) Breaking the ice: developing strategies for collaborative working with carers of older people with mental health problems, in H. Kemshall and R. Littlechild (eds) *User Involvement and Participation in Social Care*. London: Jessica Kingsley Publishers.

Rose, D. (2001) *Users' Voices: The Perspectives of Mental Health Service Users on Community and Hospital Care*. London: Sainsbury Centre for Mental Health.

Rudge, S. (2002) Age and isms: older people and power, in J. Dooher and R. Byrt (eds) *Empowerment and Participation: Power, Influence and Control in Contemporary Health Care*. Wiltshire: Mark Allen Publication Limited.

Sheffield Care Trust Council (2004) *Joint Evaluation Service User Involvement*. Sheffield: Sheffield Care Trust Council.

Shuttleworth, A. (2003) *Protocol Based Care*. London: Nursing Times/Professional Nurse.

Stevenson, O. and Parsloe, P. (1993) *Community Care and Empowerment*. York: Joseph Rowntree Foundation/Community Care.

Thorp, S. (2004) Positive engagement, *Care and Health*, 6–12 July: 22–3.

5

Legal and ethical considerations in the role of the CMHN

Dee Jones

Introduction

Law and ethics influence professional practice, shaping and forming the basis for complex decision-making for community mental health nurses (CMHNs) who often find themselves making decisions for individuals whose capacity to do so may be adversely affected by ill health or disability. These are challenging times for CMHNs, not only has the focus of practice shifted towards the care of the serious mentally ill, usually defined as younger people with schizophrenia (Keady and Ashton 2004), but also because the legislation surrounding the practice for CMHNs is in a state of flux. While a variety of legal aspects influence CMHN practice (for example, confidentiality, administration of medicines), this chapter primarily discusses the complexities of consent in relation to the Mental Health Act (1983), the Mental Capacity Act (2005) (due to come into force in April 2007) and the new Mental Capacity Act Code of Practice (due 2007). Legal responsibilities are further explored through a discussion of consent to treatment as evolved through tort law. Case studies are provided to help apply legal principles to practice. Ethical considerations are fundamental to the role of the CMHN and aspects that are considered in this chapter include, individual autonomy and practical approaches to decision-making that incorporate a utilitarian perspective. To aid understanding, law and ethics are discussed separately although the author recognizes that, at times, these issues are intertwined and complementary to one another.

What is the law?

Law is fundamentally about distributive and corrective justice. Distributive justice is political in essence, requiring no interaction between members of the community, but applies to all. Distributive justice 'defines the scope of a person's positive freedom to have access to the resources necessary to realise her humanity' (Wright 1995: 168), for example, access to health care and education.

Corrective justice 'defines the scope of a person's negative freedom not to have her person or existing stock of resources interfered with by others' (Wright 1995: 168), for example, as in the scope of consent to treatment where an individual's decisions can be overridden or decision-making over the right to one's property (see the Gage case which defines 'property' to include human bodies). Through the processes of corrective justice a benchmark for acceptable behaviour in society is defined. Those who fall short are punished either by enforcing pecuniary loss, loss of liberty or both on the perpetrator. The law in a broader sense acts as 'watchdog' over the workings of public bodies (for example, using judicial review to ensure a social services department has acted *intra vires* (within its powers)). The legislative process includes one of consultation, peer review and refinement. In addition, there are many rules and regulations that provide a framework for the whole legal system, these include; those that define court-room activities (types of court, formality of proceedings), evidence that can be submitted and considered (including the ways in which evidence can be heard which may be different depending on the age of the witness or whether it is in the interests of the public for evidence to be heard privately and not in an open court-room), the adversarial nature of proceedings in order to secure the best outcome for one's client and even the aspects of legal decisions that have to be applied (ratio) or considered (obiter) in a judgment. Legal decision-making is subject to the sort of rigorous scrutiny that allows judgments to be overruled (for example, because a judge erred in law by misunderstanding or misapplying the law to the current case). The system of precedence (where the decisions of a higher court bind those of a lower) is intended to give consistency to legal decision-making and provide guidance for judges for often emotive subjects (for example, withdrawal of treatment) yet this is flexible enough to allow for.

Legal framework for practice

CMHNs' professional practice is governed by key pieces of legislation. The Mental Health Act (1983) (MHA) and accompanying Code of Practice (1999) are currently under review and subject to pre-legislative scrutiny, the NHS and Community Care Act (1990) (NHSCCA) (which covers after-care for those discharged from mental health services under s.117; and the principles of Guardianship which incorporate the 'essential powers'), the Disability Discrimination Act (1995) (DDA), the Mental Health Patients in the Community Act (1995) (MHPCA), the Human Rights Act (1998) (HRA), and more recently the Mental Capacity Act (2005) (MCA) (due to come into force in April 2007) and Code of Practice (at time of writing before Parliament awaiting approval).

As far as consent to treatment is concerned, current law (MHA (1983)) allows for admission to hospital and treatment for mental illness (s.2, s.3) even where there has been no consent (s. 63). The MHPCA (1995) under the auspices of supervised discharge (which created s. 25 A–H of the MHA (1983)) impose on certain categories of patient (having one of the four mental illnesses listed, considered to be at risk to themselves or others, see below) explicit requirements (i.e. to attend clinic or a place of work) that stop short of compulsory treatment; although under the powers to convey, patients can be taken to a place for medical treatment to be given. Government policies behind the MHA (1983) envisaged where possible treatment would be provided outside of the hospital setting, and was endorsed by the philosophy of the NHSCCA (1990). This approach was curtailed by the death of Jonathan Zito (caused by Christopher Clunis, thereby establishing the principle of the mentally ill posing a risk to others) and the injury of Ben Silcock (by climbing into the lions' enclosure in Regent's Park Zoo, thereby establishing the principle of the mentally ill posing a risk to themselves) which resulted in the supervised discharge approach to care of the mentally ill in the community. The enduring fear the public has of attack from those with mental illness has continued to shape policy and legislation (especially for individuals who have been diagnosed with severe personality disorder) although evidence suggests that in reality attacks by the mentally ill on the public are not only very low but decreasing (Parliamentary Office of Science and Technology (2003)).

It could be argued that existing law already allows practitioners sufficient scope to carry out professional practice. Especially when the definition of treatment for what is in the best interests of patients is often given a broad interpretation (see Tameside and Glossop Acute Services Trust, below). However, the view is that the current MHA (1983) does not really reflect the current context in which care is delivered and is incompatible with the Human Rights Act (1998). The review of the MHA (1983) (Bill published Sept. 2004) received criticism with regard to a proposal to compulsorily treat patients in the community (this will now not happen (DOH 2004)), but failure to comply with the Care Programme may result in a return to a hospital setting for a patient where treatment can be given without consent. The appropriateness of this is questionable, for in certain circumstances this approach may amount to duress which negates consent and may make treatment illegal.

The MCA (2005) provisions are similar to the previous approach taken for supervised discharge. They will allow for the compulsory treatment of patients if they meet both a definition of mental disorder and a set of relevant conditions. Patients will be subject to an assessment and, upon this assessment, their care plan will include inpatient and outpatient treatment. Failure to comply with these requirements, or a change in circumstances, enables the clinical supervisor to alter the client status to that of a resident patient. Treatment included in the plan can be given without the patient's consent, but only at a hospital.

The MCA (2005) and accompanying Code of Practice (2007), developed because of the 'indefensible gap in mental health law' (Lord Shayne, H.L. v. The United Kingdom ("The Bournewood Case") [2004]), will allow for treatment for anything other than mental illness if done with the *best interests* of the patient in mind. CMHNs need to be aware that following the Bournewood case, full attention must be given to the *processes* involved in the implementation of legislation (and accompanying codes of practice) so that arbitrary decisions relating to patient care are not made that result in a direct breach of legislation.

Re. Bournewood [2004]

Mr L. was admitted to hospital under sedation under s.131 of the Mental Health Act. This was lawful under the doctrine of necessity, but keeping him there (justified, because it was necessary due to his mental state), was insufficiently underpinned by a clear procedural protection which he could have used to challenge the lawfulness of his detention at the time. This was contrary to the HRA (Article 5) which presumes that everyone has the right to liberty and security of person, deprivation of such will entitle individuals to take proceedings by which the lawfulness of detention can be decided. Mr L. did not have such recourse.

The MCA (2005) resonates with legal principles of consent to treatment that have developed through case law. The author suggests that it would therefore be useful for CMHNs to have an understanding of the *legal process* in determining;

- whether or not an individual has capacity to consent to or refuse treatment;

- the best interests of a patient or client.

This is fundamentally important to CMHN practice as the MCA (2005) states that practitioners will have to take reasonable steps to establish whether a patient lacks capacity in question to what is being proposed and, where an individual refuses treatment, the practitioner/client relationship reflects appropriate practice (for example, should a client require restraining in order to prevent sustaining harm to self or others), this does not breach other regulatory protection (for example, Article 5 of the HRA (1998)).

Tort law

Tort law gives the user (and the practitioner) of the service legal rights. Legal rights impose duties on others and there are legal sanctions where these duties have been either negligently carried out (commission) or not carried out at all (omission) (Kennedy and Grubb 1994).

Negligence is covered by three separate 'heads of claim' these are: (1) duty; (2) breach of duty; and (3) damage. In order to acknowledge that negligence has occurred, the court will assess whether the duty owed to an individual has been breached. This is done by evaluating whether the standard of care delivered was at an appropriate professional standard, if the standard of care was not at an appropriate professional standard, the court has to decide whether this breach of duty has caused the damage the individual complains of. Initially, though, the court has to ascertain whether a duty of care is owed in the first place.

Duty of care

In the first instance, the duty of care for CMHNs appears quite broad. Among other things it arises out of being contractually bound to provide services over a given geographical area to a specified case load of clients (Montgomery 1995). This view is further supported by the Care Programme Approach (CPA), intended to be the basis for the care of people with serious mental health needs outside hospital who are accepted as clients of specialist mental health services. The fact that this process is in existence creates not only the statutory duty to provide aftercare in line with s.117 of the MHA but also supports *prima facie* the tortuous liability of a duty of care on CMHNs in their role as key workers. The leading case dealing with a duty of care comes from a civil case decided in 1932. The *neighbour principle* derived from this case has been used extensively in health care to help determine the first head of a negligence claim as to whether a duty was owed to the plaintiff. The case was Donoghue v. Stevenson [1932] and the neighbour principle was set out as:

> The rule that you are to love your neighbour becomes in law, you must not injure your neighbour; and the lawyer's question, Who is my neighbour? receives a restricted reply. You must take reasonable care to avoid acts or omissions which you can reasonably foresee would be likely to injure your neighbour. Who, then, in law is my neighbour? The answer seems to be – persons who are so closely and directly affected by my act that I ought reasonably to have them in contemplation as being so affected when I am directing my mind to the acts or omissions which are called in question.
>
> (Lord Atkin)

The nature of the relationship between CMHNs and their clients will give rise to a *prima facie* duty of care as it would be reasonable to assume that certain acts or omissions of the CMHN will have an effect on the client.

Duty of care in mental health practice

The duty of care in relation to CMHN practice is such that CMHNs must give high regard to the mental *capacity* of the individuals in their care in order that decisions will have *positive outcomes* with regard to health and well-being. In Tameside and Glossop Acute Services Trust v. CH [1996], the patient was heavily pregnant and suffered from schizophrenia, the treatment being refused was a caesarean section which was *prima facie* unrelated to her mental illness and if performed could amount to the tort of battery. The court held that the operation could go ahead as the patient was deemed not to have the mental capacity to understand the implications for refusing consent. The judge accepted expert opinion that the operation had a direct bearing on the mental state of the patient (if the baby had not survived, then further treatment for schizophrenia would have been ineffective) and was in her best interests. Many individuals who are being cared for by CMHNs may not have consented or not fully consented to all of the care being provided, though this may have been done with the best interests of the patient in mind. There is a duty on CMHNs to ensure that patients have full recourse to challenge these decisions (Re: Bournewood [2004], Hockton 2002), this forms part of the duty of care for CMHNs in their role as advocate (Code of Professional Conduct 2004).

Scope of the duty of care

The scope of the duty of care is limited to the 'foreseeable victim' in as much as the duty to take care is reasonable only if the practitioner could have foreseen that their acts or omissions would have harmed this particular individual (client/other) (Donoghue v. Stevenson [1932]). A further explanation of foreseeability is provided in the case of Bolton v. Stone [1951]. The explanation is as follows:

> It is not enough that the event should be such as can reasonably be foreseen; the further result that injury is likely to follow must also be such as a reasonable man would contemplate, before he can be convicted of actionable negligence. Nor is the remote possibility of injury occurring enough; there must be sufficient probability to lead a reasonable man to anticipate it. The existence of some risk is an ordinary incident of life, even when all due care has been, as it must be, taken.
>
> (Lord Porter)

The case of A B and Others v. Leeds Teaching Hospital NHS Trust and Cardiff and Vale HNS Trust [2004] (the Gage case) raises the issue of foreseeability of harm to parents in the light of consent to the removal and use of organs of their deceased children. The claimants suffered psychiatric injury (nervous shock). Two of the claimants failed on foreseeability of harm because it would not have been reasonable for the doctors in question to have foreseen the extent of their injuries due to the fact they appeared robust, the third claimant succeeded because of her apparent vulnerability. Does this throw up the possibility that claimants who have a pre-existing mental vulnerability to harm are more likely to be successful in a negligence case? If so, any damages awarded will be reduced because a pre-existing illness makes quantifying harm very difficult through the legal principle of 'causation' (for a discussion of causation and quantum, see the case of Hotson v. East Berkshire Area Health Authority [1987] 2 All ER 909 (H.L.). In essence, with regard to consent to treatment, the CMHN duty is twofold. First, to ensure that they have not been negligent in assessing whether individuals have capacity to act in their own best interests, and, second, when acting in the best interests of their clients as advocate and making decisions on their behalf they need to consider:

- what reasonable harm may ensue from the decisions they are making;
- that the decision they are making on behalf of another truly represents what that person would have wanted and not what the CMHN may decide (Re B (Adult: Refusal of Medical Treatment) [2002]).

Standard of care

Deciding whether an acceptable standard of care has been provided is determined through analysis of the care provided and evaluating this against what should have been given at the time. For this, the court will look at:

- the legal standard (for example, precedence, legislation, codes of practice);
- the clinical standard (for example, NICE guidelines, expert witness testimony);
- the professional standard (for example, codes of conduct);
- the employer standard (employment law assumes employees are to follow reasonable requests from their employer).

This is viewed in the light of established case law (precedent) so that a coherent body of legal knowledge evolves.

Legal standard

A CMHN may be expected to ask more questions than a lay person by nature of their professional background but they would not need to have specialist knowledge relating to an intervention outside of their field (A B and Others [2004]). When acting in the best interests of clients, CMHNs will be expected not to make assumptions about the client's age, appearance, existing condition, and behaviour and must attempt to engage the client at all times in decision-making (MCA [2005] s.2 (3)). Where the client no longer lacks capacity and decisions have to be made regarding life-sustaining treatment, the CMHN will be expected to consider any past wishes, values and beliefs of the client and consult carers, designated donee, anyone who is deemed to have Lasting Power of Attorney (LPA) status or deputy appointed by the court.

The legal standard: case law

The leading case for mental capacity for consent to treatment is Re C [1994]. The patient in question suffered from schizophrenia, the treatment for which the Trust requested permission to proceed with was amputation of a gangrenous right lower leg. Mr C. did not consent and sought an injunction to stop the Trust proceeding. Thorpe J held that C. had been able to do the following:

- comprehend the information;
- balance the risks and needs;
- arrive at a choice.

He was, therefore, deemed to have mental capacity, and was competent to refuse medical treatment even despite a pre-existing mental illness.

This three-point test is echoed in the proposed Code of Practice accompanying the Mental Capacity Act (2005). The test for assessing whether a person has capacity to make decisions affecting their own well-being is one of functionality as to *how* the decision is made rather than the possible outcome of that decision. The person is deemed to have capacity if they can:

- understand the information relevant to the decision;
- retain that information;
- use or weigh that information as part of the process of making the decision;
- communicate the decision (whether by talking, using sign language (or any other means).

(MCA (2005) s.3)

The MCA s.3 also requires those assessing mental capacity to ensure information is presented in an understandable way, in the context for which the decision is required and to give regard for what is known as 'fluctuating capacity' (in which it is recognized a client's mental capacity can change due to pain and fear, Norfolk and Norwich Healthcare (NHS) Trust v. W [1996] 2 FLR 613). The MCA Code of Practice requires clinicians to do all they can to facilitate and obtain an informed consent. While the MHA (1983) and MCA (2005) do not impose a legal duty to follow the accompanying Codes, failure to do so could be referred to in evidence in legal proceedings (R v. Ashworth Hospital Authority [2005]).

Clinical standard

The role of the Supervisory Board Assessors (SBA) envisaged under the MCA (2005) will be pivotal in establishing the mental capacity of an individual. The criteria upon which assessment will be made will include:

- mental health (clinical diagnosis);
- mental capacity (subjective judgement);
- eligibility (to include age threshold and applicability of mental health provisions to individual);
- best interests to detain (treat) proportionate of possible harm if not detained (treated).

While a clinical diagnosis of mental incapacity rests primarily with the Registered Medical Officer (RMO), the role of the CMHN is vital in providing information that can sway a diagnosis on mental health and mental capacity especially if the CMHN has been working with the patient for some time and knows of any subtle changes in the mental health and well-being of the patient.

The professional standard for determining consent to treatment

Professional standards are of interest to the courts as they provide a benchmark by which to ascertain whether the practitioner has been working at an appropriate and acceptable level. For CMHNs the professional standard the courts are interested in are those set by the Nursing and Midwifery Council (NMC). The Code of Professional Conduct is the most important document published by the NMC because it sets out the standards expected of every practitioner on the register. It is the benchmark against which complaints of professional misconduct are judged. The code specifically requests the requirement on patient involvement in care delivery. In addition, with regard to information sharing, the Code of Professional Conduct (NMC, 2004) emphasizes:

> 3.1 All patients and clients have a right to receive information about their condition . . . Information should be accurate, truthful and presented in such a way as to make it easily understood.

The *Guidelines for Mental Health and Learning Disabilities Nursing: A Guide to Working with Vulnerable Clients* (United Kingdom Central Council (UKCC) 1998) states:

> You have three over-riding professional responsibilities with regard to obtaining consent.
> The first is that you must, acting in the best interests of the client, obtain consent before you give any treatment or care. Secondly, you must ensure that the process of establishing consent is rigorous, transparent and demonstrates a clear level of professional accountability. Thirdly, all discussions and decisions relating to obtaining consent must be recorded accurately. Valid consent consists of three elements:
>
> • it is given by a competent person, who may be a person lawfully appointed on behalf of the client;
> • it is given voluntarily;
> • it is informed.

Employer standard

Employers have an implied right under industrial law to make reasonable requests to employees in the fulfilment of work duties. The standard upon which the employer requires these duties to be carried out is usually in the form of employer-developed protocols, guidelines and procedures. Employers will expect staff to have a sound working knowledge of these and the national standards/reports/publications on which they are based. The court will look to employer-developed standards (whether these were followed) and conditions of employment when evaluating the standard of care delivered.

Breach of duty

The duty on the clinician is to provide an appropriate standard of care when ascertaining a patient's mental capacity to refuse or give consent to treatment and when acting in the patient's best interests. If the court has to decide whether the duty has been breached, it will do so under the auspices of 'reasonableness' and for this principle we look to the case of Bolam v. Friern Hospital Management Committee [1957].

The test is the standard of the ordinary skilled man exercising and professing to have that special skill. A man need not possess the highest expert skill at the risk of being found negligent . . . it is sufficient if he exercises the skill of an ordinary competent man exercising that particular art.

(Lord Wilberforce)

What is being stated here is that the law expects CMHNs to be working to a competent, reasonable standard. If a CMHN's practice is called into account, it may be sufficient to demonstrate that a responsible body of clinicians would have provided care to the same standard, as long as decisions are not based on a residual adherence to out-of-date ideas. Only where a lacuna is apparent in professional practice will the court intervene (Hucks v. Cole [1968]).

Causation

The last head of a negligence claim deals with causation. Negligence may be proven but it has to have caused the damage complained of for the plaintiff to be able to receive compensation. This principle is well illustrated in the case of Barnett v. Chelsea and Kensington Hospital Management Committee [1968] in which the plaintiff (represented by the deceased's widow) claimed negligence for the failure of a doctor to attend her husband at casualty when he presented with abdominal pains. The court found that the doctor had been negligent in not attending but that this did not cause the damage that ensued (the plaintiff's husband had arsenic poisoning and would have died even if the doctor had attended), therefore the widow was unsuccessful in claiming any compensation. In Bolithio v. City and Hackney Health Authority [1992], failure to attend was scrutinized for reasonableness and whether this was contrary to acceptable medical practice. In this instance, the defendant's expert witness (the deemed body of responsible medical opinion put forward by the defendant) demonstrated that failure to attend in this instance was not unreasonable and the chain of causation was broken.

Damage

If the duty of care is deemed to have been breached and that breach to have caused the damage complained of, then the chain of causation is proven and damages are paid by the defendant. Payment is based on what is known as 'quantum'. Quantum is determined by the sort of injury sustained (this includes psychiatric injury), the extent of that injury (e.g. more than one limb, brain damage), the age of the injured (this acts as a multiplier) and the profession or likely profession of the injured (this acts as a multiplier).

While this part of the chapter has focused primarily on the Capacity Act (2005) and accompanying COP (2007) tort law, CMHNs' practice will still largely be influenced by the MHA (1983) (in particular part 4 of the Act). The delay in CPA (2005) coming into force (due April 2007) has been because of a protracted consultation and legislative scrutiny to ensure compatibility with the MHA (1983) and the Human Rights Act (1998). The MHA (1983) and accompanying COP are also undergoing reform, but revised changes are not expect to go through Parliament until the end of 2007.

What are ethics?

The philosophy of ethics is about the value or quality we place on human action or thought. It is divided into three primary areas: (1) meta-ethics (the definition of ethicality); (2) normative ethics (discovering and understanding ethical truths); and (3) applied ethics (what happens when we use ethical knowledge in practice). Ethical philosophies often present an ideology of what we as humans can be: 'recognition of the inherent dignity and of the equal and inalienable rights of all members of the human family is the foundation of freedom, justice and peace in the world' (Preamble to the Universal Declaration of Human Rights, 1948).

Ethics requires practitioners to make decisions in light of the principles of reason (not unlike the concept of reasonableness in law), common sense and, dare I say it, caring. There have been various philosophical theories that have influenced health-care practice, not least Immanuel Kant (Kant 1993) whose views on autonomy are considered mainstream thinking. Kant expounded the powerful ethic of equal freedom, which he considered to be the moral foundation of rights, justice and law (Owen 1997). Kant's moral duty to act (similar to the legal duty of care) is based on acting in the interests of others and not for one's own reward (Kant 1993).

Kant's moral philosophy (Right and Virtue) specifies which moral obligations are also legal obligations, and which are enforceable through coercion by others. CMHNs involved in team decisions (for example, working with the approved social worker), that they do not ethically agree with may have to subjugate their own beliefs. This is part of an internal subjective criteria that we all make in order to 'live with' decisions.

Acting in the best interests of others in a way that limits or overrides their decision-making power is known as paternalism. Paternalism erodes individual autonomy but in certain circumstances may be necessary where the individual is unable to make value judgements about their own care. How do we determine the client's ability to make a value judgement when the values held by clients may at the very least be different from the CMHN because, if nothing else, the client has had different life experiences, let alone mental illness? In essence, the CMHN's value judgement on the mental capacity of another to determine their own decisions has to be made minus the personal values of the CMHN.

A utilitarian approach to decision-making would be to balance the interests of the client with those of the wider community. For example, under what circumstances should potentially dangerous clients (to themselves and others) be free to live out a chosen lifestyle among others? When should it be limited? And what rationale can be used to aid the CMHN in achieving a fair outcome? A utilitarian approach would require the CMHN to make a decision based on what is ultimately a cost/benefit analysis to those involved. This often comes into play where the CMHN may be called upon to breach confidentiality in order to protect some other group or individual (for example, the protection of children in the case of paedophiles).

The CMHN has to take a 'rounded view' of things and in certain circumstances, forced treatment may well be an ethically appropriate decision to make if in the long term it is in the best interests of their clients: 'Only by having regard to the whole can nurses ensure that their work is in the interests of their clients' (Cribb 1995).

The 'supplementing of a patient's ability' was recognized by Christiansen (1993) as part of the nurse–patient relationship. Taking the principle of acting in the best interests of others to a logical conclusion, Kant's moral philosophy of respect for the individual is central to ethical decision-making in health care. This is a subjective process and ultimately may rely on what the CMHN intrinsically knows to be right. Paradoxically, what the CMHN has to consider first and foremost is what the patient would consider to be right and this may land CMHNs in a decision-making loop where they have to act in the way the patient would want, even if this is in conflict to what the CMHN considers right or appropriate in the circumstances.

Ethical framework for practice

Besides paternalistic and utilitarian approaches, the four principles of health-care ethics expounded by Beauchamp and Childress (1989) and Gillon (1994) are invaluable when considering CMHN practice. These are:

1   respect for autonomy = respect autonomy
2   nonmaleficence   = avoid harming
3   beneficence   = where possible, benefit
4   justice   = consider fairly the interests of all those affected.

Aristotelian influences on CMHN's practice include being punished if you do something knowingly wrong; this suggests a move from the prevalent 'blame culture' in health care towards a 'responsibility culture' where clinicians are not able to hide behind therapeutic privilege.

Assuming the role of decision-maker for those deemed incapable is fraught with difficulties, not just in areas where consent to treatment is required but also where moral decisions may need to be made regarding ending life (Cribb 1995). Where clients present not only with incurable physical diseases such as cancer or multiple sclerosis and also advanced dementia, the author suggests that no blanket policy or guideline should be adopted and each individual case should be judged on its own merits. It may be worth remembering that while euthanasia is illegal in Britain, the giving of pain-relieving medications is legal, even if one of the consequences of this results in the shortening of a patient's life (doctrine of dual effect). Where a client has made an advanced directive, the NMC is clear in stating that the CMHN must respect the wishes of the client (Code of Professional Conduct 2004). The right to life/treatment for clients is compounded by the availability of resources; and the generic models used to distribute them are often not sensitive to mental health outcomes (Chisholm et al. 1997), leading to tensions in the scope CMHNs have in making ethically sound decisions (for example, within the four principles cited above). CMHN practice is complex and fraught with pitfalls, while Kant's espoused theory of duty is based on non-reward for the clinician, it is often the case that most CMHNs' reward is a positive outcome for their client which forms the basis of professional clinical practice.

Case example 1

Mr Peterson has advanced dementia which renders him incapable of making decisions affecting his health and well-being. He has recently been admitted to a care home environment because his elderly wife can no longer care for him at home. Mr Peterson has attempted to leave the home on several occasions and refuses to take medication (for his dementia and for a urinary tract infection). He had (while competent) written an advanced directive stating that if his condition deteriorates to the extent he has to be admitted to a care home, he should not be forced to take medication and should be allowed to die if he became physically ill.

- An advance directive is a way of prolonging autonomy. Individuals with capacity have the right to refuse treatment that may be given at a later date. An advanced directive should be followed unless it could reasonably be decided that in the present circumstances the individual would have changed their mind. Advanced directives cannot be used to ensure future treatment is provided (R (on the application of Burke) v. The GMC [2004] EWHC 1879).

- While one adult cannot legally consent for another (Hockton 2002), where the patient lacks competence, it is best practice to involve relatives to provide information to clarify what treatment the patient would have considered in the present circumstances. In addition, the CMHN should consider their own and the health-care team's knowledge of the patient's background (for example, cultural and religious beliefs).

- The CMHN should consider the quality of life for Mr Peterson. Refusing to take medication (for his dementia and for the urinary tract infection) may well be contributing to Mr Peterson's state of mind. An assessment would have to be made as to whether it would be in his best interests to give medication without his consent and, if given, reassess his mental state and/or future decision-making through open and honest discussion with him.

- Occasionally there will be a situation (for example, where the patient's capacity remains questionable or where treatment is non-therapeutic such as in withdrawal of treatment) where the CMHN may have to consider legal advice and apply to the court for a ruling.

Case example 2

A person with dementia attends a memory clinic. She is prescribed medication to help with her cognitive performance but refuses to take it. Her family have been consulted and they want her to take the medication.

- One adult cannot legally consent for another although it is evidence of good practice for CMHNs to consult carers in order to get a full and meaningful picture of the patient.

- If possible, a carer may have to be nominated as having a Lasting Power of Attorney (LPA) MCA (2005); decision-making powers over those who are regarded as not having mental capacity include those affecting health and well-being.

- A full assessment will have to be made as to whether this lady has the capacity to consent or refuse consent to treatment. This will involve first of all a clinical diagnosis of mental capacity and subsequently consideration of the legal process described above in relation to a duty of care and the standard that would be required in law, in relation to consent to treatment. The CMHN should be guided by the decision in Re C [1994] and by the Code of Practice that requires clinicians to ensure that consent is sought in the best circumstances possible (i.e. time given to a Person With Dementia (PWD) to consider what is being proposed, full and meaningful explanations given). In addition, what would have to be ascertained would be whether the lady is a danger to herself or others and whether it would be in her best interests to treat her against her wishes (i.e. would result in some improvement of condition), if this were the case, then reasonable force could be used to ensure medication is taken.

- The CMHN may also rely on the Mental Patients in the Community Act (1995) which includes the powers to convey, which allows for patients to be taken to a place for medical treatment to be given if they are deemed to be a danger to themselves (and/or others).

Case example 3

A carer is out shopping with his father who has dementia and, despite the son's best efforts to keep a close eye on his father's movements, at some stage he managed to put a digital camera into his pocket while the son was being served. Upon leaving the store, the father was approached by a security guard who has asked for the father to accompany him to the manager's office. The father becomes afraid and aggressive and physically assaults the security guard. Eventually the son is able to escort his father to the manager's office whereupon he is informed that his father may be charged with shoplifting and assault.

- *Prima facie* the PWD may be guilty of theft if it can be proven that they 'intended to permanently to deprive the owner of the property' (Theft Act s.1). However, in this instance, we are again directed to case law to determine whether the PWD has sufficient capacity to intend anything and for this we have to consider that there are two aspects to a crime. *Mens rea*, which basically means a guilty mind and refers to the state of mind of the individual at the time the proposed crime was committed, and the *actus reus* (the second aspect of a crime), which is the act of committing a crime. *Mens rea* and *actus reus* must exist at the same time for a criminal conviction.

- In the case study above, the CMHN would be able to apply the rules laid down in R v. McNaughton (1843) which are: 'Every man is presumed to be sane and possess a sufficient degree of reason to be responsible for his crimes until the contrary be proved.' To establish a defence of insanity, it must be clearly proved that at the time of committing the act the accused was labouring under 'such a defect of reason, from a disease of the mind as not to know the nature and quality of the act he was doing, or if he did know, that he did not know, he was doing what was wrong'.

- For a criminal prosecution to be successful, it would have to be proven that the PWD had full knowledge of what he was doing and intended to take the camera without paying for it. Determining the mental capacity of the PWD is vital. Both the clinical diagnosis of dementia and ascertaining whether the PWD had capacity at the time the crime was committed will define whether or not a criminal prosecution is successful.

Summary

CMHNs work in a climate where they are increasingly expected to take on complex clinical caseloads of severely ill people. This will involve ethical dilemmas that require practitioners to constantly revisit what is right, what is appropriate and what is in the best interests of individuals in their care (Mason and McCall Smith 1994). CMHNs should strive to achieve a degree of patient autonomy and consider holistically what the individual would want if they had the capacity to make decisions for themselves.

The processes involved in ensuring that a legal and ethical consent to treatment is obtained are multifaceted and there is much to remember. Where possible, the CMHNs should view these challenges as opportunities to develop practice, and place themselves central to these changes to provide the best care.

Lessons for CMNH practice

- Do ensure that the consent that you have is valid and is in line with legal requirements.

- Do make sure that any future policies and guidelines relating to consent to treatment take into account the changes envisioned in new legislation and codes of practice.

- Do ensure that professional practice is underpinned by sound ethical decision-making.

- Do make sure that your practice is of a sufficient professional standard to stand up to legal scrutiny.

- Do note that when you are ensuring you are within the legal requirements of consent to treatment that attention is paid to the processes involved so that patients retain the right to have decisions about their care challenged.

References

Beauchamp, T.L. and Childress, J.F. (1989) *Principles of Biomedical Ethics*. Oxford: Oxford University Press.

Chisholm, D., Healey, A. and Knapp, M. (1995) QALYs and mental health care, in *Mental Health Research Review* 2. 17–19.

Christiansen, J. (1993) *Nursing Partnership: A Model for Nursing Practice*. Edinburgh: Churchill Livingstone.

Cribb, A. (1995) The ethical dimension, in J. Tingle and A. Cribb (eds) *Nursing Law and Ethics*. London: Blackwell Science.

Declaration of Human Rights (1948) United Nations Department of Public Information.

DOH (2004) *Improving Mental Health Law: Towards a New Mental Health Act*. Summary Sep. 2004 www.dh.gov.uk/publications.

Gillon, R. (1994) *Principles of Health Care Ethics*. Chichester: John Wiley and Sons Ltd.

Kant, I. (1993) *Critique of Practical Reason*, edited by L.W. Beck. New York: Macmillan.

Keady, J. and Ashton, P. (2004) The older person with dementia or other mental health problems, in I.J. Norman and I. Ryrie (eds) *The Art and Science of Mental Health Nursing: A Textbook of Principles and Practice*. Maidenhead: Open University Press, pp. 552–93.

Kennedy, I. and Grubb, A. (1994) *Medical Law: Text with Materials*. London: Butterworths.

Mason, J.K. and McCall Smith, R.A. (1994) *Law and Medical Ethics*. London: Butterworths.

Montgomery, J. (1995) Negligence the legal perspective, in J. Tingle and A. Cribb (eds) *Nursing Law and Ethics*. London: Blackwell Science.

Nursing and Midwifery Council (2004) *Code of Professional Conduct*. London: NMC.

Owen, D.G. (1997) *Philosophical Foundations of Tort Law*. Oxford: Clarendon Press.

Parliamentary Office of Science and Technology (2003) Postnote number 2004. Reform of Mental Health Legislation.

Wright, R.W. (1995) Right, justice and tort law, in D. Owen (ed.) *Philosophical Foundations of Tort Law*. New York: Oxford University Press.

Cases cited

A.B. and Others v. Leeds Teaching Hospital NHS Trust and Cardiff and Vale HNS Trust [2004] QBD (The Gage case)

Barnett v. Chelsea and Kensington Hospital Management Committee [1968] 1 QB 428

Bolam v. Friern Hospital Management Committee [1957] 2 All ER 118

Bolithio v. City and Hackney Health Authority [1998] AC 232 HL

Bolton v. Stone [1951] AC 850 HL

Donoghue v. Stevenson [1932] All ER Rep 1; House of Lords

H.L. v. The United Kingdom ('The Bournewood Case') [2004]

Hotson v. East Berkshire Area Health Authority [1987] 2 All ER 909 (H.L.)

Hucks v. Cole (1968) [1993] 4 Med LR 393 (C.A.)

Norfolk and Norwich Healthcare (NHS) Trust v. W [1996] 2 FLR 613

R (on the application of Burke) v. The GMC [2004] EWHC 1879

Re B (Adult: Refusal of Medical Treatment) [2002] EWHC 429 (Fam)

Re C [1994] 1 All E.R. 819
R v. Ashworth Hospital Authority (now Mersey Care National Health Service Trust) (Appellants) ex parte Munjaz (FC) (Respondent) HOUSE OF LORDS [2005] UKHL 58
R v. Mc'Naughten (1843) 10 CI and Fin 200; 4 State Trials (New Series) 847–934
Tameside and Glossop Acute Services Trust v CH [1996] 1 FCR 753,766

Legislation

Disability Discrimination Act (1995)
Human Rights Act (1998)
Mental Capacity Act (2005)
Mental Health Act (1983)
Mental Health Patients in the Community Act (1995)
National Assistance Act (1948)
NHS and Community Care Act (1990)

6

Ethnic minority communities and the experience of dementia

A review and implications for practice

Jenny Mackenzie

Introduction

In the past 10 years, marked changes in the tone of health and social care policy documents have generated an increased awareness among formal care providers that diverse populations have different health and social care needs. Increased awareness that difference and diversity in a population of potential service users require a flexible approach to service provision, however, does not automatically lend itself to increased understanding at the client interface, with professionals often left lacking confidence about how well they engage with clients whose cultural life ways are different to their own.

I will begin this chapter by considering what 'ethnic minority community' has come to mean in Britain and how social and political meanings create for all those thus classified an imposed identity. Connections will be drawn between this imposed identity and the different ways that growing old as a pioneer migrant in Britain have been constructed, based on the experience of migration and the struggle for citizenship rights. This leads to a consideration of how regarding people as individuals alongside knowledge of the social and political influences on their lives rather than regarding them simply members of 'other' groups can open the way to mutually satisfying user/provider relationships.

What is meant by 'ethnic minority community'?

To begin, the word 'ethnic' is derived from the Greek word 'ethnos' meaning 'nation' and in its original use, to be 'ethnic' meant to be 'heathen' (Smaje 1995). Over the past 40 years the world has witnessed the decolonization process in Africa and Asia and new nation states being created. As a result, the meaning of the word 'ethnic' has drifted away from its connections to membership of a given nation to being understood as a recognized symbol of belonging and grouping e.g. Guibernau and Rex (1997) who identified 'positive feelings of belonging' to be a fitting description of 'ethnic', and Spoonley (1993) who concluded that 'ethnic' meant 'positive feelings of belonging to a cultural group'. Even earlier, Weber (1922) had proposed that a 'subjective belief in a common descent' typified the pattern of ethnic groupings, membership of which might be determined by shared physical attributes, shared customs and/or a shared political structure.

These rather comforting 'belonging' definitions of ethnicity unfortunately lose their appeal when we consider how 'belonging' also tends to act as a boundary marker and a mechanism for separating people into groups, particularly according to their apparent, and usually visible, differences as proffered by Weber. Consequently, the word 'ethnic' as used today tends to slide into the vocabulary as a replacement for the now contested term 'race' as a classificatory device to unite others in their differences, which establishes an 'us and them' understanding of the meaning of 'ethnic' that automatically sets a subjective distance between us as people as we systematically categorize one another into groups.

Being 'ethnic' as in belonging to an 'other' group is a theme Mason (2000) developed as he concluded that white British people tend to see themselves as individuals, whereas they tend to see 'ethnic' people as others who belong to a group descended from the former British colonies. It goes without saying that this assumption also conflates 'ethnic' with skin colour, and has come to refer to anyone who is not white, a trend identified as being prevalent in the health service by De Bono (1996). The intervening years have seen little improvement in this rather ethnocentric meaning of 'ethnic', which appears to be widespread across the Western world where the majority ethnic populations are white. Zapf Creations provide us with a wonderful example of this in the marketing of their internationally popular white doll 'Baby Annabell', as they promote their black edition of the doll as 'Baby Annabell Ethnic', while an online search for 'ethnic products' in the UK reveals a myriad of importers and traders of 'ethnic' craft, home wares and cosmetics, mostly from Africa and the Indian subcontinent.

The ease with which we conflate ethnic and non-white skin colour underpins a great deal of misunderstanding about what constitutes ethnic identity and indeed minority ethnic status. Mason (2000) offers as examples the offensiveness of being a black British person seen as culturally exotic because of their skin colour, and white European people who are culturally diverse and distinct from the white British majority, who are seldom included in considerations of the needs of ethnic minorities. Indeed, such a common and falsely assumed level of cultural proximity based on a person's appearance contributes to yet another cycle of marginalization of minority ethnic service users, which has been, and remains, to a large extent unexplored in medical research (Aspinall 1998) and in ethnicity politics in general (Anthias and Yuval-Davies 1992). The primacy of the 'white' ethnic category on most ethnic monitoring forms and in research in health and social care disciplines renders white minority groups in Britain invisible (Aspinall 1998) and hides the existence of significantly high morbidity and mortality ratios compared to the majority white population (Abbotts 2001).

Minority ethnic people in Britain then have come to be understood as being black or Asian and belonging to a group where their shared and individual differences are all contained by their ethnicity. This is an imposed identity that has been generated by the majority over time and applied to the minority. Thankfully, despite the prevalence of this standpoint, it is also contested by Mason and others who see ethnic status as only one facet of all of our individual and complex identities, rather than as the social glue which bonds others into out-group classifications by virtue of their appearance. Gerrish et al. made the point that 'We are all ethnic, yet our ethnicity does not define us. We all need our ethnic identity to be respected, yet we cannot be adequately understood solely in terms of our ethnicity' (1996: 19).

If we cease to determine that ethnic identity is the leading category by which 'others' are defined and accept that ethnic identity is only one component of our complex and multi-faceted social identities, then like other components of ourselves, we can all bring our ethnic identity into play to present aspects of ourselves, either in celebration of, or in defence of, our individuality. If ethnicity is judged in this context, we can all generate our own understanding of what our ethnicity means to us, as well as being aware of the constraints of imposed definitions.

However, imposed and self-generated meanings of ethnic identity are connected by the ways in which a person engages with society and how society controls the person's social interactions. Hence, no consideration of the meaning of 'ethnic' can be removed from what we think we mean when we refer to 'community', which is a term that, like 'ethnic', infers belonging. For example, people, who describe themselves in terms of their ethnicity, are expressing a part of their identity they share with others – a consciousness of kind – 'wrapping their sense of *me* within a powerful shared *we*' (Burkitt et al. 2001: 39). It is through applying this consciousness of kind that individuals express a sense of collective identity (Wallman 1986; Husband 1996). We have come to expect that institutional structures, including religion, culture, leisure and family, interacting with social, economic and geographical dynamics, both symbolize and preside over our collective identities and, therefore, our membership of a community. Such institutional structures are essential to the existence of a community as we imagine it ought to be and yet, regardless of what our ethnic identity is, we accept our individual right to opt in and out of such institutional structures while imagining that members of other communities remain cohesive and committed to their own such structures at all times.

To illustrate, television soaps reinforce our sense of how we imagine other communities exist by depicting small communities centred on institutional structures, e.g. pubs, cafés, a place of worship, which provide the mechanisms through which we, the viewers, are able to observe all the characters and how they interact with one another. The structure of the television soap demonstrates how any attempt to define a community can only be successful if it and its members are simplified beyond possible reality. Where in the world does everyone living on one street meet several times daily in the same place, enjoy endless job opportunities within walking distance from their homes, where colleagues are also neighbours and family members and where no one ever watches television soaps? I would suggest nowhere, and yet, if viewing figures are to be believed, hundreds of thousands of us tune in and get lost in the story lines, as if the communities presented and their characters were real. Irresistible as television soap communities may be, we are all individuals and our collective identities and, therefore, our community memberships are as multi-faceted as our social identities. Any one individual will have a place in more than one community as that individual may take part in paid work, a family, a neighbourhood, all spaces where collective or 'communal' identity becomes real, and as a consequence, fragmented.

Communities then can mean more than geography and assumptions about what really constitutes 'community' are explored and critiqued by a number of commentators, including Barth (1969), Cohen (1982, 1985) and Jenkins (1996), who proposed that communities are defined by boundaries between similarity and difference, bringing into play the in-group/out-group dynamics present in the imposed 'ethnic' identity above. In-group/out-group dynamics are informed by the ways in which a community constructs its institutional structures as symbols that define its boundaries. In the case of diverse communities, boundary symbols may be read inaccurately by those outside of the community, or deliberately constructed by a threatened community driven by pride to project a more favourable public image than the reality of private experience.

Cohen (1985) attempted to unravel many of the discrepancies in the meaning of community, arguing, as above, that the symbolism apparent at community boundaries is a reflection of the meaning members and non-members give to a community and its population. As in the notion of ethnicity above, Britons tend to regard only themselves as individuals, expecting 'others' to be part of a group where they all share significant similarities. The danger in this thesis is that we can all make assumptions about the beliefs and values of a community of people and load it with expectations about cultural lifestyles that we imagine correspond to that ethnic type, through a combination of what we assume we see in boundary symbols and the subjective distancing which comes about from popular definitions of ethnic identity.

This takes us back to the notion of the television soap as a mentally constructed, or fictional, community. The ways in which people imagine communities has been extensively argued by Anderson whose work has been frequently referred to in support of arguments that communities don't exist as one analytic construct, or, if they do, are 'conceived as a deep, horizontal comradeship' (1991: 7).

It is a combination of the symbolic construction of boundaries and the 'deep horizontal comradeship' notion of community that poses particular problems for minority ethnic citizens in that their perceived identities and their needs are understood to be a reflection of how their ethnicity and culture are symbolically constructed at the boundaries of their communities. If the recognized institutional structures that bind a community together, such as places of worship and family, are in place and visible as symbols at the boundary of that community, does that mean all members of a community are welcome to participate in those institutional structures, or even want to participate? The answer of course is no, but an outsider might form the impression that inside all is well, because our received understanding of other people's communities and their ethnic identities convinces us of their similarity and their shared belonging.

In some respects the British approach to multiculturalism since the 1960s presupposes that all individuals are able to maintain their own identities in separate communities while also being part of society at large, which compounds the kind of assumptions we all make about how one another live. In the way of multi-cultural politics, it is proposed that cultural diversity can exist within one society as a collection of 'communities', but that people are equal in the public arena (Kelly 2003). Hence cultural diversity becomes both an individual and a shared issue (Rex 1996).

While emphasizing the important role of communities, British politics has also highlighted self-help, and encouraged the generation of formal community associations providing tailored services to community members (Candappa and Joly 1994; Kelly 2003) as essential facets of community development. Just as television soaps broadcast a community that is far from real, our expectation of one another's communities are similarly idealized, based on the judgements we make about each community's institutional structures. Therefore, we can be misled into thinking that where a large church, temple, synagogue or mosque is sited, the populations in those communities are all devout worshippers. Or, that a predominance of family and community centres within a short radius means that members of the surrounding community live in harmony and cohesion.

Concepts of community and ethnic identity are areas that dementia research in Britain has not yet fully addressed. In essence, although difference and diversity have begun to be recognized in older people's policy frameworks, what goes on beyond the boundaries of minority ethnic communities and how, in turn, old age and dementia are conceptualized by people within such communities have yet to be fully explored. An understanding of how individuals' life histories, including their migration experiences, have conspired with social and political influences on the imposed understanding of ethnic identity begins to yield insights into how and when people from minority ethnic communities engage with mainstream health and social care services.

Experiences of migration

The migration period relevant to today's older minority ethnic service users stretches from the Second World War and the post-war years into the 1960s. This was when mass migration from Europe and the colonies took place – something that directly affects people with dementia and family carers today, as their experiences of migration and their rights as citizens have shaped their social status, their identities and their view of the world. So in keeping with the broader understanding of ethnic identity, let us focus on the differing migration experiences of today's Eastern European and South Asian older people.

Eastern European military personnel came to Britain ahead of their families during the Second World War. They were assisted to settle in Britain after the war by a government programme designed to facilitate integration in British society (Rees 1982; Mason 2000). Those not so fortunate were the European Volunteer Workers (EVWs), who entered Britain from displacement camps after the war (Mason 2000). Following the redrawing of political boundaries in Europe, several camps for displaced persons and refugees existed in Germany and Austria, which became recruitment resources for Ministry of Labour officials (Solomos 1989). Thus, a new scheme developed, wherein the British State met the costs of recruitment, transport and repatriation of personnel from such camps to participate in Britain's rebuilding process (Solomos 1989). EVWs were categorized as alien and had to comply with a number of conditions of entry that placed restrictions on where they could work and what types of jobs they could engage in (Phizacklea and Miles 1987). While some regulations, such as being paid the same as British workers benefited the EVWs, others, such as being the first to be made redundant, restrictions on promotion, being admitted for one year only and not being allowed to change jobs without Ministry of Labour approval (Tannahill 1958) placed considerable restrictions on any prospect of early settlement. Furthermore, settlement was further constrained by conditions of employment stipulating that EVWs could only work in areas and jobs where British labour was unavailable and that they were not allowed to bring their families/dependants to Britain after 1947 (Mason 2000). Although in subsequent years a slow moderation of restrictions meant many EVWs were joined by their families (Rees 1982; Solomos 1989), the organization of similar guest worker schemes in countries such as South Africa, Canada and Australia inevitably meant that many families became globally dispersed.

An interesting distinction was made between the refugee/asylum seeker status of the people recruited, and the 'volunteer worker' title chosen for them, as it seemed less demeaning than 'displaced person'. As indicated above, those who migrated to Britain under this scheme were not in effect volunteers, but were allocated to manual employment, e.g. mining, textiles and menial jobs in the NHS, regardless of their qualifications or past work histories (McDowell 2003). McDowell also highlights the dearth of evidence about the lives and status of European Volunteer Workers, which leaves us with very little in the way of an analysis of how they constructed their identity in Britain during a period of assimilation rather than multi-cultural policy.

However, there are some clues to their experiences. Tannahill (1958) argues that the EVW scheme created racial and gender divisions in the labour force and McDowell (2003) points out that the EVW scheme was implemented by the British government against the wishes of the trades union movement. Taken alongside Zubrzycki's (1956) record of Polish immigrants in Britain, the indications are that these workers endured a period of tension and conflict that posed significant hurdles to their adjustment and assimilation to life in Britain.

Zubrzycki's account tells of hostile reactions from the British towards the Poles after Russia's entry into the war, spurred on by media reports that stereotyped Poles as 'Jew baiters and fascist reactionaries'. Hostility continued in the post-war period, fuelled by views – expressed both at the TUC Congress and in the media – of foreign labour taking British jobs, undermining standards of living and exacerbating the housing shortage. For Polish exiles in Britain, gratitude turned to distrust following the Warsaw uprising in 1944 and Britain's consent in yielding half of Poland's pre-war territory to Soviet Russia at the Yalta Conference of 1945. According to Zubrzycki, this also significantly impeded the subsequent assimilation and amalgamation of Polish EVWs as the Polish community became even more determined to 'uphold their cultural and national distinctiveness' (1956: 84).

The period of compulsory assigned labour for volunteer workers lasted for two years, during which time the majority of workers resided communally in hostel accommodation managed by the state or their employers. There they tended to meet and marry co-nationals (McDowell 2003). Social mobility as well as class mobility was restricted through geographical allocation and also restrictions on promotion (Tannahill 1958). Until regulations regarding aliens were relaxed, rights of nationalization, political involvement and welfare privileges were limited (Mason, 2000). In the various migrant communities involved in the EVW scheme, people pooled resources to acquire property and construct self-sufficient communities (Smith and Jackson 1999; McDowell 2003).

Many of the allied and EVW migrants to Britain during that period had been subjected to unimaginable physical and emotional trauma in their homelands, something frequently played out in old age, and particularly distressing for people with dementia and their carers (Alzheimer Scotland 2000). An extract from Alzheimer Scotland's newsletter illustrates this:

> Lothian has a substantial Polish population; many came in the 1940s to join the armed forces, and are now reaching their 80s. Polish Outreach Worker . . . has already received 35 referrals. She described two particularly disturbing examples. In one, a Polish woman with dementia, confined to a hospital bed with her leg in plaster and a feeding tube, was terrified that she was back in a concentration camp and saw the doctors and nurses as commandants. In another case, an elderly Polish person with dementia had returned, mentally, to refugee status, keeping belongings in a case under the bed and suffering constant agitation.
>
> (Alzheimer Scotland – Action on Dementia 2000)

It is important to bear in mind that many of the transit hostels where EVWs were accommodated on arrival were in hospitals, with the result that hospitals may have significant memories and meanings for older Eastern Europeans. A further aspect of

Eastern European migrant history is that women were frequently posted to work as cleaners or auxiliaries in hospitals. This may account for their apparent familiarity with the health and welfare system in the UK, in comparison to the documented under-use of services by South Asian families.

Regrettably, and perhaps as a function of the conflation of 'ethnic' and skin colour in British thinking, post-war Eastern European migration and the experience of being a refugee did not sustain the interest of scholars and researchers (Stein 1986). As a result, the heritage and cultural lifeways of these older people are somewhat hidden from service providers and the construction of EVW identities in terms of their 'labour' (McDowell 2003), and the assumption that Eastern European migrants and their subsequent generations are 'just like us' on the basis of their skin colour and religion, have combined to draw a veil over the impetus to investigate the needs of older Eastern European people. Nevertheless, it is reasonable to conclude that as service users, older Eastern European people are unlikely, because of their history of dispersal, to have extended family support networks, while their health and social care needs may be significantly altered by the ways in which many survived earlier life trauma.

The migration history of South Asian older people in the post-war years contains some marked differences to the experiences of Eastern European migrants described above. Unlike their Eastern European counterparts, South Asian and Caribbean post-war migrants were, according to the British Nationality Act of 1948, free to enter Britain and settle with their families as members of Commonwealth countries. In addition, unlike the EVWs, whose migration was determined by a combination of push and pull factors by virtue of their displacement, Black and South Asian migrants were actively recruited to fill Britain's labour shortages. Again, available work consisted of manual labour, and geographical patterns of settlement were dependent on labour demand, such as manufacturing in London and the West Midlands and the textile industries in Lancashire and Yorkshire. Subsequent waves of immigrants from the Commonwealth tended to settle in the same areas as the original pioneers who facilitated their search for employment and housing, even though restrictions on access to social housing placed these migrant groups in the least desirable accommodation as well as the least desirable jobs (Mason 2000). These beginnings have laid the foundation for today's demographic trends, despite industrial recession in many cities and towns.

The response to meeting labour shortages with migrant labour aroused a wave of white British hostility, culminating in the Notting Hill riots of 1958 (Solomos 1989; Mason 2000), which led to the Commonwealth Immigrants Act of 1962 that sought to impose restrictions on the movements of Commonwealth citizens into Britain (Mason 2000). The history of immigration control from 1962 until now might suggest that the years between 1945 and 1962 constituted a period of openness in which the state facilitated the migration and settlement of black and Asian workers. In his account of the politics of migration, Solomos (1989) illustrates how the period above was in reality a time in which political ideologies became inherently racialized. Citing Carter et al. (1987), Solomos describes how, by 1952, successive Labour and Conservative Governments had created administrative policies to actively discourage black immigration. As McDowell's (2003) study also shows, the attitude of government and the host population towards Commonwealth immigrants was less than welcoming and it is during this period that the link between race relations and immigration control was forged, in that the state response to controlling the 'colour' problem was to look to ways to limit the immigration of black workers, which by the 1950s had begun to gather momentum (Joshi and Carter 1984; Rich 1986; Solomos 1989).

The Commonwealth Immigrants Act of 1962 imposed strict control on the number of black labour migrants coming into Britain by implementing a system of vouchers allocated to applicants:

- Category A vouchers issued to people with a job to go to
- Category B vouchers issued to those with qualifications or skills in short supply.
- Category C vouchers issued on a first come first served basis in deliberately limited supply.

Subsequently, the Category C voucher was revoked altogether in 1965, following continuing concerns about the number of black and Asian migrants entering Britain (Mason 2000: 26), which impeded women and children's ability to join their husbands and fathers.

Tightening immigration control was, however, not to appease social concerns over the 'colour' problem in Britain. Enoch Powell's famed 'Rivers of Blood' speech in 1968 warned of the 'total transformation of Britain' and the long-term risk of increasing racial tension, which brought into play debates about forced repatriation (Solomos 1989).

The hostile social and political environment described above has direct relevance to the older pioneer migrants who are potential service users today. The impacts of immigration controls have had profound consequences for South Asian family life in Britain, as Ahmad (1996) examines in his appraisal of family obligations in the face of social change in Britain. Economic and kinship obligations meant that sending money to families still residing in the Indian sub-continent consumed the majority of what was already a poor income. This delayed the process by which families could be reunited and the immigration controls of 1962 put a further obstacle in the way of unification. Once families were reunited, financial remittance to remaining relatives waned, despite being 'a significant source of financial support to a large number of families in the sub-continent' (Ahmad 1996: 60).

South Asian migration history gives some valuable insight into the way in which post-war labour migrants from the Indian sub-continent had to struggle to negotiate their citizenship and livelihood in the face of social and political racism. These are the roots of a discriminatory system that conspired to exclude today's South Asian older people from social participation and, despite the current shift in political focus from exclusion towards inclusion, the memories of being victims of state-organized xenophobia will have impacted on their willingness to engage fully with health and welfare services.

Implications for service development

Despite policy recognition that flexible provision is the key to meeting diverse needs, the system of care in the UK is still one that expects users to present themselves to services in the first instance on recognizing a health need. In the case of older people with dementia, this presupposes that the dementia experience can be generalized across the multi-ethnic population, and that all members of the population are able to and will connect with the relevant service within the system. This creates an impasse between service providers and potential users, because while the need for multi-ethnic services has been recognized, before such services can be designed to provide for a multi-ethnic population, there needs to be a comprehensive understanding by service developers and providers of the ways they and their services are conceptualized by diverse populations.

Valle (1998) suggests that to recognize the ways services are conceptualized interculturally:

> [service providers] generally have to step outside of their own cognitive and emotional home base. They have to leave the relative comfort of their own formal training backgrounds to see their own service organizations through the eyes of very needy but interculturally confused individuals and family groups coming for help.
>
> (1998: 23)

There is therefore a requirement for service providers not only to recognize the ways in which their services may be perceived, but also to determine how they can communicate more effectively what needs their services seek to address within conceptual frameworks that can be understood by diverse users.

This type of comprehensive understanding also applies at the individual professional/ user interface, for example, Kleinman (1988) suggested that an understanding of the user's experiences required the professional to engage in mini-ethnographies, as a mechanism for translating the user's understandings of their illness, and consequently their health need, to the professional's perspective. This is no more important than in dementia care where it is recognized that an element of regression is an aspect of the dementia process. To this end, Valle also argued that service providers need to be able to develop a flexible understanding of the person with dementia's culture of origin, given that the process of dementia:

> forces the affected person farther and farther back into his or her long-term memory, where the culture-of-origin orientations still reside. The family members seeking to accommodate the dementia-affected elder are likewise forced back into this more traditional cultural orientation, as are practitioners.
>
> (1998: 23)

This underlines the importance of understanding the history of the groups being targeted for service provision and consequently becomes a vital component of cultural competence. In the case of the Eastern European and South Asian older people's history of migration considered above, the dementia process itself could be contributing to the factors that make these groups 'hard to reach', in that their early experiences of being 'ethnic minority' people in Britain have, for many, been marginalizing and consequently discriminatory. Valle's (1998) assumption, written from a US perspective, was that the culture of origin could take on primary importance in the person with dementia's life. Given the number of years that today's pioneer migrant populations have resided in Britain, combined with their diverse early life experiences, for some users, reliving resistance to hostile power structures rather than traditional cultural orientations is equally possible. What is also required, therefore, within the development of flexible approaches to service provision is the willingness to adapt the principles of the service culture to address the perceptions of potential users and to ensure that alternative illness narratives proffered by users are recognized.

Summary

This chapter began by referring to contemporary advances in health and social policy that require older people's service providers to recognize the way cultural life ways and ethnic identities influence user needs. The onus is placed on service providers to meet the needs of diverse populations and we can see how such policy advances have opened the door to a more inclusive philosophy of service provision. Herein lies a tension in older people's services, though, as the problem for minority ethnic older people in connecting with this now inclusive philosophy is their experience of having had their ethnic identities defined and redefined through half a century of state control over the ways that they as pioneer migrants and their communities interact with society.

For many older people, the experience of being the 'ethnic other' has been marginalizing and discriminatory. Their experience has been constructed through migration as a process that encompasses political and state control over early citizenship rights, social and economic immobility and the experience of racism and xenophobia. These influences have shaped their social identities and as Jenkins (1996) argued, social identity has no meaning in isolation, it is dependent upon interaction and is mediated by internal (how we see ourselves) as well as external (how others see us) factors.

For Eastern European and the South Asian older people, the above influences that shaped their social identities represent powerful forces that have impinged on their life experiences. The external factors mediating their social identities have contributed to a labelling process (Becker 1963). Far from being passive recipients of this labelling process, the nature of community construction means that people are able to internalize some aspects of their imposed identity and construct resistance to other aspects, to protect a strong sense of belonging to their respective cultural groups. This is in part an expression of impression management (Goffman 1969) wherein pioneer migrants strive to project an aspect of their identity they wish to share, which communicates their status in relation to their place in Britain. In another sense, this acts as a strategy that masks the experience of being victimized, which is a contributing factor to the reluctance some older people with dementia may feel about engaging with support services. For South Asian elders, the reluctance to engage with services may be traced to their experience of being marginalized linguistically, culturally, religiously, on the grounds of colour, and an expectation that their cultural and religious needs will not be catered for, nor their kinship obligations understood. For the older Eastern European people with dementia, their reluctance may be similarly related to language and culture, but also to refugee and war experiences, through which being moved or transported to care facilities or being separated from loved ones can be extremely distressing.

The history of strong kinship networks in minority ethnic communities is also born of internalization and resistance that preserves a personal and also a social identity, grounded in ethnic, religious and cultural heritage. The need to recreate a former social world was integral to survival and a sense of security as 'ethnic other' for pioneer migrants and has, through the generations, been a sustaining factor in the continuation of cultural lifeways.

In effect, older minority ethnic service users have become expert transcultural communicators over the years, having negotiated white British and their own culture in a manner that has enabled them to survive in an often hostile social and political climate. However, for some minority ethnic service users, the dementia process itself may undermine their ability and indeed their willingness to engage with services. Consequently, dementia itself may be a contributing factor to making minority ethnic older people a 'hard-to-reach' group.

For service providers, an awareness and appreciation of all of the above factors and how they have impacted on the lives of users individually are integral to the success of transcultural communication and care delivery. We have only considered the major social and political influences on the lives of South Asian and Eastern European older people in this chapter as exemplars. This, however, is a process practitioners need to engage in with their own local populations in order to begin to break down the subjective distancing that arises between practitioners and users whose ethnic identities and experiences of living in Britain are different from each other, and whose experience of dementia may encompass revisiting the traumas of earlier life.

Lessons for CMNH practice

- Advances in health and social policy require service providers to recognize the influences that ethnicity and culture have on user needs and to work towards ensuring services are socially inclusive.

- The ways in which old age and dementia are conceptualized in minority ethnic communities in Britain have yet to be fully explored.

- Beginning to understand older minority ethnic users as individuals whose life histories and migration experiences have contributed to their social identities is fundamental to the development of cultural competence in dementia care.

- If practitioners are able to recognize the social and political factors that may have influenced users' experiences of living in Britain, this facilitates a greater understanding of how older minority ethnic users might perceive their dementia and mainstream services.

- A consideration of the above factors helps to break down the subjective distancing that arises between practitioners responsible for supporting service users with different ethnic identities to their own.

References

Abbotts, J. (2001) Morbidity and Irish Catholic descent in Britain: Relating health disadvantage to socio-economic position, *Social Sciences and Medicine*, 52(7): 999–1005.

Ahmad, W.I.U. (1996) Family obligations and social change among South Asian communities, in W.I.U. Ahmad and K. Atkin (eds) *Race and Community Care*. Buckingham: Open University Press.

Alzheimer Scotland – Action on Dementia (2000) Minister launches minority ethnic services, Newsletter.

Anderson, B. (1991) *Imagined Communities*. London: Verso.

Anthias, F. and Yuval-Davies, N. (1992) *Racialised Boundaries: Race, Nation, Gender, Colour and Class and the Anti-racist Struggle*. London: Routledge.

Aspinall, P.J. (1998) Describing the 'white' ethnic group and its composition in medical research, *Social Science and Medicine*, 47(11): 1797–808.

Barth, F. (1969) Introduction, in F. Barth (ed.) *Ethnic Groups and Boundaries: The Social Organisation of Culture Difference*. Oslo: Universitetsforlaget.

Becker, H.S. (1963) *Outsiders: Studies in the Sociology of Deviance*. New York: Free Press.

Burkitt, I., Husband, C., Mackenzie, J., Torn, A. and Crow, R. (2001) *Nurse Education and Communities of Practice*. Cambridge: English National Board for Nursing Midwifery and Health Visiting.

Candappa, M. and Joly, D. (1994) *Local Authorities, Ethnic Minorities and Pluralist Integration*. Coventry: Centre for Research in Ethnic Relations, University of Warwick.

Carter, B., Harris, C. and Joshi, S. (1987) The 1951–55 Conservative government and the racialisation of black immigration, *Policy Papers in Ethnic Relations*, 11. Coventry: Centre for Research in Ethnic Relations, University of Warwick.

Cohen, A.P. (1982) Belonging: the experience of culture, in A.P. Cohen (ed.) *Belonging: Identity and Social Organisation in British Rural Cultures*. Manchester: Manchester University Press.

Cohen, A.P. (1985) *The Symbolic Construction of Community*. London: Routledge and Kegan Paul.

De Bono, D. (1996) White populations also need to be accurately described, *British Medical Journal*, 313: 425.

Gerrish, K., Husband, C. and Mackenzie, J. (1996) *Nursing for a Multi-ethnic Society*. Buckingham: Open University Press.

Goffman, E. (1969) *The Presentation of the Self in Everyday Life*. London: The Penguin Press.

Guibernau, M. and Rex, J. (1997) *The Ethnicity Reader*. Cambridge: Polity Press.

Husband, C. (1996) Defining and containing diversity: community, ethnicity and citizenship, in W.I.U. Ahmad and K. Atkin (eds) *Race and Community Care*. Buckingham: Open University Press.

Jenkins, R. (1996) *Social Identities*. London: Routledge.

Joshi, S. and Carter, B. (1984) The role of Labour in the creation of a racist Britain, *Race and Class*, 25(3): 53–70.

Kelly, L. (2003) Bosnian refugees in Britain: questioning community, *Sociology*, 37(1): 35–9.

Kleinman, A. (1988) *The Illness Narratives: Suffering, Healing and the Human Condition*. New York: Basic Books.

Mason, D. (2000) *Race and Ethnicity in Modern Britain*, 2nd edn. Oxford: Oxford University Press.

McDowell, L. (2003) The particularities of place: geographies of gendered moral responsibilities among Latvian migrant workers in 1950s Britain, *Transactions of the Insitute of British Geographers*, 28(1): 19–34.

Phizacklea, A. and Miles, R. (1987) The British trade union movement and racism, in G. Lee and R. Loveridge (eds) *The Manufacture of Disadvantage*. Buckingham: Open University Press.

Rees, T. (1982) Immigration policies in the United Kingdom, in C. Husband (ed.) *Race in Britain: Continuity and Change*. London: Hutchinson University Library.

Rex, J. (1996) *Ethnic Minorities in the Modern Nation State*. Basingstoke: Macmillan.

Rich, P. (1986) *Race and Empire in British Politics*. Cambridge: Cambridge University Press.

Smaje, C. (1995) *Health, 'Race' and Ethnicity*. London: King's Fund Institute.

Smith, G. and Jackson, P. (1999) Narrating the nation: the 'imagined community' of Ukrainians in Bradford, *Journal of Historical Geography*, 25: 367–87.

Solomos, J. (1989) *Race and Racism in Contemporary Britain*. Basingstoke: Macmillan Publishers Ltd.

Spoonley, P. (1993) *Racism and Ethnicity*. Oxford: Oxford University Press.

Stein, B.N. (1986) The experience of being a refugee: insights from the research, in C. Williams and J. Westermeyer (eds) *Refugee Mental Health in Resettlement Countries*. London: Taylor and Francis.

Tannahill, J. (1958) *The European Volunteer Workers*. Manchester: Manchester University Press.

Valle, R. (1998) Caregiving across cultures, in *Working with Dementing Illness and Ethnically Diverse Populations*. Washington, DC: Taylor and Francis.

Wallman, S. (1986) Ethnicity and the boundary process in context, in J. Rex and D. Mason (eds) *Theories of Race and Ethnic Relations*. Cambridge: Cambridge University Press.

Weber, M. ([1922] 1968) *Economy and Society*. Los Angeles: University of California Press.

Zubrzycki, J. (1956) *Polish Immigrants in Britain: A Study of Adjustment*. The Hague: Martinus Nijhoff.

7

An inclusive and relationship-centred approach to community mental health nursing to people with dementia and their family carers

Trevor Adams and Paula Gardiner

Introduction

Community mental health nursing care to people with dementia is primarily undertaken by community mental health nurses to older people (CMHNs). The speciality emerged in the 1970s and 1980s through the development of a number of innovative community-based teams that shifted the focus of mental health care for older people from the institution to the community. Excellent accounts of the development of early CMHN services to older people are provided by Barker and Black (1971), Leopoldt et al. (1975), Ainsworth and Jolley (1978) and Lancaster (1984).

The focus of community mental health nursing to people with dementia has always been problematic. The underlying issue is, who should receive CMHN care? Traditionally, within hospitals, it was the person with dementia who was considered the main recipient of care. While recognizing the centrality of the person with dementia, mental health nursing or, as it was then called, psychiatric nursing, often positioned visiting relatives as marginal and at worst, an intrusion to nursing care. However, nurses working within innovative community mental health nursing services to older people realized that this understanding 'of relatives' was not appropriate in community and domiciliary-based settings and that relatives should be seen as joint recipients of care alongside the person with dementia. Returning to the key issue of who should receive community mental health nursing care, the approach adopted by innovatory community mental health nursing services suggested that the person with dementia *and* their carer should be the joint recipients of community mental health nursing care (Barker and Black 1971).

This dual focus within community mental health nursing work to people with dementia did not last very long. This was due to an increased recognition that family carers experienced emotional and physical burden and was reflected in empirical research and government policy towards older people (DHSS 1981; Heaton 1999). Increasingly, in the 1980s, family members (now transformed into 'family carers') were seen as the primary recipients of community mental health nursing care. This approach was similar to trends within other professions working in dementia care and may be called 'care for the carer approach'.

In the late 1980 and 1990s, however, a new set of ideas flowed into dementia care that provided an alternative to the dominant 'care for the carer approach'. Underlying this new approach was the centrality of 'the person with dementia' (Downs 1997). The approach argued that service provision to people with dementia should focus on the person with dementia and that health and social professionals should hear the voice of people with dementia and help them make decisions about the sort of care they wanted to receive. These ideas are seen in the work of Kitwood (1997) who developed the idea of 'person-centred care'; Goldsmith (1996) who argued that people with dementia have a voice that should be heard, and Keady and Gilliard (1999) who described the inner subjective experience of people with dementia. This new approach highlighted the marginalization of people with dementia that had occurred in community mental health nursing as a result of the 'care for the carer approach'. Thus returning to the key question 'Who should receive community mental health nursing care?', it was gradually recognized that family carers could not be seen as the sole focus of care and that there was a need to return to the earlier idea of the dual focus of community mental health nursing practice in which family carers *and* people with dementia were the joint recipients of community mental health nursing care.

In the early to mid-1990s, mental health nursing went through a period of rigorous self-examination as it sought to define itself within the context of multi-disciplinary mental health care (Department of Health 1993). This self-examination led, in part, to a greater recognition of the subjective experience of mental health nurses that may be seen in the increased recognition of transference and counter-transference processes (Butterworth and Faugier 1997) and also the ability of mental health nurses to critically reflect upon their practice (Rolfe et al. 2001). Acknowledgement of these processes contributed to the development of clinical supervision within mental health nursing.

The problematic nature of CHMN practice, together with an appreciation of the usefulness of clinical supervision, corresponds very well with developments that were occurring within dementia care. In the 1990s, clinical areas in dementia care were increasingly seen as problematic. As Morris noted:

> Working with people with dementia at all stages of the disease, but perhaps particularly so in the more advanced stages, is stressful. Staff recruitment and retention problems are pervasive, and low morale and burn-out are the norm in the many of the care facilities.

(2004: 67)

As recognition of the intrapersonal and interpersonal nature of dementia care increased in the 1980s and 1990s, the use of defensive mechanisms by dementia care workers in practice settings was recognized. To address these processes, Kitwood (1997) commends the use of clinical supervision and identifies it as an important feature of the 'new culture of dementia care' and Carradice et al. (2003) and Holman (2003) describe its use within dementia care.

Thus, rather than conceptualizing mental health nursing to people with dementia in dyadic terms – the person with dementia and their carer – it became common to see community mental health nursing practice in triadic terms – people with dementia, their informal family carer(s) and the CMHN. We would suggest the term 'dementia care triads' can be adopted to describe these relationships. We should, however, point out that there may be more than one informal carer involved in the provision of community mental health nursing to people with dementia and that there are also likely to be other dementia care workers involved. Nevertheless, the term 'dementia care triad' is useful as frequently the primary relationship within community mental health nursing practice comprises the person with dementia and their family carer.

Dementia care triads

The idea of 'dementia care triads' originated in the late 1980s. This idea developed through the work of Doherty and Baird (1983) that outlined the therapeutic triangle within chronic health care between the patient, the physician and the family, although they did not use the term 'dementia care triad'. This term, however, was applied to dementia care by Silliman (1989) and later was incorporated into the work of Adams and Clarke (1999) on 'partnerships', Fortinsky (2001) on 'triadic interaction', Adams (2003) on 'inclusion' and Keady and Nolan on 'relationship-centred care' (2003). The underlying idea within this work is that three people or agencies are usually involved in the care of people with dementia: the person with dementia, their informal carer and their paid-for carer, and that an important feature of the delivery of good dementia care is the maintenance of good relationships between each participant (Davis 1992). This understanding of the importance of the interactive and relational nature of 'dementia care triads' raises important questions about the nature of interaction in groups of three, or 'triadic interaction'.

Theoretical basis

Early thinking about triadic interaction was developed by the German sociologist Georg Simmel who argued that the size of social groups affects their structure and functioning. Simmel identified three 'types' of role played by the third person within triads: the mediator, the exploiter and the oppressor. Additional roles were developed by Caplow (1968) who identified eight possible coalitions within three-person groups. He argued further that coalitions arise as a result of members seeking to increase their own power and control within the group. This understanding of triadic interaction was later developed within family therapy by Haley (1977) and also by Hoffman (1981) who identified the occurrence of 'pathological triads' within families.

This theoretical position was supported by various empirical studies that examined the relationship between doctors, older people, and their informal family carers (see Hasselkus 1994; Haug 1994). Roscow (1981) examined different coalitions within triadic medical encounters: (1) patient and carer versus doctor; (2) doctor and carer versus patient; and (3) doctor and patient versus carer. In the first coalition, there is an alliance between the patient and the carer which may limit the power of the doctor. In the second coalition, the doctor and the carer form an alliance against the patient. In this coalition, the wishes of the patient may be ignored, dismissed or undermined. In the last coalition, the doctor and the patient form an alliance that outbalances the power held by the carer.

The problematic nature of triadic interaction in service delivery has been noted by other professional groups. Within social work, Biggs et al. highlighted the collusive alliances that frequently develop between professionals, family carers and older people and argue that 'the triangle of professional helper, carer and elder is thus the primary relation arising from community care' (1995: 73). They suggested that '[L]ike all triangular relationships it is inherently rivalrous, as there is always the possibility of two members pairing off, thus forming a collusive alliance that to some extent excludes the third party' (1975: 73). Biggs (1993, 1994) proposed three types of collusive alliance. In the first, the informal carer and the professional helper excluded the older person. In the second, the informal carer and the older person allied together against the professional helper. In the third, the professional helper and the older person allied against the informal carer.

A similar understanding is shared by Twigg and Atkin who acknowledged the 'ambiguous position' (1994: 11) of family carers within community care. Twigg and Atkin outlined various types of the relationship between service agencies and family carers that represent family carers as acting either as resources, co-workers, co-clients or superseded family carers, where a disabled person has no need of the carer. Twigg and Atkin argued that, due to their cognitive impairment, some people with dementia are unable to fully negotiate their own package of care and that some family carers may collude with their confused relative.

Relationship-centred care

As we have already identified, Nolan et al. (2004) develop a model of health-care inter-action which highlights the importance of relationships in the provision of health and social care and thus describe it as 'relationship-centred care'. Relationship-centred care is much broader than person-centred care and allows broader consideration of the contribu-tion and experience of the informal carer and the paid-for carer (Kitwood 1997). As with any new model, aspects of it need to be refined. For example, Nolan et al. (2004) only talk about the existence of different senses such as the sense of security, belonging and con-tinuity, and say little about how relationships develop and this raises the need to develop a more satisfactory understanding of what is meant by 'relationship'. And, second, there is a need to recognize the problematic and unstable nature of relationships within dementia care triads that often leads to coalitions and alliances and the marginalization of people with dementia. We would argue that a social constructionist perspective offers scope for a more conceptual, analytical and thorough account of interaction within dementia care triads.

Social constructionism is particularly suited to an understanding of interaction in dementia care triads because it takes the view that the social order, for example, who is who and what is what, arises out of social practices such as what people say (verbal language) and what people do (non-verbal and body language) (Burr 2003; Tuffin 2005). In this way, social practices shape social situations and organize who it is that has the power to make things happen. As Dallos and Draper note, 'Social constructionism emphasises that interactions are invariably connected to power and that language use defines power' (2000: 95). This perspective has been used in a range of studies on dementia care and has provided many worthwhile insights. Sabat and his colleagues, for example, have shown how talk within dementia care affects the personhood of people with dementia and also contributes to their sense of awareness (Sabat and Harré 1992; Clare 2004). Moreover, Adams (2001c) has shown how participants within dementia care settings construct what they consider to be a 'risky situation' through conversational and interactive processes.

Two ideas drawn from social constructionism are particularly useful when considering how identity and the meaning of particular events are reproduced within dementia care triads. The first idea is 'subject position' (Wetherell 1998; Burr 2003). This idea draws on the notion of 'interpellation' developed by Althusser (1971) in which ideology summons or hails people to listen and act in certain ways that cause them to take on a particular social identity. Positioning theory (Harré and van Langenhove 1999) argues that interactive and conversational practices such as those within dementia care triads call upon people to take up specific social roles that provide them with particular rights, duties, entitlements and obligations. Positioning has been found to be an important way for people to manage their own and each other's identity within partnerships between health-care providers and their clients (Cheek 2003) and also within dementia care triads (Sabat 2001; Adams 2000, 2001a). Thus, while a conversation is unfolding, triad members offer each other different subject positions that, if accepted, make available various inferences about their own identity and that of other triad members.

The second idea relates to the inferential nature of communication. This approach to communication explains how meaning is constructed through the skilful use of inter-action. The key idea is that social practices, what people do and say, make various inferences possible within the communication that allows certain 'truths' to be heard (Potter 1996; Hutchby and Wooffitt 1998). This idea provides a more sophisticated, though more realistic, model of communication than either 'channelling' models of communica-tion (Thwaites et al. 2002) or the use of symbolic interactionism that have often been used within dementia care (Kitwood 1997). In addition, the inferential model of communica-tion adopts 'a critical stance to "truths" and "realities" ' (Forbat 2003: 70) that provides worthwhile insights into the inclusion and exclusion of particular triad members. Through the inferential model of communication, therefore, social practices such as talk are under-stood in terms of 'constructing understandings, identities, relationships and even dementia itself' (Forbat 2003: 71).

Inferential communication within dementia care triads

The use of subject position and the inferential nature of communication to understand the dynamics of dementia care may be seen in the following extract which provides an example of a typical CMHN consultation between members of a dementia care triad, comprising a CMHN, a person with dementia, John, and, John's wife, acting as an informal family carer. The extract illustrates how inference, body language and spoken language allow different sets of meaning to emerge about what has, what is, and what will happen within particular dementia care settings.

CMHN looks towards John who has dementia.

1. CMHN: John, what tablets are
2.   you taking now?
3. John: Oh he is on them white
4.   tablets, he has them before he

5.   goes to bed.
6.   CMHN: Oh.
7.   John: He has them after a drink.
8.   CMHN: A drink?
9.   John: He has a scotch before he goes
10.   to sleep. He always has done.
11.   It helps him to go to sleep.

First, communication not only comprises what participants say to each other but also what they do. Note therefore that the CMHN looks towards John and addresses what he says to 'John' (lines 1 and 2). He thus allows John to believe the CMHN wants him to respond to what he has just said. However, the CMHN reinforces that inference by making the bodily action of looking at John.

Second, while the question is directed towards John, the carer responds to the question. This allows various inferences. The first inference is that John's wife is involved in giving her husband the tablets. The second is that John does not know what drug he is taking. And the third is that John cannot say how much medication he is having and allows the further inference that he is confused. This latter inference may impair John's participation in the consultation and identify him as not being able to contribute very much to the consultation. This may push him out and he may be sidelined in the discussion. In addition, John may internalize the inference and this can affect his sense of well-being and feelings that he will not be taken seriously in the consultation. He may just give up, particularly if the inference is repeatedly made within the consultation by what is said and done. John's inferred inability to contribute in the consultation may well be exacerbated by his diminished cognitive ability (Bryan and Maxim 2003).

Finally, the carer says that John has 'a drink' (line 7). This utterance allows the possibility that the 'drink' may be an alcoholic drink that might have an adverse effect on John and constitute a risk (Adams 2001c). This possibility is recognized by the CMHN who makes the utterance 'a drink' (line 8) that may be heard as a question and constructs the carer's reference to 'a drink' (line 8) as 'a risk'. The carer responds to the possibility that the drink may be a risk, by making two utterances that prevent the inference being made that John is doing something risky. First, that he has 'always' has had a drink (line 10). Note that the carer uses an exaggerated form that strengthens her point and says that John 'always' has a drink. The use of the utterance 'always' is interesting. It is difficult to imagine that the carer remembers every night and that on each night he had 'a drink'. The use of the term 'always', however, is not used as a statement of fact but rather as an 'extreme case formulation' (Pomerantz 1986) that strengthens the carer's case. Second, the carer makes the utterance that it helps John 'go to sleep' (line 11). This utterance allows other members of the dementia care triad to make the inference that 'a drink' helps John's well-being and therefore should be supported by the CMHN.

Inclusion and exclusion within dementia care triads

Shakespeare (1998), as part of a wider project, describes the conversational processes that occur within dementia triads comprising people with dementia, their family carers, and a researcher. Shakespeare describes dementia care triads that occur in two different groups of clients: 'minimally active confused speakers' and 'moderately active confused speakers'. With respect to 'minimally active confused speakers', Shakespeare identifies various conversational practices that are displayed by family carers when acting as an interlocutor within these triads. With 'moderately active confused speakers', Shakespeare identifies the ways in which family carers may act as an interlocutor who answers for the confused speaker, promoting and giving their opinion of some issue that is being discussed within the triad, discussing and acting as an informant.

Drawing on the work of Shakespeare (1998), Kitwood (1997), Sabat (2001) and Forbat (2005), together with discussion with health and social care professionals, and also our own clinical practice, we would identify two overall types of communication that may, and frequently do, occur within dementia care triads. The first type of communication is 'enabling dementia communication'. This form of communication occurs when family carers or CMHNs either help the person with dementia express their views, feelings and wishes or represent the person with dementia as someone who is able to make decisions about their own care. The second type of communication is 'disabling dementia communication'. This occurs when informal family carers or CMHNs either prevent the person with dementia from expressing their views, feelings and wishes or represent them as unable to participate in decisions. It should be noted that sometimes people with dementia display disabling dementia communication, perhaps through verbal threats or aggressive behaviour.

Within this context, we have identified types of enabling and disabling dementia communication that occur within dementia care triads. In conversational exchanges we found that people with dementia, family carers and CMHNs frequently locate themselves in powerful subject positions in triads that provide them with particular rights within the decision-making process. In addition, we found that as a result of their neurological impairment and perhaps also because of the respect and deference given to CMHNs in society, we found that people with dementia may experience difficulties gaining and holding on to strong subject positions. The examples that follow that are taken from practice have been supported by a NHS local ethics committee.

Enabling dementia communication

Enabling dementia communication comprises bodily or verbal communication that allows the person with dementia and their family carer(s) to make their feelings, views and wishes known within dementia care settings. Note that not only will enabling dementia communication promote feelings of well-being within triad members but they will also ensure that the voices of all triad members will be heard in assessment, care-planning and decision-making meetings, including the person with dementia.

To enable dementia communication, the following are useful:

- removing unwanted stimuli;
- getting in the right position;
- promoting equal participation;
- promoting and enabling meaningful communication;
- being sensitive to non-verbal cues;

- valuing and respecting contributions;
- overcoming disabling dementia communication;
- promoting joint decision-making and care planning.

Removing unwanted stimuli

This form of enabling dementia communication occurs when the CMHN or the family carer reduces the stimuli a person with dementia is receiving and the amount of information they need to comprehend. This helps the person with dementia to gather their thoughts together and allows them to make a more appropriate response to what is being said.

Case example 1

While Mr Amy was telling the CMHN about the successful trip he and his wife had had to the cinema, Mrs Amy was watching the television. The CMHN was unable to engage Mrs Amy in their conversation. The CMHN explained that it was difficult for Mrs Amy to join in the conversation while the television was turned on and asked if it could be turned off. After Mr Amy turned off the television, Mrs Amy was able to join in the conversation.

Getting in the right position

Where people stand or sit will affect the effectiveness of communication within dementia care triads. Often when CMHNs are about to leave a house, the CMHN will leave the living room and go to the front door with the family carer. Family carers often use this time to say a few things to the CMHN. This provides the family carer with the opportunity to share information with the CMHN. However, it may allow the person with dementia to think their relative and the CMHN are in league together and against them. Getting in the right position allows each member of the triad to communicate and thus constitutes an enabling dementia communication.

Case example 2

Mr Beaton, the family carer, sat in a chair on the other side of the room while the CMHN and his wife talked. It felt as though he was being aloof, supervising the conversation rather than contributing to it. Mrs Beaton kept looking to her husband to complete her sentences for her. The CMHN suggested that it would be helpful if Mr Beaton would move his chair towards them so they could talk more easily. Mrs Beaton appeared more relaxed sitting closer to her husband and her conversation became less hesitant. Mrs Beaton did not now need to shout across the room and was more able to help her husband say what she wanted to the CMHN.

Promoting equal participation

This occurs when CMHNs encourage the person with dementia or their family carers to express their views and opinions about either what is happening or what they want to happen and thus facilitates better communication.

Case example 3

The CMHN asked Mr and Mrs Connor what they were expecting from the CMHN's visit. Mr Connor thought the CMHN would monitor Mrs Connor's response to the medication the consultant had prescribed her. Mrs Connor said that she thought so too. The CMHN explained that people who had recently developed memory problems often wanted more information about what is happening to them and that members of their family often wanted to know how best to support them. Mrs Connor replied that she wondered what made her memory problems any worse than other people's and her husband wanted to know how they could cope with her forgetfulness.

Promoting and enabling meaningful conversation

This occurs when CMHNs encourage the person with dementia to say more in discussions and promote more appropriate conversation between all the participants. The CMHN asks the person with dementia or their family carer questions that allows them to talk more fully about issues that are important to them. Through the use of short, simple sentences and slow-paced conversation the person with dementia is engaged in conversation. Family carers are encouraged to express their views to improve the plan of care. In this way, the CMHN acts as a role model for enabling good communication.

Case example 4

Mr East complained that his wife never talked to him any more and 'doesn't do anything all day and just sits there'. The CMHN turned to Mrs East, gently touched her hand, and said her name. Mrs East looked first at her hand, then looked up to the eyes of the CMHN saying 'Oh, hello, dear.' The CMHN asked Mrs East what she does to pass the time. Mrs East replied, 'Every day is much the same, I just sit here and wait.' When asked what she was waiting for Mrs East replied, 'Something to do.' When asked what she would like to do, Mrs East said she loved to knit. Mr East complained she had said that before and he tried giving her knitting materials but she 'didn't even attempt it'. The CMHN asked Mrs East what she liked about knitting and replied that she loved the colours and textures of the wool. When she was given her knitting box, she appeared happy touching and rearranging the materials in her knitting box.

Being sensitive to non-verbal cues

This occurs when CMHNs observe the person with dementia making bodily movements or facial expressions that may indicate they want to say something.

Case example 5

Mrs Field was saying that she felt anxious about her husband's recent aggressive outbursts when she tried to wash him. As she was saying this, Mr Field's relaxed posture became more rigid and his face became more sullen. The CMHN asked Mr Field if he had felt angry recently. Mr Field said he got upset when he thought people were treating him like a child.

Valuing and respecting contributions

This occurs when triad members show their appreciation at hearing the views of other members of the triad.

Case example 6

The CMHN asked Mr Gray's son to say why he had asked that his father should have an assessment. The son said that it was because he was worried about his father's safety after incidents involving door-to-door salesmen, leaving his credit card in public places and getting lost when he goes out for walks on his own. The CMHN turned to Mr Gray and asked him how he felt about his son's concerns. Mr Gray replied that he knew his memory was bad and that he had no recollection of the events his son had just described. The CMHN asked Mr Gray how he thought his son's fears might be reduced. Mr Gray then outlined some practical changes he could make to his life that would help reduce risk. The CMHN praised Mr Gray for his ideas and helped Mr Gray and his son develop a care plan based on Mr Gray's comments.

Overcoming disabling dementia communication

This occurs when disabling dementia communications within meetings are ignored and enabling communication is modelled, allowing the continuing needs of the person with dementia to be addressed.

Case example 7

Mr Howe was telling the CMHN about the impact of his wife's illness upon their life. Mrs Howe asked him to repeat what he had said because she had not heard it properly. Mr Howe turned towards Mrs Howe and said, 'I wasn't talking to you, I was talking to the nurse.' Mrs Howe replied, 'I know, but I still want to hear what you say.'

Promoting joint decision-making and care planning

This occurs when CMHNs encourage the person with dementia and their family carer to work together to develop care plans and make decisions. In this way, the facilitation of joint-care planning and decision-making occurs through the use of enabling dementia communication.

Case example 8

Mr Irons expressed his increasing frustration about coping with the changes in his wife's personality and behaviour. The CMHN turned to Mrs Irons saying, 'It looks like things have been difficult between you and your husband.' Mrs Irons replied, 'You can say that again!' The CMHN asked them both if they could think of anything that could help them cope with their current difficulties. Mrs Irons replied, 'I wish I could just get away, it's all too much.' Mr Irons agreed that a break would do them both good.

Disabling dementia communication

Disabling dementia communication comprises bodily or verbal communication that inhibits the person with dementia or their family carer(s) making their feelings, views and wishes heard within dementia care. Not only will disabling dementia communication promote feelings of ill-being and powerlessness in either people with dementia or their family carers, it will also marginalize their voices within meetings where assessment, care-planning and decision-making is taking place. The person with dementia is particularly likely to find themselves marginalized as a result of disabling dementia communication as their dementia may impair their ability to communicate.

To prevent disabling dementia communication, the following behaviours should be avoided:

- interrupting;
- speaking on behalf of;
- reinterpreting;
- using too technical or complex language;
- talking out of earshot;
- taking sides;
- ignoring;
- ridicule;
- not inviting the person with dementia to meetings.

Interrupting

This occurs when a CMHN or their family carer interrupts a person with dementia while they are expressing their views.

Case example 9

Mrs Johnson was talking about the jobs she had had when Mr Johnson challenged her about how long she had worked in a shop. He cut in, saying, 'How long did you say you worked for Smeaton's? Oh, never mind, you won't remember that anyway.'

Speaking on behalf of

This occurs when the CMHN or the family carer talks about a person with dementia having views and opinions that they have not expressed themselves.

Case example 10

The CMHN asked Mr Jones whether he would like to stay in the hospital for two weeks. His wife answered and said he would.

Reinterpreting

This occurs when CMHNs or family carers rephrase or change the meaning of something that has been said by the person with dementia.

Case example 11

Mrs Lorentz was explaining to the CMHN how she disliked the home family carers coming into her house and taking her jobs away from her. Mr Lorentz interrupted saying, 'You don't mean that, you love the family carers visiting. You spend the whole time that they are here following them around and chatting to them.'

Using too technical or complex language

This occurs when the CMHN or the family carer use words or phrases the person with dementia finds difficult to understand.

Case example 12

The CMHN was talking to a person with dementia and their daughter. Every time the daughter wanted to refer to a local residential home she was wondering might be suitable for mother, she spelt out the word H-O-M-E. The CMHN later talked to the daughter about how this prevented her mother joining in the discussion. At the next meeting, the daughter started using the word 'home' and allowed her mother to hear what was being said and join in the discussion.

Talking out of earshot

This occurs when the CMHN or the family carer turns their body away from the person with dementia and lowers their voice so that the person with dementia cannot hear what they are saying.

Case example 13

Mr Nicholas had been discussing his frustration caused by the combination of his congenital hearing impairment and memory problems. Mr Nicholas's wife kept interjecting comments to the CMHN, but not so that Mr Nicholas could hear her. Mr Nicholas appeared to be getting irritated by his wife's behaviour. The CMHN asked Mrs Nicholas if she could speak up so that Mr Nicholas could hear the whole of the conversation. 'Oh, I can't do that, he'd accuse me of interfering.'

Taking sides

This occurs when the CMHN or the family carer make either a verbal utterance or a bodily movement that allows either the CMHN or the family carer to think that they agree with each other.

Case example 14

Mrs Oliver introduced the CMHN to Mr Oliver saying, 'Darling, do you remember I took you to your doctor and he agreed you have a problem with your memory? This nurse has come to do the memory tests and help me to look after you.'

Ignoring

This occurs when no effort is made to listen to the person with dementia within the dementia care triad.

Case example 15

As the CMHN arrived for the first meeting with Mr and Mrs Peters, she saw that Mrs Peters was sitting in the corner of the room staring into space. Before she could introduce herself to Mrs Peters, Mr Peters started a lengthy description of Mrs Peters' unusual behaviours. The CMHN asked Mr Peters if he felt comfortable talking about the issues when his wife was there. Mr Peters replied, 'Oh, yes, it's fine. We always talk in front of her. She never pays any attention anyway.'

Ridicule

This occurs when family carers say or do something that identifies the person with dementia as foolish, silly, or childish.

Case example 16

Following a lengthy discussion, Mrs Quinne became agitated, saying that she had to go and visit her mother. Her daughter said to her, 'Don't be silly, mum, we buried Nan years ago.' Mrs Quinne told her daughter off for being cruel. Mrs Quinne's daughter laughed and challenged her mother by saying that if her Nan was still alive she would be in the record books as the oldest woman in the world.

Not inviting the person with dementia to meetings

This occurs when the person with dementia is not invited to meetings when decisions about their own care are being discussed.

Case example 17

Mr Richards' son requested that the Care Programme Approach meeting should be held in Mr Richards' absence, so that he and his mother could talk to the psychiatrist openly about their concerns.

Summary

This chapter has developed a number of innovative ideas that may be used to enhance community mental health nursing practice to people with dementia. It has argued first of all that the idea of dementia care triads is worthwhile and able to help practitioners understand how situations in dementia care are developed and shaped. Of course, it is easy to forget that many people with dementia live alone and have little access to a family carer. For these people, a modified version of this approach may be implemented that focuses on the dyadic relationship between the person with dementia and the CMHN.

Second, the chapter has argued that identity and order within dementia care arise out of social practices: what people say and what people do. This perspective allows a more critical understanding of power and its distribution within dementia care triads, than that offered by writers such as Nolan et al. (2004). It is frequently noted that triadic interaction is inherently problematic and frequently leads to the formation of coalitions and alliances between two members of the triad that marginalizes the third. We would argue that this occurs through social processes within dementia care triads as triad members find themselves occupying subject positions that either lead to their inclusion or exclusion from decision-making processes.

We would also argue that this chapter raises the possibility that different triad members may have different beliefs, stories and accounts of what is happening to them. This raises a practical problem for CMHNs relating to which version of the world they should work with – the version belonging to the person with dementia, the carer's, or their own. We would suggest that through the interaction that occurs within the triad, an agreed version of what is happening is negotiated and co-constructed. As Paré notes in the context of dyadic relationships within families, social constructionism 'references knowledge neither in the observer nor the observed, but rather in the place between the two, in the social area among participating subjects' (1995: 5).

Lessons for CMHN practice

- Community mental health nursing for people with dementia and their family carers has a dual focus and views each of them as joint recipients of their care.
- Communication within dementia care triads allows various inferences and different subject positions that construct clinical settings.
- Communication between triad members may lead to either the inclusion or exclusion of each participant within the dementia care triad.
- Enabling dementia communication comprises bodily or verbal communication that allows the person with dementia or their family carer(s) to make their feelings, views and wishes known within dementia care settings.
- Disabling dementia communication comprises bodily or verbal communication that inhibits the person with dementia or their family carer(s) to make their feelings, views and wishes heard within dementia care.

References

Adams, T. (1999) Developing partnership in dementia care: a discursive model of practice, in T. Adams and C. Clarke (eds) *Dementia Care: Developing Partnerships in Practice*. London: Baillière Tindall, pp. 37–56.

Adams, T. (2000) The social construction of identity by community psychiatric nurses and family members caring for people with dementia, *Journal of Advanced Nursing*, 32: 791–8.

Adams, T. (2001a) The construction of moral identity within accounts of informal family carers for people with dementia, *Education and Ageing*, 16: 39–54.

Adams, T. (2001b) The conversational and discursive construction of community psychiatric nursing for chronically confused people and their families, *Nursing Inquiry*, 8: 98–107.

Adams, T. (2001c) The social construction of risk by community psychiatric nurses and family carers for people with dementia, *Health, Risk and Society*, 3(3): 307–19.

Adams, T. (2003) Developing an inclusive approach to dementia care, *Practice*, 15: 45–56.

Adams, T. and Bartlett, R. (2003) Constructing dementia, in T. Adams and J. Manthorpe (eds) *Dementia Care*. London: Arnold, pp. 3–21.

Adams, T. and Clarke, C. (eds) (1999) *Dementia Care: Developing Partnerships in Practice*. London: Baillière Tindall.

Ainsworth, D. and Jolley, D. (1978) The community psychiatric nurse in a developing psychogeriatric service, *Nursing Times*, 74(21): 873–4.

Althusser, L. (1971) *Lenin and Philosophy and Other Essays*. London: New Left Books.

Barker, C. and Black, S. (1971) An experiment in integrated psychogeriatric care, *Nursing Times*, 67(45): 1395–9.

Biggs, S. (1993) User participation and interprofessional collaboration in community care, *Interprofessional Care*, 7(2): 151–60.

Biggs, S. (1994) Failed individualism in community care: the case of elder abuse, *Journal of Social Work Practice*, 8(2): 137–50.

Biggs, S., Phillipson, C. and Kingston, P. (1995) *Elder Abuse in Perspective*. Buckingham: Open University Press.

Bryan, K. and Maxim, J. (2003) Managing language and communication difficulties in Alzheimer's dementia: the link to behaviour, in *Dementia Care*. London: Arnold, pp. 69–85.

Burr, V. (2003) *An Introduction to Social Constructionism*, 2nd edn. London: Routledge.

Butterworth, C.A. and Faugier, J. (eds) (1997) *Clinical Supervision and Mentorship in Nursing*. Cheltenham: Stanley Thornes.

Caplow, T. (1968) *Two Against One: Coalitions in Triads*. Englewood Cliffs, NJ: Prentice Hall.

Carradice, A., Keady, J. and Hahn, S. (2003) Clinical supervision and dementia care, in J. Keady, C.L. Clarke, and T. Adams (eds) *Community Mental Health Nursing and Dementia Care*. Maidenhead: Open University Press, pp. 215–35.

Cheek, J. (2003) Negotiated social space: a relook at partnership in contemporary health care, *Primary Health Care Research and Development*, 4: 119–27.

Dallos, R. and Draper, R. (2000) *An Introduction to Family Therapy*. Maidenhead: Open University Press.

Davis, L.L. (1992) Building a source of caring for caregivers, *Family and Community Health*, 15(2): 1–9.

Davis, S. and Nolan, M. (2003) 'Making the best of things': relative's experience of decisions about care-home entry, *Ageing and Society*, 23: 429–50.

Department of Health and Social Security (1981) *Growing Older*. London: HMSO.

Department of Health (1993) *Working in Partnership*. London: The Stationery Office.

Department of Health (1995) *Carer's (Recognition and Services) Act*. London: The Stationery Office.

Department of Health (1999) *The Carer's National Strategy*. London: The Stationery Office.

Department of Health (2001) *The National Service Framework for Older People*. London: The Stationery Office.

Doherty, W.J. and Baird, M.A. (1983) *Family Therapy and Family Medicine*. New York: Guildford Press.

Downs, M. (1997) The emergence of the person within dementia research, *Ageing and Society*, 17: 597–607.

Feinberg, L.F. and Whitlatch, C.J. (2001) Are persons with cognitive impairment able to state consistent choices? *The Gerontologist*, 41(3): 374–82.

Forbat, L. (2002) Tinged with bitterness: re-presenting stress in family care, *Disability and Society*, 17(7): 759–68.

Forbat, L. (2003) Relationship difficulties in dementia care: a discursive analysis of two women's accounts, *Dementia*, 2(1): 67–84.

Forbat, L. (2005) *Talking about Care: Two Sides of the Story*. Bristol: Policy Press.

Fortinsky, R.H. (2001) Health care triads and dementia care: integrative frameworks and future directions, *Aging and Mental Health*, 5(1): S35–S48.

Goldsmith, M. (1996) *Hearing the Voices of People with Dementia*. London: Jessica Kingsley Publications.

Haley, J. (1977) Toward a system of psychological systems, in P. Watzlawick and J. Weakland (eds) *The Interactional View*. New York: Norton.

Harré, R. and van Langenhove, L. (1999) Introduction to positioning theory, in R. Harré and L. van Langenhove (eds) *Positioning Theory*. Oxford: Blackwell.

Hasselkus, B.R. (1994) Three-track care: patient, family member and physician in the medical visit, *Journal of Aging Studies*, 8(3): 291–307.

Haug, M.R. (1994) Elderly patients, caregivers, and physicians: theory and research on health care triads, *Journal of Health and Social Behaviour*, 35: 1–12.

Heaton, J. (1999) The gaze and visibility of the carer: a Foucauldian analysis of the discourse of informal care, *Sociology of Health and Illness*, 21: 759–77.

Henderson, J. and Forbat, L. (2002) Relationship-based social policy: personal and policy constructions of 'care', *Critical Social Policy*, 22(4): 669–87.

Hofman, L. (1981) *Foundations of Family Therapy*. New York: Basic Books.

Holman, M. (2003) Supporting and supervising in dementia care, in T. Adams and J. Manthorpe (eds) *Dementia Care*. London: Arnold, pp. 213–24.

Hutchby, R. and Wooffitt, R. (1998) *Conversation Analysis*. London: Polity Press.

Keady, J. and Gilliard, J. (1999) The early experience of Alzheimer's disease: implications for partnership and practice, in *Dementia Care: Developing a Partnership in Practice*. Edinburgh: Churchill Livingstone.

Keady, J. and Nolan, M. (2003) The dynamics of dementia: working together, working separately, or working alone, in M. Nolan, U. Lunth, G. Grant and J. Keady (eds) *Partnerships in Family Care: Understanding the Caregiving Carer*. Maidenhead: Open University Press, pp. 15–32.

Keith, C. (1995) Family caregiving systems: models, resources and values, *Journal of Marriage and the Family*, 57: 179–89.

Killick, J. and Allen, K. (2001) *Communication and the Care of People with Dementia*. Buckingham: Open University Press.

Kitwood, T. (1997) *Dementia Reconsidered: The Person Comes First*. Buckingham: Open University Press.

Lancaster, C. (1984) Community psychiatry in Bloomsbury. 2. Adjusting to old age, *Nursing Times*, 80(43): 26–7.

Leopoldt, H., Robinson, J. and Corea, S. (1975) Hospital-based community psychiatric nursing, *Nursing Mirror*, 141(25): 54–6.

Lloyd, L. (2000) Caring about family carers: only half the picture? *Critical Social Policy*, 20(1): 136–50.

Morris, C. (2004) Personal-construct psychology and person-centred care, in G.M.M. Jones and M.M.L. Miesen (eds) *Care-Giving in Dementia: Research and Applications*. London: Routledge.

Morris, J. (1991) Us and them? Feminist research, community care and disability, *Critical Social Policy*, 33: 223–9.

National Heath Service (2001) *National Service Framework for Older People*. London: The Stationery Office.

Nolan, M.R., Davies, S., Brown, J., Keady, J. and Nolan J. (2004) Beyond 'person-centred' care: a new vision for gerontological nursing, *Journal of Clinical Nursing*, 13, s1, 45–53(9).

Paré, D.A. (1995) Of families and other cultures: the shifting paradigm of family therapy, *Family Process*, 33: 217–31.

Pomerantz, A. (1986) Extreme case formulations, *Human Studies*, 9: 219–30.

Potter, J. (1996) *Representing Reality: Discourse, Rhetoric and Social Construction*. London: Sage.

Rolfe, G., Freshwater, D. and Jasper, R. (2001) *Critical Reflection for Nursing and the Helping Professions: A User's Guide*. London: Palgrave.

Roscow, I. (1981) Coalitions in geriatric medicine, in M.R. Haug (ed.) *Elderly Patients and their Doctors*. New York: Springer, pp. 137–46.

Sabat, S.R. (2001) *The Experience of Alzheimer's Disease: Life through a Tangled Veil.* Oxford: Blackwell.

Sabat, S.R. and Harré, R. (1992) The Construction and deconstruction of self in Alzheimer's disease, *Ageing and Society*, 12: 443–61.

Shakespeare, P. (1998). *Aspects of Confused Speech: A Study of Verbal Interaction between Confused and Normal Speakers.* Mahwah, NJ: Lawrence Erlbaum Associates Publishers.

Silliman, R.A. (1989) Caring for the frail older patient: the doctor patient caregiver relationship, *Journal of General Internal Medicine*, 4: 237–41.

Thwaites, T., Davis, L. and Mules, W. (2002) *Introducing Cultural and Media Studies.* London: Palgrave.

Tuffin, K. (2005) *Understanding Critical Social Psychology.* London: Sage.

Twigg, J. and Atkin, K. (1994) *Family Carers Perceived: Policy and Practice in Informal Care.* Buckingham: Open University Press.

Wetherell, M. (1998) Positioning and interpretative repertoires: conversation analysis and post-structuralism in dialogue, *Discourse and Society*, 9: 387–412.

PART TWO

Professional role and clinical work

8

The Alzheimer's Medication Service

Developing an early intervention service
in a rural community

Diane Beavis

Introduction

The introduction of the acetylcholinesterase inhibitor medications (AChEIs), Donepezil®, Rivastigmine® and Galantamine® has opened up new avenues of treatment for people in the early to moderate stages of Alzheimer's disease. As a consequence, a number of nurse-led 'treatment services' have been developed to implement and monitor the effectiveness of the medicines (see, for example, Beavis and Simpson 2003; Page 2003). These 'treatment services' provide community mental health nurses (CMHNs) with an opportunity to engage with people in the early stages of Alzheimer's disease (Adams and Page 2000; Page 2003), often at an earlier stage than when the more traditional community services would begin. As such, this may be viewed as an ideal time for CMHNs to offer early interventions that seek to promote health, identify and pre-empt potential risk areas and most importantly, empower the person with Alzheimer's disease to be an active participant in his/her care.

The aim of this chapter is to explore the range of early interventions and health promoting strategies that can be incorporated into the work of CMHNs and to demonstrate how these strategies have been developed as part of a treatment service (the Alzheimer's Medication Service – AMS) in West Dorset. Beginning with a brief overview of the AMS, the chapter will broaden out to discuss the role of CMHNs in the implementation of early interventions for people with dementia and their families and the wider use of a health promotion strategy within community practice. Case studies illustrating the use of these approaches will be provided. The chapter concludes by making a number of recommendations for CMHN practice.

Setting up the AMS: principles in practice

In 2001, the National Institute for Clinical Excellence (NICE) (2001, Technology Appraisal Guidance No. 19) recommended the use of the AChEIs for people with mild to moderate Alzheimer's disease. The main clinical trials (Corey-Bloom et al. 1998; Rogers et al. 1998; Burns et al. 1999; Raskind et al. 2000; Wilcock et al. 2000) have demonstrated that the AChEIs can enhance cognitive abilities and lead to global improvements in areas

Table 8.1 Percentage of older people by local authorities

	West Dorset	North Dorset	Weymouth and Portland
Ages 60–75	18.3	15.5	15.0
Aged 75 and over	12.3	9.8	9.8

Source: National Statistics website: www.statistics.gov.uk

Note: Crown copyright material is reproduced with the permission of the Controller of HMSO and the Queen's Printer for Scotland.

of functioning, such as daily living skills (Corey-Bloom et al. 1998; Wilcock et al. 2000) and problem solving (Rogers and Friedhoff 1998). Further studies suggest that they may reduce the frequency of behavioural symptoms, see, for example, Cummings et al.'s (2000) study using Donepezil®, or slow down the progression of these symptoms; see Rösler et al.'s (1998/1999) study using Rivastigmine®. They may also be of benefit to other types of dementia such as dementia with Lewy Bodies (Rivastigmine®, McKeith et al. 2000), or vascular dementia (Galantamine®, Erkinjuntti et al. 2002).

In West Dorset the publication of the NICE (2001) recommendations led to the Dorset and Somerset Strategic Health Authority agreeing to fund the development of the AMS. Central to the AMS was the generation of a Specialist Nurse post that would enable the case-load to be managed effectively and efficiently, while also complementing the work of existing CMHNs.

The North Dorset Primary Care Trust (NDPCT) (for mental health) and the AMS cover three local authorities: North Dorset, West Dorset and Weymouth and Portland. The area spans almost 700 square miles (Dorset County Council 2004), much of which is rural in nature, making it the most popular retirement destination in England (Dorset County Council 2004). This is reflected in the age distribution, with all three local authorities having higher percentages of older people when compared to the national average of 13.3 per cent (ages 60–74) and 7.6 per cent (aged 75 and over) (Office for National Statistics – ONS 2001), see Table 8.1.

Within the NDPCT there are six separate CMHTs. Each team has a designated consultant psychiatrist (who may cover more than one CMHT), CMHNs, occupational therapists (OT), health care assistants and support from a clinical psychologist for older people. At present, one specialist nurse, one health care support worker and a part-time secretary (job shared between two people) staff the AMS.

The primary function of the AMS is to provide information about the medicines, conduct assessments to determine efficacy (see Box 8.1) and monitor the person's progress throughout the duration of treatment (Beavis and Simpson 2003). Physical assessments are

---

Box 8.1 Assessments completed to determine efficacy of the AChEIs

- The Mini-mental State Examination (Folstein et al. 1975);
- The Alzheimer's Disease Assessment Scale – Cognition (Rosen et al. 1984);
- The Bristol Activities of Daily Living Scale (Bucks et al. 1996);
- The Neuropsychiatric Inventory (Cummings et al. 1994).

also completed prior to treatment with the AChEI. This includes a 12-lead electro-cardiogram (ECG) at baseline and blood pressure, pulse and weight measurements at all visits.

Initially, the AMS began as a 'clinic'-based service. However, it gradually became apparent that a clinic-based system was problematic, with concerns about poor access, travelling difficulties and long waiting times for clinic appointments being raised. From a nursing perspective, the Specialist Nurse also felt that assessing people in a clinic setting was restricting the application of a fully 'person-centred' approach to patient care. Consequently, the structure of the AMS was altered to a more flexible appointment system, enabling people to choose whether to be seen at home or in a clinic. In practice, this means that the emphasis of the appointment is moved away from a clinical setting and into the person's own home, which in turn encourages a more person-focused, less medically orien-tated appointment. It also enables the Specialist Nurse to complete more accurate assess-ments. For example, during the process of recording an ECG, the nurse is able to observe a wide range of skills and abilities (see Box 8.2), many of which would not be captured by a clinic environment.

Early interventions and health promotion: role of the CMHN

The AMS has been in operation since 2003 and during this time the role of the Specialist Nurse has developed beyond the remit and scope of the original clinic-based model of care. In addition to implementing and monitoring the effectiveness of the medications, the Specialist Nurse also provides advice and information on a range of psychosocial and healthy life-style issues. This includes giving:

1   Information on healthy eating, nutritional requirements and dietary supplements. In some cases, referrals can be made (with the person's permission) to the community dietician for more detailed dietary advice.

2   Guidance on moderating alcohol consumption and cigarette smoking.

Box 8.2 Areas observed during a home visit

- *Orientation* – can the person find his way around his home and to his bedroom?

- *Short-term memory* – Can the person follow a short set of instructions?

- *Mobility* – Is the person fully ambulant, can he/she climb the stairs with ease?

- *Environment* – Are there any potential hazards, such as objects left on the stairs, loose rugs and carpets, portable electric fires or paraffin heaters being used for heating? Is the home in satisfactory condition?

- *Economic factors* – Is the heating adequate? Is there evidence of poverty?

- *Personal care* – Can the person dress and undress without help? Is the person dressed appropriately? Is there evidence of self-neglect, or poor hygiene?

- *Physical health* – Are there any concerns about the person's physical health e.g. checking skin integrity – are there any bruises, lesions or skin complaints? Does the person become short of breath when lying down?

3 Financial information, in particular, details concerning enduring power of attorney, the attendance allowance and other financial benefits.

4 Recommendations for the safe administration and storage of medicines, advice on the use of compliance aids and referral to the community pharmaceutical services, if necessary.

5 Advice on risk management, in particular, giving information regarding the legal requirements and responsibilities related to continued driving.

6 Advice on preventing falls.

7 Support for psychological interventions and therapeutic activities that encourage the person to maintain existing skills. This may include referral to an early memory loss group.

8 Contact details for voluntary, statutory and private agencies in the area, including local carers' support groups and carer education programmes (run by the CMHTs).

9 Support to the person with dementia, his/her family, relatives, friends and other informal carers.

While some of these interventions feature in the regular work of CMHNs and form a key component of the local memory clinics (Simpson et al. 2004), it would be fair to say that within the AMS they have developed on an 'ad-hoc' basis rather than by following a defined, evidence-based protocol. However, the introduction of Clinical Governance (Department of Health 1997) has altered the way health-care professionals view service developments. In particular, the emphasis now placed upon increased accountability, efficiency, effectiveness and standardization of care practices means that it is no longer acceptable to develop services in an 'ad-hoc' manner. For the AMS, it is particularly important to address these issues because for many of the people referred to the service, this will be their first contact (other than during the diagnostic period) with the mental health services for older people. Therefore, it is essential that any information, advice or care given is up-to-date and evidence-based (as far as possible) and most importantly, that it is offered at an appropriate time and reflects the person's individual needs and wishes.

Consequently, the development of the AMS has begun to focus upon incorporating the key areas of practice (points 1–9) into an evidence-based and person-centred frame-work of care, specifically tailored towards early interventions and health promotion activities relevant to people with dementia. Needless to say, this is not as straightforward as it seems. First, developing evidence-based practice requires considerable investment in time, money and resources. As poignantly argued by Woods (2003), it is difficult, and in many cases not appropriate, to apply the 'gold standard' randomized controlled trials (frequently used as a method of generating evidence-based practice) to the investigation of interventions that are predominately psychological or social in nature. For example, gaining sufficient sample numbers, the lack of suitable control groups and variability to external factors including researcher bias are all factors that are likely to impede the success of quantitative research studies when applied to early psychosocial interventions for people with dementia (Woods 2003). Second, until recent years, much of the research in dementia care has avoided the direct involvement of people with dementia (Cotrell and Schulz 1993), concentrating primarily on the needs of carers (Pusey and Richards 2001 provide a comprehensive review of psychosocial interventions for carers), factors related to carer burden (Zarit et al. 1986; Donaldson et al. 1997) and stress (Donaldson et al. 1998) or obtaining 'by proxy' reports such as Albert et al. (1996).

Nevertheless, over the past decade, alternative research methods such as single case studies (Clare et al. 2003), qualitative interviews (Werezak and Stewart 2002) and evidence collected from existing memory clinics (Moniz-Cook and Woods 1997) have gained considerable momentum and support the potential benefits of early interventions in dementia care. Moreover, there is a growing body of evidence to demonstrate that not only is it *possible* to include people with dementia in research (Goldsmith 1996; Allen 2001), but that when they are included they can provide a valuable insight into the experience of dementia – Elaine Robinson (2002) and James McKillop (2002) provide illuminating accounts of how they (as people with Alzheimer's disease) have participated in research studies. Other studies (Keady et al. 1995; Gillies 2000) support these findings and further research (Sperlinger and McAuslane 1994; Sutton and Fincham 1994; Reid et al. 2001) also suggests that when asked, people with dementia *can* provide feedback on the quality of care and type of services they would like to receive.

In light of this evidence, it would seem appropriate to adopt a similar approach to the development of a health promotion strategy within the AMS. As suggested by Page (2003), the 'post-diagnostic' period can be a useful time for CMHNs to work therapeutically with people in the early stages of Alzheimer's disease. Equally, it may also be an ideal time to thoughtfully engage them in the advancement, implementation and evaluation of the AMS, in particular, evaluating the benefits of an early intervention and a health promotion strategy. However, before moving into a description of how this can be achieved, it is important to establish what is actually meant by the term 'health promotion'.

The concept of 'health' itself is not easy to clarify and is open to various interpretations (Naidoo and Wills 2000), which can vary according to personal values, beliefs and life experiences (Ewles and Simnett 2003). Similarly, Maben and Macleod Clark (1995) suggest that the term 'health promotion' is difficult to define and in a concept analysis they conclude that:

> Health promotion is an attempt to improve the health status of an individual or community, and is also concerned with the prevention of disease, though this is not its only purpose, as health is not merely the absence of disease.
>
> (1995: 1163)

They go on to say 'health promotion is in itself an approach to care through empowerment, equity, collaboration and participation, and may involve social and environmental change' (1995: 1163).

In contrast to this broad definition, the traditional medical approach views health promotion as a three-tiered process, namely, primary, secondary and tertiary prevention (Naidoo and Wills 2000). Primary level interventions are generally applied to the detection and prevention of specific illnesses, for example, mass screening or immunization programmes; secondary interventions are usually concerned with the instigation of early interventions that seek to prolong the progression of a condition and improve well-being; and, finally, tertiary interventions, which are aimed at maximizing the quality of life in the latter stages of an illness or disease process (Naidoo and Wills 2000).

Using this delineation, early interventions form only one component of health promotion activities and do not encompass the breadth and depth of possible interventions open to CMHNs working with people who have dementia. Additionally, Lyman (1989) suggests that by concentrating upon medical interventions alone, there is a temptation to lose sight of the social context of dementia and to view the person affected in isolation from his family, life history and social biography. Lyman argues that while the application of a 'staging' process to dementia may ameliorate the caring role, giving the carer a guide to the timescale involved in the progression of the illness, it does little to support the person with dementia. Consequently, the development of a health promotion strategy in dementia care must look further afield, to a more inclusive and person-centred model of care that spans the entire journey along the course of dementia.

Perhaps, then, it is useful to begin by providing a global picture of the policies that inform health promotion. From this perspective, the World Health Organization (WHO) has paved the way for the development of health promotion programmes. By endorsing the principles of the Jakarta Declaration ('leading health promotion into the 21st Century'), the WHO has made a firm commitment to promoting health as a *'basic human right'* (WHO 1997: 261), whereby individuals and communities are encouraged and empowered to actively shape the factors, which influence their health. In conclusion, the WHO identifies a number of key priorities that are required to advance health promotion at a global level. This includes creating collaborative networks, generating knowledge and sharing best practice and strengthening a commitment to health promotion policies that are clear and publicly accountable.

In the UK, the National Service Framework for Older People (NSF-OP, Department of Health 2001) has embraced these principles. This is reflected by the four core themes that run through it: 'respecting the individual, intermediate care, providing evidence-based specialist care and promoting an active healthy life' (2001: 12–14). Within these themes, eight specific standards are identified, six of which can be linked to health-promoting activities for older people with dementia:

- minimizing age discrimination;
- enhancing person-centred care;
- reducing the incidence of strokes;
- reducing the incidence of falls;
- promoting mental health;
- encouraging health and activity in older life.

These standards provide a useful starting point from which to develop a health promotion strategy for the AMS. However, a clear philosophical and theoretical basis for health promotion for people with dementia is still required. From this stance, the work of Professor David Seedhouse (2000, 2004) and his 'foundations theory of health' have been inspirational to the Specialist Nurse for the AMS. Seedhouse (2000, 2004) suggests that the aim of health-promoting activities should be to enable each person, or group of people to reach their ultimate human potential within the realistic boundaries of day-to-day life. Seedhouse (2004) proposes that there are four essential foundations to maintaining health; these are illustrated in Box 8.3.

Using this approach, the health professional acts a 'facilitator', offering help and advice *only* when one or more of the foundations become damaged or unfulfilled (Seedhouse 2004). In essence, it is an empowering theory, a theory that places the understanding of health firmly in the hands of the people concerned, namely, people with dementia and their family members.

Box 8.3 The essential foundations of health

1   Providing for basic needs, including the provision of essential materials such as food, fluids and warmth, but also maintaining a sense of hope.

2   Awareness and understanding of information that might impact upon one's health.

3   The ability to adequately interpret information, thus enabling a person or people to make balanced and appropriate decisions.

4   An acknowledgement of the interrelatedness that exists between individuals, their family members and society as a whole.

Source: Seedhouse 2000, 2004

However, in order to develop the facilitator role and a health promotion strategy, Seedhouse urges all health professionals to closely examine the values that underpin their work, to be open and explicit about these values and to recognize how they influence or hinder their ability to implement a health promotion strategy. To this end, the AMS has undoubtedly been led by the medical approach to care, largely because of the rigorous, scientific development of the AChELs through randomized controlled trials (as cited earlier). However, it could equally be argued that the *emerging* service is being driven by a more person-centred approach, which is heavily influenced by the social-psychological theory of dementia care (more commonly referred to as the 'person-centred theory of dementia care') developed by the late Professor Tom Kitwood (1990, 1993, 1997; Kitwood and Bredin 1992). Central to this theory is a commitment to maintaining personhood and improving the well-being of people with dementia. Kitwood defines personhood as 'a standing or status that is bestowed upon one human being, by others, in the context of relationship and social being' (1997: 8).

Kitwood and Bredin (1992) suggest that there are four components essential to personhood and well-being. First, personal worth, that is a feeling of being valued by others; second, a feeling of being in control of one's destiny and able to influence the course of one's life; third, social confidence, being able to reach out and know that others will respond positively, and finally, a sense of hope that all will be well, no matter what happens. Kitwood's theory has gained widespread support from CMHNs and its principles form the basis of the philosophy of care for the AMS and the Practice Development Unit, which represents mental health services for older people across the NDPCT (Beavis 2004).

It is envisaged that the ongoing development of the AMS will gradually combine the theoretical frameworks suggested by Kitwood (1990, 1993, 1997; Kitwood and Bredin 1992) and Seedhouse (2000, 2004) into a health promotion strategy that is sensitive to the needs of people with dementia and their relatives and values their contribution towards its future development. The following two case studies illuminate the potential benefits of combining these theories.[1]

Case example 1

Mrs Cunningham is a 78-year-old widow, who lives on her own in a terraced house in the county town of Dorchester. She has one son who is married and lives in Birmingham. He is unable to visit his mother on a regular basis owing to his hectic work schedule. However, he calls his mother on the telephone daily and ensures that groceries are delivered to her every week. Mrs Cunningham has lived in Dorchester all her life and has several good friends. However, she no longer sees them because of her increasing frailty and loss of confidence – the last time she went shopping she couldn't find the supermarket (which has been relocated out of the town centre) and had to be 'escorted' home by a local shopkeeper. Not long after this event (and after the accumulation of several similar incidents), Mrs Cunningham was given a diagnosis of Alzheimer's disease and referred to the AMS. Her son fully supported the referral and was keen to pursue treatment having read a lot of information about the AChEIs.

The first appointment was scheduled at Mrs Cunningham's house. On arrival, Mrs Cunningham's son greeted the nurse at the door and immediately directed her into the kitchen. Once here, it quickly became evident that although Mrs Cunningham was well supplied with groceries, most of them had been left to waste. Her son was visibly concerned about the situation, but when he asked his mother about the food, she replied rather curtly, 'I'm eating well, I haven't lost any weight, I've always been about eight stone.' Unfortunately, this was not reflected in her appearance – she looked emaciated and pale, her skin was dry and her clothing hung loosely around her body. Her weight was recorded as 39 kilograms (just over 6 stone). In a state of panic, her son started demanding that his mother be taken into residential care.

In this scenario, the nurse needs to remain calm and focus upon using her knowledge and skills of both Kitwood's and Seedhouse's theories to navigate an appropriate and safe course of action for Mrs Cunningham. Using Seedhouse's foundations of health theory it is evident that her son needs more information about the options available to his mother (foundation 2) before an informed decision about her future can be made (foundation 3). However, from Mrs Cunningham's perspective, it is clear that the first foundation of health, namely, the provision of basic needs is not being adequately fulfilled and her well-being will be compromised by taking such rash and sudden decisions. Thus, the main priority for the nurse is to restore Mrs Cunningham's basic needs as far as it is possible within existing resources. While the option of residential care would ensure that her basic needs are met, and it would relieve her son's understandable anxiety, it is likely to have a negative impact upon Mrs Cunningham's ability to remain in control of her own destiny, which in turn, may also prevent her from restoring the remaining three foundations of health.

At this stage the role of the nurse becomes pivotal to the decision-making process; by using knowledge acquired from both Kitwood's and Seedhouse's theories, the nurse can attempt to create a more positive, person-centred approach to Mrs Cunningham's future – crucially it must reflect her wishes, enable her to be in control of her future, and thereby regain a sense of hope and well-being.

After discussion with Mrs Cunningham, it transpired that she desperately missed her old friends and being in the company of others. She was not overly concerned about her weight loss, but admitted that she often felt very tired and couldn't be bothered to cook for herself. With these issues in mind the following action plan was agreed between all parties:

Mr Cunningham

1   To contact his mother's closest friend and arrange weekly get-togethers if possible.
2   To liaise with the local Social Services department to organize home care visits three times a week (to help with meal preparation) and a meal delivery system four days a week.
3   To apply for the attendance allowance.

Specialist Nurse

1   To refer Mrs Cunningham to the local Social Services department to provide assistance and advice regarding the implementation of home care.
2   To refer Mrs Cunningham to the occupational therapist for a home/kitchen assessment.
3   To visit fortnightly to check on physical health and monitor weight.
4   To liaise with Mrs Cunningham's general practitioner and ensure that her physical health is fully investigated.
5   To refer Mrs Cunningham to the community dietician for assessment and dietary advice.

Outcome

Two months later, Mr Cunningham had contacted an old friend of his mother's who was delighted to have the opportunity of reacquainting herself with Mrs Cunningham. It emerged that her friend regularly attended the local community centre for a luncheon club, followed by bingo and presentations by guest speakers and was more than happy to take Mrs Cunningham to these events. Physically, Mrs Cunningham was beginning to benefit from the regular meals and had gained 6 kilograms in weight. The GP completed a full physical examination, but could not find any physical ailments. Nonetheless, after a home visit from the community dietician a prescription for regular meal supplements was provided. The OT completed a kitchen assessment and found that with a few simple modifications Mrs Cunningham was able to safely prepare herself a light snack. On this basis, an OT assistant was assigned to visit weekly and observe/assist in meal preparation.

Final comments

Although Mr Cunningham initially felt uneasy about the care plan, after two months he began to appreciate how important it was to understand his mother's view of the situation. Mrs Cunningham had been equally sceptical about having carers coming into her home, but these feelings soon evaporated when she met the carers and realized that they could also become her friends. She was clearly benefiting from the increased social contact and stated on many occasions how content and happy she was, particularly now that she had rekindled an old friendship.

From a nursing perspective, having restored Mrs Cunningham's basic needs, she was able to move towards the second and third foundations of health, namely to assimilate and understand information about her health. Although, Mrs Cunningham had difficulty retaining information, she was able to understand information given to her at the time, and consequently was able to make a decision about treatment with the AChEIs.

Case example 2

Mr and Mrs Hartley are a married couple who retired to live in an idyllic village in West Dorset approximately 15 years ago. Prior to their retirement Mrs Hartley had been employed as a 'pastry chef' and Mr Hartley had been a surveyor. Mrs Hartley was very 'houseproud' and enjoyed indoor hobbies such as jam making, knitting and sewing. In contrast, Mr Hartley spent his spare time pottering around in the garden. They have three children, the eldest two live abroad and the youngest lives in the neighbouring county of Somerset, a distance of approximately 40 miles. Despite living in the village for a long time, they have kept themselves to themselves and have very few close friends.

Over the past year, Mr Hartley has gradually become aware of his wife's inability to complete her usual daily chores. For example, on several occasions she has hung dirty washing on the line, or has served up inappropriate combinations of food, much of which had either been overcooked, or partially raw. The situation finally came to a crisis point during a weekend away, when Mrs Hartley was found lighting a gas ring to boil water in an electric kettle. After seeking advice from their GP, Mrs Hartley was seen in the outpatient department by the consultant psychiatrist and a diagnosis of probable Alzheimer's disease was given. Mrs Hartley was then referred to the AMS.

At the first AMS appointment, Mrs Hartley warmly welcomed the nurse into their home, which was noted to be in an immaculate condition. Mr Hartley busied himself making coffee, while Mrs Hartley anxiously began to explain that although her memory wasn't as good as it used to be, she thought it was 'just old age'. She concluded by saying, 'My mother had the same problem and we didn't have any help then, we just got on with it.' Mr Hartley entered the room just at the end of this conversation and replied, 'Things are different now, you can take some tablets to make you better, and that's why the nurse has come today.'

As the interview progressed, it gradually emerged that Mr Hartley had a very limited understanding of Alzheimer's disease and believed that the medicines would 'solve all their problems'. Additionally, he had become so anxious about his wife's safety that he had taken over all the domestic chores and was even beginning to answer for her in conversation. As a result, Mrs Hartley had become withdrawn and despondent and looked unhappy. Mr Hartley commented, 'She's often like this, I don't know why, I do everything for her.'

Again, in this scenario, the nurse can draw upon Seedhouse's foundations theory and Kitwood's person-centred theory of care to guide Mr and Mrs Hartley in a more positive direction. In this case, it was quickly established that Mrs Hartley's basic needs (the first foundation of health) were being met, even if her husband was completing most of them. Nevertheless, the nurse sensed that although his intentions were good, Mr Hartley's actions were having a negative impact on his wife, gradually eroding away her self-esteem, her sense of control over the situation and optimism or hope for the future. Thus, her personhood and well-being were both being compromised.

By examining the remaining foundations of health (Box 8.3), it was evident that a significant improvement to the situation could be made, first, by providing Mr and Mrs Hartley with information about Alzheimer's disease and the AChEIs. Second, by helping Mr Hartley recognize that although his wife has an illness that is likely to impair her previous level of functioning, it does not necessarily mean that she is unable to participate at all. As a result, the following actions were agreed.

The Specialist Nurse

1   To provide information about Alzheimer's disease and the local support group.
2   To register Mr Hartley for the next Carers' Education Group.
3   To provide ongoing support to both Mr and Mrs Hartley. In particular, to examine ways in which Mrs Hartley could be safely encouraged to participate in household chores, even if this means that their previous high standards might not be attained.
4   To refer Mrs Hartley to the day hospital and OT to develop a range of therapeutic activities that can be easily replicated in the home.

On the face of it, the action plan seems fairly straightforward. However, the nurse will have to tread very carefully in this situation to avoid devaluing Mr Hartley's contribution to his wife's care, while also demonstrating ways of keeping Mrs Hartley involved with her care and their domestic arrangements. This is a delicate situation, and the nurse will need to use expert communication skills to negotiate a positive outcome for both Mr and Mrs Hartley.

Outcome

Six weeks later, Mrs Hartley has started attending the activities session at the local day hospital one afternoon a week. So far she has enjoyed these afternoons tremendously, often using the opportunity to demonstrate her baking skills to the other group members. While Mrs Hartley attends the group, Mr Hartley uses his time positively by going to the carers' group, held in the adjacent building. He is still struggling with the home situation, but has begun to involve his wife in preparing the vegetables for their evening meal and washing up after tea. He also realizes that he does not need to answer for his wife and although he finds it difficult to stop himself, on several occasions he has cut himself off mid-sentence to allow his wife to answer. The AChEI medications have been started, but efficacy has yet to be determined. Nonetheless, subsequent visits have been encouraging with Mrs Hartley seeming to be less anxious and more animated in conversation.

Discussion

Over the past decade there has been a gradual shift in the focus of dementia care services towards developing effective interventions for people in the early stages of dementia. In some areas this has taken the form of memory clinics (Moniz-Cook and Woods 1997; Simpson et al. 2004), which seek to provide early diagnosis, offer early treatment with the

AChEIs if indicated, and facilitate a range of psychosocial interventions. These early psychosocial interventions (whether through a memory clinic or a traditional outpatient service) are typically orientated towards providing information, support and advice to the person with dementia and his/her relatives. This might include providing advice on the management of memory difficulties experienced, making simple modifications to the home environment to overcome practical problems (Wilson and Evans 2000 provide a useful overview of these interventions), giving information on a range of subjects including financial matters such as enduring power of attorney and the attendance allowance, the availability of local services and national organizations and if necessary, discussing safety issues, for example, continued driving, living alone and managing medication. Additionally, formal carer-based educational programmes (e.g. Brodaty et al. 1997) may be offered at this stage and more recently, memory-retraining programmes (see, for example, Moniz-Cook and Woods 1997; Clare et al. 2003) have started to feature in the post-diagnostic period.

While any developments which have the overarching aim of improving the quality of life and well-being of the person with dementia are welcomed, one is perhaps left, still feeling that the *person* with dementia is somewhat marginalized from the equation. Furthermore, many of these early interventions have only a limited application and duration and although Simpson et al. (2004) found that there was greater involvement with the services available following a memory clinic appointment (compared to a domiciliary appointment), it remains the case that finite resources dictate the level of input from community services (whether health or social care), with those who have the greatest needs understandably receiving the greatest amount of care (Hunter et al. 1997). In terms of the CMHT, anecdotally, it would appear that there is a gap between the early diagnosis stage and people being taken onto caseload by the CMHNs, with many CMHTs only becoming more intensely involved with the person when his/her level of impairment becomes more apparent or with the manifestation of 'problem behaviour(s)'. As a result, the role of CMHNs during the early stages may be limited to assisting with the memory clinics and subsequent follow-up work after the clinic appointment. Arguably, there are some exceptional examples of work done by the CMHNs following the early diagnostic phase (Page 2003), but as indicated by the literature cited in this chapter, much of the research and development in this area of dementia care has been led by other professional groups, rather than by CMHNs, whose role appears to have been subsumed into the whole process.

In summary, three particular issues are raised: (1) the early interventions currently available to people with dementia are limited in their application, focus and duration; (2) these interventions fail to capture the 'wider picture' of what is meaningful to the person with dementia (and his/her relatives); and (3) there is a lack of clarity surrounding the role and value of CMHNs during these early interventions.

In an attempt to address these issues, the emphasis of this chapter has been to demonstrate how an alternative approach to care can be implemented, whereby, instead of focusing upon 'early interventions' *per se*, *all* health professional groups involved in the care of people with dementia begin to adopt a 'health-promoting' approach to the services that they offer. This means that instead of viewing the person in terms of being in different stages of dementia, with certain interventions being applied according to the 'problems' encountered during these 'stages', the person is viewed as being on a journey, or continuum whereby support, encouragement and advice may be requested or required at any time along the journey. The foundations theory of health (Seedhouse 2000, 2004), described in this chapter, demonstrates how a health promotion strategy can be incorporated in this manner. Furthermore, as the case studies illustrate, Seedhouse's (2000, 2004) theory enables health-care practitioners to focus upon what is truly important for the person and his/her family members, rather than offering a preset range of interventions that may, or may not, be of any value to the person. In essence, Seedhouse's theory provides a logical, straightforward, but dynamic approach to care. A theory, which when overlaid with Kitwood's person-centred theory of care, enables the health-care professional to adopt a more positive way of thinking about the *person* with dementia.

In this last paragraph, I have deliberately talked about 'health-care professionals', as a way of referring to all health-care disciplines, the point being that we all have a valuable role to play and must work together towards a common goal, namely to improve the quality of care provided to people with dementia. However, as exemplified in the case studies, it is CMHNs who are able to acts as the 'lynchpin' to the success (or failure) of these interventions and who possess the skills and tenacity to deliver a health promotion strategy of this nature. It is these skills which shine through the examples given; skills that are grounded in the experiences gained by consistently working alongside people with dementia. Thus, CMHNs are ideally placed (and ideally suited) to develop and instigate a new approach to dementia care, whether this is through specialist medication services (as described in this chapter) or through the work of local CMHTs.

Summary

In this chapter I have discussed the development of the Alzheimer's Medication Service within the North Dorset Primary Care Trust. To a large degree, the ongoing development of the service has been dictated by the results of randomized controlled trials using the AChEI medications and the guidelines for the use of the AChEIs produced by NICE (2001). However, I have also endeavoured to illustrate how a service of this nature can also provide CMHNs with an opportunity that is rarely available in traditional CMHT work, namely, to work alongside people with dementia before 'problems' occur, or crisis interventions are necessary and to offer an alternative model of care based on a health promotion strategy. By using a combination of Seedhouse's foundations of health theory (2000, 2004) and Kitwood's (1990, 1993, 1997; Kitwood and Bredin 1992) person-centred theory of dementia care, I have demonstrated how these theories can work together to keep *the person* at the centre of his/her care and obtain the best possible outcome for the person with dementia and his/her relatives. This new approach is not merely an 'adjunct' to existing psychosocial interventions, but represents a whole theory of care, which follows the person along his/her personal journey through dementia. CMHNs can (and should) play a pivotal role in the implementation of this new health-promoting approach to care and should take steps to ensure that they are at the forefront of service provision for people with dementia.

Lessons for CMHN practice

- The recent emergence of treatment services provides a welcome addition to the range of services available for people with dementia. The fundamental challenge facing

CMHNs is how to turn a medically based service into a more complete 'health-orientated' and person-centred approach to care.

- Early psychosocial interventions form a valuable component of memory clinics during the early diagnostic period. However, the aim of developing a 'health promotion' strategy, as opposed to just early interventions is to embrace the concept of promoting health and well-being along a continuum, rather than at just one point, or stage in time.

- Health promotion encompasses all dimensions of health, but most importantly, it should reflect what the person and his/her family want and feel is necessary to enhance their sense of well-being.

- CMHNs have the skills, training and experience to deliver a health promotion strategy as described in this chapter and should be at the forefront of care provision and future developments in dementia care.

- The next step is for CMHNs to explore what people with dementia want in the way of early interventions or health promotion (*if anything*), to establish when and where they want to receive the services (*if at all*) and finally, to discover how the services (*if required*) can be best delivered.

Note

1   The case studies included in this article are hypothetical but reflect the reality of the author's day-to-day practice.

References

Adams, T. and Page, S.C. (2000) New pharmacological treatments for Alzheimer's disease: implications for dementia care nursing, *Journal of Advanced Nursing*, 31(5): 1183–8.

Albert, S.M., Del Castillo-Castaneda, C., Sano, M., Jacobs, D. M., Marder, K., Bell, K., Bylsma, F., Lafleche, G., Brandt, J., Albert, M. and Stern, Y. (1996) Quality of life in patients with Alzheimer's disease as reported by patient proxies, *Journal of American Geriatrics Society*, 44(11): 1342–7.

Allen, K. (2001) *Communication and Consultation: Exploring Ways for Staff to Involve People with Dementia in Developing Services*. Bristol: The Policy Press and the Joseph Rowntree Foundation.

Beavis, D. (2004) The Practice Development Unit Submission Document: mental health services for older people, unpublished report, North Dorset Primary Care NHS Trust.

Beavis, D. and Simpson, S. (2003) Monitoring medication: the development of a specialist medication service for people with Alzheimer's disease, *Journal of Dementia Care*, 11(2): 16–17.

Brodaty, H., Gresham, M. and Luscombe, G. (1997) The Prince Henry Hospital dementia caregivers' training programme, *International Journal of Geriatric Psychiatry*, 12: 183–92.

Bucks, R.S., Ashworth, D.L., Wilcock, G.K. and Siegfried, K. (1996) Assessment of activities of daily living in dementia: development of the Bristol Activities of Daily Living Scale, *Age and Ageing*, 25: 113–20.

Burns, A., Rossor, M., Hecker, J., Gauthier, S., Petit, H., Möller, H.-J., Rogers, S.L. and Friedhoff, L.T. and the International Donepezil Study Group (1999) The effects of Donepezil in Alzheimer's disease: Results from a multinational trial, *Dementia and Geriatric Cognitive Disorders*, 10: 237–44.

Clare, L., Wilson, B.A., Carter, G. and Hodges, J.R. (2003) Cognitive rehabilitation as a component of early intervention in Alzheimer's disease: a single case study, *Aging and Mental Health*, 7(1): 15–21.

Corey-Bloom, J., Anand, R. and Veach, J. for the ENA 713 B352 Study Group (1998) A randomized trial evaluating the efficacy and safety of ENA 713 (rivastigmine tartrate) in patients with mild to moderately severe Alzheimer's disease, *International Journal of Geriatric Psychopharmacology*, 1: 55–65.

Cotrell, V. and Schulz, R. (1993) The perspective of the patient with Alzheimer's disease: a neglected dimension of dementia research, *The Gerontologist*, 33(2): 205–11.

Cummings, J.L., Donohue, J.A. and Brooks, R.L. (2000) The relationship between Donepezil and behavioural disturbances in patients with Alzheimer's disease, *American Journal of Geriatric Psychiatry*, 8(2): 134–40.

Cummings, J.L., Mega, M., Gray, K., Rosenberg-Thompson, S., Carusi, D.A. and Gornbein, J. (1994) The Neuropsychiatric Inventory: comprehensive assessment of psychpathology in dementia, *Neurology*, 44: 2308–14.

Department of Health (1997) *The New NHS: Modern and Dependable*. London: HMSO.

Department of Health (2001) *The National Service Framework for Older People*. London: HMSO.

Donaldson, C., Tarrier, N. and Burns, A. (1997) The impact of the symptoms of dementia on caregivers, *British Journal of Psychiatry*, 170: 62–8.

Donaldson, C., Tarrier, N. and Burns, A. (1998) Determinants of carer stress in Alzheimer's disease, *International Journal of Geriatric Psychiatry*, 13: 248–56.

Dorset County Council (2004) *The Dorset Data Book: Data and Statistics for the County of Dorset*. Dorset: Research and Information, Dorset County Council.

Erkinjuntti, T., Kurz, A., Gauthier, S., Bullock, R., Lilienfeld, S. and Damaraju, C.V. (2002) Efficacy of galantamine in probable vascular dementia and Alzheimer's disease combined with cerebro-vascular disease: a randomised trial, *The Lancet*, 359(9314): 1283–90.

Ewles, L. and Simnett, I. (2003) *Promoting Health: A Practical Guide*. London: Baillière Tindall.

Folstein, M.F., Folstein, S.E. and McHugh, P.R. (1975) Mini-mental state: A practical method for grading the cognitive state of patients for the clinician, *Journal of Psychiatric Research*, 12: 189–98.

Gillies, B.A. (2000) A memory like clockwork: accounts of living through dementia, *Aging and Mental Health*, 4(4): 366–74.

Goldsmith, M. (1996) *Hearing the Voice of People with Dementia*. London: Jessica Kingsley Publishers.

Hunter, R., McGill, L., Bosanquet, N. and Johnson, N. (1997) Alzheimer's disease in the United Kingdom: developing patient and carer support strategies to encourage care in the community, *Quality in Health Care*, 6: 146–52.

Keady, J., Nolan, M. and Gilliard, J. (1995) Listen to the voices of experience, *Journal of Dementia Care*, May/June: 15–17.

Kitwood, T. (1990) The dialects of dementia: with particular reference to Alzheimer's disease, *Ageing and Society*, 10: 177–96.

Kitwood, T. (1993) Person and process in dementia, *International Journal of Geriatric Psychiatry*, 8: 541–5.

Kitwood, T. (1997) *Dementia Reconsidered: The Person Comes First*. Buckingham. Open University Press.

Kitwood, T. and Bredin, K. (1992) Towards a theory of dementia care: personhood and well-being, *Ageing and Society*, 12: 269–87.

Lyman, K.A. (1989) Bringing the social back in: a critique of the biomedicalization of dementia, *Gerontologist*, 29(5): 597–605.

Maben, J. and Macleod Clark, J. (1995) Health promotion: a concept analysis, *Journal of Advanced Nursing*, 22: 1158–65.

McKeith, I., Del Ser, T., Spano, P., Emre, M., Wesnes, K., Anand, R., Cicin-Sain, A., Ferrara, R. and Spiegel, R. (2000) Efficacy of rivastigmine in dementia with Lewy bodies: a randomised, double-blind, placebo-controlled international study, *Lancet*, 356: 2031–6.

McKillop, J. (2002) Did research alter anything?, in H. Wilkinson (ed.) *The Perspectives of People with Dementia: Research Methods and Motivations*. London: Jessica Kingsley Publishers.

Moniz-Cook, E. and Woods, R.T. (1997) The role of memory clinics and psychosocial intervention in the early stages of dementia, *International Journal of Geriatric Psychiatry*, 12: 1143–5.

Naidoo, J. and Wills, J. (2000) *Health Promotion: Foundations for Practice*. London. Baillière Tindall in association with the Royal College of Nursing.

National Institute for Clinical Excellence (2001) *Technology Appraisal Guidance on the Use of Donepezil, Rivastigmine and Galantamine for the Treatment of Alzheimer's Disease*, No. 19. London: HMSO.

Office for National Statistics (2001) *Census 2001*, available at: http://www.statistics.gov.uk/ neighbourhood.

Page, S. (2003) From screening to intervention, in J. Keady, C.L. Clarke and T. Adams (eds) *Community Mental Health Nursing and Dementia Care: Practice Perspectives*. Maidenhead: Open University Press.

Pusey, H. and Richards, D. (2001) A systematic review of the effectiveness of psychosocial interventions for carers of people with dementia, *Aging and Mental Health*, 5(2): 107–19.

Raskind, M.A., Peskind, E.R., Wessel, T. and Yuan, W. and the Galantamine USA–1 Study Group (2000) Galantamine in AD: a 6-month randomised, placebo-controlled trial with a 6-month extension, *Neurology*, 54(2 of 2): 2261–8.

Reid, D., Ryan, T. and Enderby, P. (2001) What does it mean to listen to people with dementia?, *Disability and Society*, 16(3): 377–92.

Robinson, E. (2002) Should people with Alzheimer's disease take part in research?, in H. Wilkinson (ed.) *The Perspectives of People with Dementia: Research Methods and Motivations*. London: Jessica Kingsley Publishers.

Rogers, S.L. and Friedhoff, L.T. (1998) Long-term efficacy and safety of Donepezil in the treatment of Alzheimer's disease: an interim analysis of the results of a US multicentre open label extension study, *European Neuropsychopharmacology*, 8: 67–75.

Rogers, S.L., Farlow, M.R., Doody, R.S., Mohs, R., Friedhoff, L.T. and the Donepezil Study Group (1998) A 24-week, double-blind, placebo-controlled trial of Donepezil in patients with Alzheimer's disease, *Neurology*, 50: 136–45.

Rosen, W.G., Mohs, R.C. and Davis, K.L. (1984) A new rating scale for Alzheimer's disease, *American Journal of Psychiatry*, 141: 1356–64.

Rösler, M., Retz, W., Retz-Junginger, P. and Joachim Dennler, H. (1998/1999) Effects of two-year treatment with the cholinesterase inhibitor rivastigmine on behavioural symptoms in Alzheimer's disease, *Behavioural Neurology*, 11: 211–16.

Seedhouse, D. (2000) *Practical Nursing Philosophy: The Universal Ethical Code*. Chichester. John Wiley and Sons, Ltd.

Seedhouse, D. (2004) *Health Promotion, Philosophy, Prejudice and Practice*. 2nd edn. Chichester. John Wiley and Sons, Ltd.

Simpson, S., Beavis, D., Dyer, J. and Ball, S. (2004) Should old age psychiatry develop memory clinics? A comparison with domiciliary work, *Psychiatric Bulletin*, 28: 78–82.

Sperlinger, D. and McAuslane, L. (1994) Listening to users of services for people with dementia, *Clinical Psychology Forum*, Nov: 2–4.

Sutton, L.J. and Fincham, F. (1994) Clients' perspectives: experiences of respite care, *PSIGE Newsletter*, 49: 12–15.

Werezak, L. and Stewart, N. (2002) Learning to live with early dementia, *Canadian Journal of Nursing Research*, 34(1): 67–85.

Wilcock, G.K., Lilienfeld, S. and Gaens, E. on behalf of the Galantamine International–1 Study

Group (2000) Efficacy and safety of galantamine in patients with mild to moderate Alzheimer's disease: multicentre randomised controlled trial, *British Medical Journal*, 32: 1445–9.

Wilson, B.A. and Evans, J.J. (2000) Practical management of memory problems, in G.E. Berrios and J.R. Hodges (eds) *Memory Disorders in Psychiatric Practice*. Cambridge: Cambridge University Press.

Woods, B. (2003) Evidence-based practice in psychosocial intervention in early dementia: how can it be achieved?, *Aging and Mental Health*, 7(1): 5–6.

World Health Organization (1997) The Jakarta Declaration on Leading Health Promotion into the 21st Century, *Health Promotion International*, 4: 261–6.

Zarit, S.H., Todd, P.A. and Zarit, J.M. (1986) Subjective burden of husbands and wives as caregivers: a longitudinal study, *The Gerontologist*, 26(3): 260–6.

9

Nurse prescribing and the CMHN
Assuming new responsibilities in dementia treatment

Sean Page

Introduction

The concept of nurse prescribing within the National Health Service (NHS) is relatively new and its introduction, over two decades, has been ponderously slow and at times frustrating. Despite this, there is now a real opportunity for nurses to engage fully with the prescribing process and to influence it in such a way as to benefit the patient. However, within the field of community mental health nurse (CMHN) practice and dementia care there is a paucity of available literature to guide practice and to comment on the efficacy of this role extension. In many ways this chapter builds upon the author's contribution to the first book (Page 2003) – and Chapter 8 in this book – and the overview of the nursing role in a Dementia Treatment Clinic (DTC), with specific reference to his own practice in South Manchester. Instead, this time, the chapter will explore the main mechanisms for delivering non-medical prescribing and consider possible relationships with dementia care. More specifically, a case study will be introduced that compares and contrasts some of the dilemmas faced in (the author's) practice when a person with dementia wished to take a cholinesterase inhibitor (ChEI) and was happy for the CMHN to be involved as a prescriber, but required further information and guidance before agreement was reached. Steps and dilemmas faced by all parties in this process are rehearsed. Before this is introduced, however, the chapter will set the case study in context by rehearsing some of the policy and procedural landmarks in nurse prescribing and provide an overview of its constituent elements.

Background

The introduction of a nurse-prescribing programme to the NHS was first proposed by the Cumberledge Report (Department of Health and Social Security 1986). Requested to review community nursing provision in England, and to make recommendations regarding future provision, Baroness Cumberledge found that the prescribing process led to both unnecessary delays in patients receiving treatment and the inefficient use of community nurses' time. Later, Baroness Cumberledge (2003) reflected:

> the vision was simple, that nurses should be allowed to prescribe because we knew that people were waiting in pain and discomfort, waiting for prescriptions. Nurses were

being humiliated, knowing exactly what the patient needed but they had to wait outside the GP's door to get a signature.

While Cumberledge had a vision for 'a prescribing pad for every nurse', her eventual recommendation, that qualified community nurses should be permitted to prescribe from 'a limited range of medicines, appliances and dressings' was, perhaps, more pragmatic. However, the recommendation was warmly received by the then Conservative government and debated rigorously between the professional groups involved, culminating a few years later with the commissioning of the Crown Report with a remit of 'advising the Secretary of State . . . how arrangements for the supply of drugs, dressings, appliances and chemical reagents . . . might be improved by enabling such items to be prescribed by a nurse' (Department of Health 1989: 3). The Crown Report recommended that suitably qualified community nurses, i.e. those with a district nurse or health visitor qualification, should, in certain circumstances, be permitted to prescribe appropriate items from a restricted formulary. The appropriate legislation to enable this, the 'Medicinal Products: Prescription by Nurses Act', was given Royal Assent in 1992. This first mode of independent nurse prescribing was then piloted in 1993 across eight sites in England and subsequently extended further by 1997. Political support waned due to Treasury concerns about the costs associated with nurse prescribing. A sense of frustration regarding the speed of the process started to emerge with the pilot sites being more commonly referred to by practitioners as 'demonstration sites' particularly following the positive evaluation by Luker et al. (1997). Reflecting later on this development, Cumberledge (2003) suggested that:

> The evaluations were very encouraging because we found, as we had thought, that nurse prescribing wouldn't be more expensive. We also found that it was safe and that patients approved. In fact, patients couldn't understand why there was an issue at all.

Pressure increased on the Department of Health to fully implement the nurse-prescribing programme in a timely manner and, in responding to the growing evidence and pressure from nursing's professional bodies, Frank Dobson, the then Labour government Secretary of State for Health, committed himself to the introduction of independent nurse prescribing by the year 2000 and to further consider ways in which non-medical prescribing could be extended.

To pursue this agenda, a second Crown Report (Crown II) was commissioned and reported at the end of the last century (Department of Health 1999). Primarily, Crown II addressed the legal position of nurses administering medication under a group prescribing protocol and, second, it recommended the extension of prescribing modalities. In so doing, the role of the extended nurse prescriber, armed with a right to prescribe from the Nurse Prescribers Extended Formulary (NPEF), was proposed alongside the new concept of the 'dependent prescriber' which opened the door for 'supplementary prescribing'.

As the 1990s drew to a close, the move towards 'nurse prescribing' had gained significant momentum and the Department of Health, concerned about falling numbers of medical practitioners, and the impact this might have upon satisfaction expressed by health-care consumers, roundly endorsed the recommendations of Crown II through the NHS Plan (Department of Health 2000a). It was then enacted through the Health and Social Care Act (2001).

In the new millennium the scope of the NPEF continued to increase but it was not until the spring of 2006 that a change of seismic proportions occurred when the DOH legislated that all nurse prescribers be re-registered with the Nursing and Midwifery Council as Independent Nurse Prescribers (INP) (Department of Health 2006).

Mechanisms for nurse prescribing

There are currently three mechanisms by which an appropriately qualified registered nurse may prescribe a medicinal product; each will be briefly discussed in turn:

1   *Independent nurse prescribing (INP)*. The original mechanism by which a registered nurse practising as a district nurse or health visitor could legally prescribe a medicinal product to a patient. Generally an extremely limited mechanism focused around a very restricted Nurse Prescribers Formulary (NPF) and principally aimed at improving the management of minor conditions requiring dressings, or appliances, to be supplied to the patient. However, under new legislation from May of 2006, all nurse prescribers are now registered as an INP and the definition has changed significantly. The INP is now legally permitted to prescribe any drug from the British National Formulary in their own right as a fully autonomous and accountable prescriber, bound only by their level of competency and Code of Conduct (NMC 2002a).

2   *Patient Group Directive*. The first Crown Report (DOH 1989) had included in its recommendations that, at a local level, doctors and nurses could collaborate in developing 'group protocols'. Such protocols offered an arrangement whereby a nurse could select and administer drugs without assessment or prescription by a doctor. As an expedient mechanism group protocols were used by a variety of nursing practitioners but mostly adopted by practice nurses and used primarily for the administration of vaccines to children.
      Concerns regarding the legality of group protocols were raised by the Royal College of Nursing in 1996 and after due consideration the DOH was ultimately unwilling to support their use despite the threat to the entire national immunization programme (Jones 1999). The second Crown Report was therefore additionally charged with reviewing the group protocol process and recommended their continued use, as potential methods for good practice, provided specific standards in respect of their content, development and implementation were met (DOH 1998). The concept of the group protocol was relabelled as Patient Group Directive (PGD) and defined specifically as 'written instructions for the supply or administration of medicines to groups of patients who may not be individually identified before presentation for treatment' (DOH 2000b).

3   *Supplementary prescribing*. As part of the second Crown Report's recommendations regarding the extension of non-medical prescribing, the concepts of the 'independent' and 'dependent' prescriber were first introduced. The independent prescriber is described as being responsible for: 'the assessment of patients with undiagnosed conditions and for decisions about the clinical management required, including prescribing' (DOH 2003), while the dependent prescriber is described as being responsible for 'the continuing care of patients who have been clinically assessed by an independent prescriber. This continuing care may include prescribing' (DOH 2003).
      The DOH re-badged the concept of 'dependent' prescribing as 'supplementary'

prescribing and defined the whole process as 'a voluntary partnership between an independent prescriber and a supplementary prescriber, to implement an agreed, patient-specific, clinical management plan with the patient's agreement' (DOH 2003).

Supplementary prescribing is therefore all about a relationship between the doctor, nurse and patient, each of whom has a contribution to make, and each of whom must agree with the clinical management plan (CMP) which will be used to articulate the prescribing process, and through which the supplementary prescriber may prescribe any licensed medication which is prescribable at NHS expense, with the exception of controlled drugs. The current DOH template for a clinical management plan is shown in Figure 9.1.

The independent prescriber must be a doctor, or dentist, and should ideally be the clinician responsible for the individual patient's care. The independent prescriber has responsibility for the assessment and diagnosis of the condition that is to be treated. The supplementary prescriber has responsibility for the ongoing care of that individual patient and, through the CMP, may use their discretion regarding choice of product, dosage, frequency or other variables that have been agreed. The patient must be in agreement with the CMP, otherwise it cannot come into operation.

The CMP is regarded by the DOH as being the 'foundation stone' of supplementary prescribing, it is a legal obligation and must be specific to a named patient. Furthermore, it must include:

(a) The specific illness or condition that is to be treated.

(b) The date on which the CMP takes effect and when it is to be reviewed.

(c) Reference to the class or description of medicines that may be prescribed or administered.

(d) Any restriction or limitation as to the strength or dose of medicines that may be prescribed.

(e) Warnings about known sensitivities for that individual patient.

(f) The means by which an adverse drug reaction is to be notified.

The CMP is to be kept as simple and straightforward as possible. It comes to an end either on the date specified for its review, at the request of the supplementary prescriber or the patient, at the discretion of the independent prescriber or where, for whatever reason, the independent prescriber is replaced.

Even with the arrival of INP, the supplementary prescribing mechanism remains both viable and valuable. This is particularly so for the newly qualified INP who may wish to have a period of supervised prescribing, to develop their experience and competency, before electing to embark on the independent role.

Finding a mechanism for mental health

Until fairly recently it has been difficult to find a mechanism whereby the CMHN could assume anything more than de facto prescribing responsibility. Patient group directives exist to treat those patients who may not be identified before presenting for treatment and

NAME OF PATIENT:	PATIENT MEDICATION SENSITIVITIES/ALLERGIES:

PATIENT IDENTIFICATION E.G. ID NUMBER, DATE OF BIRTH:

INDEPENDENT PRESCRIBER(S):	SUPPLEMENTARY PRESCRIBER(S)

CONDITION(S) TO BE TREATED	AIM OF TREATMENT

MEDICINES THAT MAY BE PRESCRIBED BY SP:			
PREPARATION	INDICATION	DOSE SCHEDULE	SPECIFIC INDICATIONS FOR REFERRAL BACK TO THE IP

GUIDELINES OR PROTOCOLS SUPPORTING CLINICAL MANAGEMENT PLAN:

FREQUENCY OF REVIEW AND MONITORING BY:

SUPPLEMENTARY PRESCRIBER	SUPPLEMENTARY PRESCRIBER AND INDEPENDENT PRESCRIBER

PROCESS FOR REPORTING ADRS:

SHARED RECORD TO BE USED BY IP AND SP:

AGREED BY INDEPENDENT PRESCRIBER(S)	DATE	AGREED BY SUPPLEMENTARY PRESCRIBER(S)	DATE	DATE AGREED WITH PATIENT/CARER

Figure 9.1 The CMP template (DOH recommended)

are largely inappropriate for mental health settings in which that person, being treated by the nurse, is already known, assessed and diagnosed. At the time of writing (July 2006), INP is a newly introduced mechanism and it is too early to say how many mental health INPs will choose to practise, or how many mental health trusts will provide indemnity should they wish to do so.

Without doubt, over the next few years INP will come to dominate and will invariably be evaluated and discussed. However, at this time, of all the mechanisms available it is supplementary prescribing which best fits with mental health services and which has the most to offer the mental health nurse. This is particularly so as not only would that nurse be otherwise unable to take a more active role in the prescribing process, but also the fact that many will already do the following:

- have an ongoing relationship with a psychiatrist, which is based on the most expedient means of delivering care and treatment to the patient;
- have a high profile role in services such as memory clinics or dementia treatment services;
- have a sound knowledge of the medicinal products commonly used in their speciality.

Consequently, it is supplementary prescribing which will now be explored further and related specifically to the use of ChEI therapy, although the issues discussed are equally relevant to other classes of medication used with this client group.

The prescribing process

Diagnosis and decision-making

The first stage in any prescribing strategy is diagnosis of the particular illness or condition that is to be treated. By the time a person is approached by the DTC, the diagnosis of Alzheimer's disease has already been made by a specialist. This specialist, acting in the role of independent prescriber, may decide that it is appropriate for the individual patient's condition to be treated through supplementary prescribing and consequently through a CMP. An element of the decision to draft a CMP will be information obtained through a suitability assessment regarding the safe and potential use of a ChEI.

Suitability assessment is based upon considering each individual patient's medical and drug history alongside their social circumstances and expectations for treatment. Considering the patient's medical history, current physical health and drug history is crucial to the safe prescribing of any medication to older people, as it is recognized that as a group they experience a greater number of health problems and consume a greater number of medications than other groups in the general population (Helling et al. 1987). Indeed, all ChEIs are, to a greater or lesser extent, metabolized by the liver through the P450 enzyme system and therefore careful note needs to be taken of any historical or current liver failure or impairment. Caution is advised for all drugs in this class. In a similar way ChEIs are excreted through the kidneys and their treatment is not recommended for those with a severe renal impairment. Additionally, as the cardiac and digestive systems also contain cholinesterase receptors, caution is advised if there is any history of cardiac conduction disorders, significant heart block or gastric ulceration.

Although ChEIs are regarded as having only limited interactions with other classes of medication, it remains prudent to take a full drug history. In part, this may be an opportunity to identify specifically what medications are being taken and how they are being used and to identify specific interactions between prescribed medications and those obtained in other ways. Further consideration of the patient will encompass their willingness to take the medication and to comply with the required regime. Many people have high, often unrealistic, expectations for treatment with a ChEI and when one considers the impact of diagnosis, it may be regarded as natural for those affected to hope for a return to normality or other significant benefit. Unless these expectations are addressed honestly at this stage they will come to challenge concordance, as the expected improvement does not occur and patient or carer becomes disheartened.

Consultation

The role of the patient in the prescribing process has historically been clearly defined and understood as one of 'passive recipient' of a treatment. Such treatments are usually selected by a medical practitioner, with only a limited dialogue and involvement of the person concerned, and then this is normally to be sure that the person is able to follow instructions. It is the accepted role of the patient to comply with these instructions, with failure to do so being the fault of the patient, not the prescriber. In recent years it has become recognized that such a view is inadequate and, that in a successful prescribing process, the patient has to be a much more active and empowered participant. Seedhouse (1991) was one of the first academics and commentators to propose a more inclusive approach as being one in which the prescriber acknowledges his or her own limitations and uncertainties and invites the patient to collaborate much more in the prescriptive process. Treatment therefore becomes a matter of negotiation rather than instruction and the role of patient expands to one in which they not only collaborate but also assume a degree of responsibility for their own health. In order to promote such a model, it becomes important to negotiate with the patient, the intention being to gain informed consent and achieve concordance.

Such a premise fits smoothly with the ideals of the 'new culture of dementia care' as proposed by Kitwood and Benson (1995). Under the 'old culture' of care, people with dementia were treated with little regard, often being relegated to the status of 'infant' or perceived as an object to which one did things without the need to obtain consent. The 'new culture' is rooted in the belief that people with dementia have a right to be as involved as possible in their own care and treatment; the prescribing process is no exception to this. Ideally, a triadic relationship should exist between the person with dementia, their carer/supporter and the doctor/nurse taking prescribing responsibility (see Figure 9.2 as a heuristic of this relationship). Such a relationship is influenced by the new culture and each party is seen as not only having a role to play but as an equal partner in the process. In the past, triadic relationships have functioned in a somewhat pathological manner in dementia care. Usually this is because the person with dementia is excluded from the relationship, which becomes dominated by the health-care professional interacting only with a less powerful carer. Where this occurs, the role of the patient is simply to take the medication given to them by the carer who in turn follows the instructions of the professional. The patient's act of swallowing medication is taken to imply consent with that treatment.

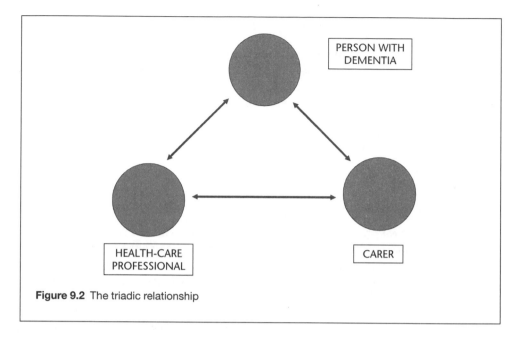

Figure 9.2 The triadic relationship

Consent

If the goal is for a more egalitarian and negotiated partnership, as displayed in Figure 9.2, then it must be accepted that the patient has a dynamic, rather than a passive, role. The old assumption that passive acceptance of a prescription equates with consent to treatment must be vigorously challenged and there must be an acknowledgement that the patient has a choice and is not obliged to consent to receive treatment (Preece 2002). The role of the prescriber is to provide sufficient information to assist in the decision-making process while respecting that the patient is empowered to make a decision. Involving nurses more actively in the prescribing process has been shown to have benefits in respect of information giving (Luker et al. 1997). A number of reasons are suggested for this, including the nurse having an existing relationship with the patient; having more time available; visiting the patient at home; and the belief that nurses are much more a social equal and consequently more approachable and easier to talk to. These advantages all suggest that making the consultation more convenient, and less anxiety-provoking, for the patient assists in the process of consenting to treatment.

Prescribing for people with dementia needs to be sensitive, as comprehension will be affected by both the setting in which information is imparted and the manner in which it is imparted. In early dementia retention of information is possible, but it is negatively affected by anxiety, which may be experienced in a clinical setting. Additionally, where information is not retained, the person with dementia, operating at an emotional level, usually recalls the way in which it was imparted. Failing to establish rapport, belittling or diminishing the patient's involvement or adopting an authoritarian approach will generally fail to achieve consent.

The process of nurse supplementary prescribing is focused on strategies aimed at patient empowerment and naturally includes consideration of consent to treatment. The patient is regarded as an equal partner who makes a decision based upon the information presented by the nurse prescriber. The nurse is challenged to present information in a way that the patient may understand, retain and recall. If the patient consents to treatment, then the CMP becomes the contract that may be ended at any time if the patient withdraws consent. The situation is less clear in respect of people who lack the capacity to make informed decisions and current good practice guidelines (Department of Health 2004) to proceed in the best interests of the patient are tempered by the caution that to do so, in relation to supplementary prescribing, is 'untested in law'.

Compliance and concordance

Those who do not consent to treatment are subsequently unlikely to achieve compliance, particularly in respect of chronic disease management. Those who do consent may fail to comply due to the effect of their cognitive impairment. There is a significant cognitive component involved in the process of compliance and this has been highlighted within the Cognitive Hypothesis Model of Compliance (Ley 1988). This suggests that a person's level of compliance may be broadly predicted by assessing not only their satisfaction with the consultation but also their understanding of any information given and their ability to recall that information. This is important as evidence exists to suggest that, following the traditional style of consultation, patients, who have a low level of understanding regarding their illness, often fail to achieve compliance (Boyle 1971). Furthermore, Bain (1982) found in studies of non-cognitively impaired individuals, that over a third could not recall the name of their treatment while a quarter could not recall the frequency or duration of the treatment.

People with dementia may be at increased risk of non-compliance by virtue of their cognitive impairment and the National Institute of Health and Clinical Excellence (2006) have recommended that the patient be supported by a compliance mechanism before any prescribing of a ChEI takes place. While this is helpful, the person with dementia continues to be regarded as a passive recipient of treatment and a more effective mechanism would be one that aims to promote the active involvement of that person in the whole process. Failing to accept the patient as partner in the process serves only to deny any regard for the individual psychological factors which impact upon the level of concordance. Rosenstock (1990) has captured these factors in the Health Belief Model that proposes that an individual will engage in behaviours aimed at 'protecting' their health and that this is based upon two assumptions. First, there is the individual's evaluation of the threat they are faced with. This leads to an approach whereby the seriousness of the threat, or the necessity of treatment, is questioned and their answers determine the extent of compliance. These answers may not always be achieved rationally. In the case of the person with dementia, the psychological stage of their lived experience influences the evaluation process. This is a contentious issue as some people may not have reached a stage of psychological adjustment in which they are prepared to accept their diagnosis; consequently, the threat is denied and the need for treatment minimized (see Keady and Nolan 1994). Second, there is an assumption that individuals undertake a 'cost–benefit analysis' before deciding whether or not to take the treatment offered. Factors related to cost may include the side effect profile, complexity of regime or acceptance of reality of illness. Those relating to benefit may include the possibility of symptom control or improved quality of life. This analysis is ongoing and the cost–benefit ratio may be recalculated at any time. In the case of dementia, calculations will be influenced by a variety of factors but most importantly will be those related to expectations and locus of control.

It has been suggested (Page 2003) that some people with dementia, and their families, have unrealistically high expectations of treatment with a ChEI. This means that they commence treatment with the potential benefit outweighing the costs, with a high locus of control and with robust, positive metaphors. For many these expectations will not be met, locus of control subsequently drops, metaphors become more fatalistic and the cost–benefit ratio is recalculated in such a way that non-compliance is more probable. Interestingly, the concept of compliance is rooted in a pejorative attitude towards those who do not comply and has recently been superseded by the more socially oriented belief in 'concordance', which is evidenced by the greater involvement of the patient and articulated through a collaborative style of consultation.

Promoting concordance in chronic disease management is aided by strategies aimed at patient convenience, quality of information, ongoing negotiation and effective communication. Convenience may be in respect of prescribing a once daily drug or introducing another person, be it spouse or district nurse, who can assist in the effective administration of medication. Quality of information provision is important particularly as understanding and recall of that information are influential in achieving concordance. Clarity in verbal information has been seen to achieve compliance rates of 52 per cent, this increases to 66 per cent where it is reinforced with written information and increased further to 75 per cent where the information is in some way personalized (Ley and Morris 1984).

Ongoing negotiation and communication are achieved through regular contact with the nurse, particularly if the nurse is acting as supplementary prescriber, at which point the subjective and objective aspects of treatment can be discussed and the patient is encouraged to continue with further treatment. Supplementary prescribing can further assist in this process as the nurse can immediately act upon any negotiated change to medication, which falls within the remit of the clinical management plan. This not only prevents unnecessary delays and expedites the process but also allows the patient to witness the immediate outcome of their involvement in that process. Such actions enhance the experience for the patient promoting greater satisfaction and concordance.

Using the CMP

Under supplementary prescribing both nurse and doctor are responsible for drafting the CMP and for agreeing its scope. First choice of treatment is specified by the independent prescriber but subsequent management is largely the responsibility of the nurse. To illustrate this, and to articulate the points made in earlier sections, the following case study is provided.

Case example 1

Beryl is 72 and lives with her husband, Barry, in a small town near Manchester. Twelve months ago, Beryl, who had noticed changes in her memory for about two years, was referred to the local memory clinic and subsequent assessment led to a diagnosis of mild to moderate Alzheimer's disease. Suitability assessment identified no reason why Beryl could not be treated with a ChEI and her consultant recommended using the supplementary prescribing process.

The memory clinic nurse visited Beryl at home one week after diagnosis to discuss that diagnosis, its implications and to consider treatment options. The outcome of this meeting was that Beryl wished to take a ChEI and was happy for the nurse to be involved as a prescriber. She was, however, very worried about side effects and therefore her first line treatment needed to have a short half life and flexible dose regime. The nurse discussed this with the consultant and together they drew up a CMP (Figure 9.3) that Beryl subsequently agreed to.

Treatment was commenced and Beryl revisited after four weeks. At that meeting she was pleased to have experienced no side effects and agreed to the dose being increased. The nurse wrote a prescription and Barry took it to the chemist later that day. A month later the nurse visited again and the dose was increased again.

Ten days later Beryl rang the nurse complaining of feeling unwell with nausea and headaches. The nurse visited that afternoon and discussed the symptoms with Beryl and Barry and on detailed questioning the symptoms seemed to be related to side effects of the drug. The nurse outlined the choices available to Beryl, she could:

- Persevere with treatment as the side effects may ease.
- Take a reduced dose of the drug.
- Switch to a different drug.
- Stop treatment.

Beryl decided to take a reduced dose of the drug, as she knew it could be tolerated, and expressed a willingness to try a higher dose at a later time. The nurse agreed, wrote a new prescription for a lower dose of the drug and the prescribing actions were recorded in the case records. Beryl remained on this lower dose for a further three months at which point the nurse repeated the clinics efficacy tests, which revealed a picture of clinical stability. Despite this, both Beryl and Barry cited a number of day-to-day examples that indicated change was occurring, they discussed this with the nurse and asked to try the higher dose again. The nurse agreed and issued a prescription.

Five days later Beryl experienced the same side effects. The nurse visited the next day, discussed the options, and Beryl asked to try a second ChEI, the nurse issued a new prescription and recommended starting it a few days later. Prescribing actions were recorded and discussed with the independent prescriber who agreed. Beryl remained in touch with the nurse who titrated the dose upwards, with no side effects and efficacy tests after six months suggested clinical improvement. Beryl and Barry felt that the illness was under control and expressed satisfaction with the supplementary prescribing process.

Beryl's experience is not uncommon and many people being treated with a ChEI will experience some changes with titration or choice of drug. Having contact with a nurse supplementary prescriber brought about a range of benefits for Beryl. She was able to spend time talking through treatment, especially her concerns about side effects, a written CMP showed her that these concerns had been listened to and built into the plan. Prescriptions were provided immediately, there was no delay when changes had to be made, and Beryl was very much involved in deciding what to prescribe. Beryl was able to phone the nurse who was subsequently able to provide her with a timely and responsive service.

Governance issues

Accountability

A fundamental basis of nurse prescribing is the acceptance of responsibility and accountability for prescribing actions by the individual nurse concerned and for some this increased liability has been a reason for not prescribing, even when registered to do so (Nolan et al. 2004). It is therefore prudent to briefly explore some aspects of liability and accountability.

NAME OF PATIENT:	PATIENT MEDICATION SENSITIVITIES/ALLERGIES:
BERYL BROWN	NONE KNOWN

PATIENT IDENTIFICATION E.G. ID NUMBER, DATE OF BIRTH:

11-11-1934   P999999

INDEPENDENT PRESCRIBER(S):	SUPPLEMENTARY PRESCRIBER(S)
DR. DOLITTLE	NURSE DOITALL

CONDITION(S) TO BE TREATED	AIM OF TREATMENT
MILD TO MODERATE ALZHEIMER'S DISEASE	SLOW PROGRESSION OF ILLNESS

MEDICINES THAT MAY BE PRESCRIBED BY SP:

DONEPEZIL, RIVASTIGMINE, GALANTAMINE, OR MEMANTINE WITHIN BNF DOSING REGIMES
Discontinuation of above treatments in accordance with current guidelines and practice within MMHSCT

PREPARATION	INDICATION	DOSE SCHEDULE	SPECIFIC INDICATIONS FOR REFERRAL BACK TO THE IP
RIVASTIGMINE	TO SLOW PROGRESSION OF ILLNESS	1.5MG B.D INCREASING TO MAXIMUM OF 6MG BD DEPENDENT UPON RESPONSE	CONCORDANCE NOT ACHIEVED. SEVERE ADVERSE REACTION. COMPLETES TWELVE MONTHS ON TREATMENT. MMSE FALLS BELOW 12/30
LACK OF RESPONSE TO RIVASTIGMINE AT 6mg BD OR INTOLERANT TO RIVASTIGMINE	ALTERNATIVE Cholinesterase Inhibitor AS PER PROTOCOL	UP TO MAXIMUM FOR BNF AND IN ACCORDANCE WITH TITRATION REGIME SPECIFIED IN MMHSCT GUIDELINES.	CONCORDANCE NOT ACHIEVED. SEVERE ADVERSE REACTION. COMPLETES TWELVE MONTHS ON TREATMENT. MMSE FALLS BELOW 12/30

GUIDELINES OR PROTOCOLS SUPPORTING CLINICAL MANAGEMENT PLAN:

NATIONAL INSTITUTE FOR CLINICAL EXCELLENCE: GUIDANCE ON THE USE OF DONEPEZIL, RIVASTIGMINE AND GALANTAMINE FOR THE TREATMENT OF ALZHEIMER'S DISEASE. TECHNOLOGY APPRAISAL GUIDANCE NUMBER 19.

FREQUENCY OF REVIEW AND MONITORING BY:

SUPPLEMENTARY PRESCRIBER	SUPPLEMENTARY PRESCRIBER AND INDEPENDENT PRESCRIBER
INITIALLY MONTHLY, SUBSEQUENTLY THREE TO SIX MONTHLY OR AS REQUIRED BASED UPON PATIENT NEED. REPORTING TO TREATMENT CLINIC MDT	SIX MONTHLY OR AS REQUIRED BASED ON PATIENT NEED.

PROCESS FOR REPORTING ADRS:
BNF ELECTRONIC YELLOW CARD SYSTEM FOLLOWING REPORT TO IP AND PATIENTS GP.

SHARED RECORD TO BE USED BY IP AND SP:
PATIENT'S CASE NOTES

AGREED BY INDEPENDENT PRESCRIBER(S)	DATE	AGREED BY SUPPLEMENTARY PRESCRIBER(S)	DATE	DATE AGREED WITH PATIENT/CARER

Figure 9.3   A CMP for Alzheimer's disease

Caulfield (2004) defines liability as the legal term for responsibility and accountability as the professional term. If harm occurs because of the nurse's prescribing action, then that nurse may be subject to criminal, civil or professional action to determine the extent of responsibility. Criminal liability is enshrined within the 1968 Medicines Act, which states the actions that clinicians may legally undertake in the supply of medications and the penalties applicable when the provisions of the act are not followed. Civil liability is through action initiated by a patient, suing for negligence, on the basis of harm occurring as a direct consequence of a failure in the standard of care.

Professional accountability is enshrined within the Code of Conduct (Nursing and Midwifery Council 2002a) and guidelines related to the administration of medication (Nursing and Midwifery Council 2002b). Both outline the behaviour expected of those involved in the professional practice of nursing and deviation from these expectations may lead to disciplinary action. Where the nurse prescriber acts within agreed protocols, including the CMP, that nurse is protected from litigation by virtue of vicarious liability, that is, the employer takes responsibility for the actions and omissions of the employee.

Competence

Making use of a behavioural competency approach, the National Prescribing Centre (NPC 2001) have identified the specific competencies, required by all nurse prescribers, who will be required to both ask and answer the question: 'How do I know that I am carrying out the prescribing aspect of my job effectively?' The NPC offer a straightforward framework that seeks to address the three main areas of prescribing competence in relation to:

- the consultation;
- prescribing effectively;
- prescribing in context.

Essentially nurse prescribers must be able to communicate effectively with each individual patient who is to be regarded as very much a partner in the prescribing process. To enable this, the nurse must possess up-to-date clinical and pharmaceutical knowledge that is sufficient to both make a diagnosis and to establish treatment options for the patient. To prescribe 'effectively', the nurse must do so in a professional manner, working within their sphere of competence and code of conduct. In addition to this, the nurse prescriber is expected to prescribe safely by recognising their personal limitations, never compromising patient safety and acting to constantly improve their prescribing practice. To prescribe 'in context' the nurse is required to have an understanding of the impact of the multidisciplinary team on the prescribing process, to be familiar with local and national guidelines and have the ability to access and critically appraise information related to the products, which are being prescribed.

All prescribing actions must be recorded in the patient's case notes. For nurse prescribers these actions must be recorded in a way that conforms to expected professional standards (Nursing and Midwifery Council 2002c) and also incorporates advice from locally agreed policies. Accurate record keeping is evidenced through a contemporaneous account being entered within 48 hours of a prescribing action and will include objective reporting of any information given to the patient and any changes to treatment which fall within the remit of the clinical management plan. The Nursing and Midwifery Council regard effective record keeping as being an indicator of effective professional practice and it is also a safeguard in respect of accountability for the degree of autonomous practice experienced by nurse prescribers.

The argument against nurse prescribing

It has been claimed that nursing has always sought to improve its professional standing by becoming more technical and taking on activity previously within the scope of the medical profession (McCartney et al. 1999). The development of nurse prescribing is simply a further expression of this strategy and although both nurses and patients are seen to benefit, there is the concern that nursing is naively allowing itself to be exploited. The first exploitation is by the medical profession, which has been able to abandon mundane tasks and consequently reduce both workloads and levels of inconvenience (McNamara 2000). The second and subtler exploitation was the use of nurse prescribing as a political pawn in the Conservative government's battle with the medical profession, allowing them a relatively inexpensive means of 'sending a message to a powerful profession that power and privilege can be deregulated away' (McCartney et al. 1999: 353).

It has also been argued that the nurse prescribing programme is potentially divisive to the unity of the nursing profession. Skidmore makes an analogy with Orwell's *Animal Farm*, stating that 'All nurses are equal, but some are more equal than others' (Skidmore 2002: 133). The suggestion is that prescribing was initially restricted to only those possessing a DN or HV qualification and even now, despite government targets, the right to prescribe will not be available to all nurses for some time to come. Potentially, this sets apart not only groups of nurses but also individuals within teams.

Perhaps a more pertinent argument in respect of dementia care is the perceived threat posed to the evolving influence of the social model of care. By allowing nurses to adopt a more significant role around pharmacological interventions they will be seduced to return back to the influences of the medical or organic model. The counter-argument, and the hope, is that involving nurses as prescribers will have the opposite effect and that the prescribing of drugs will be influenced by a social model leading to greater patient involvement, empowerment, satisfaction and concordance.

The patient perspective

In evaluating the initial nurse prescribing pilot sites, Luker et al. (1997) stated a number of benefits identified by patients who broadly welcomed the initiative (Box 9.1). Some of these are fundamental to understanding the patient perspective and are worthy of further consideration.

Patients perceive advantages occurring by virtue of their relationship with the nurse whom they regard as having more time to devote to the consultation which is further enhanced by usually occurring at home and being characterized by clear, jargon-free, information. People with mental health problems comment that they enjoy more frequent and prolonged contact with their CMHN than their psychiatrist and that the nurse possesses greater interpersonal skills than the psychiatrist and is certainly more person-centred and holistic (Harrison 2003).

Box 9.1 Patient perceived advantages

- Nurses have more time to explain medication and answer questions.
- Prescriptions can be made available much more quickly.
- Nurses know more about their patients and their needs.
- Nurses are more the social equal to the patient.
- Nurses are more approachable and have better interpersonal skills.
- Nurses listen to the views of patients.
- Much more convenient for the patient.
- Increased confidence in treatment.
- More accessible safety net if problems occur.

Source: Adapted from Harrison (2003) and Brooks et al. (2001)

In addition to this, patients cite the very fact that Cumberledge believed to be the real advantage of non-medical prescribing, nurses are usually more responsive and the patient experiences timely access to treatment without the need to wait for a GP appointment. This is mirrored in mental health practice when the CMHN, acting as supplementary prescriber, and working within the framework of the CMP, is able to respond to identified needs. This is perhaps the long-awaited acknowledgement of those things such nurses have been doing for years, the de facto prescribing and influencing of regimes for the benefit of those people who experience an enduring or severe mental illness.

In some instances the nurse is regarded as having a superior knowledge than the doctor regarding a particular clinical area, most commonly cited being the areas of wound care or care of infants. This is, however, not replicated when one moves away from the early independent nurse-prescribing programme and particularly into more complex areas where patients have a greater preference for medical rather than nurse prescribing (Brooks et al. 2001), while Harrison (2003) questions whether there are any areas in mental health where the nurse is superior to the psychiatrist. In part, the concerns of patients in this area are, perhaps rightly, about knowledge and educational preparation underpinning prescribing actions, a concern recognized by the Crown II Report, which recommended the need just for not initial educational preparation but continuing professional development (DOH 1999) enshrined in the standards of competency for the INP (NMC 2006).

Summary

For too long the expectation has been that people with dementia are passive participants of treatment and incapable of understanding or retaining information related to that treatment. There have consequently been few opportunities for people with dementia to participate in the prescribing process in any way that reflects the ideals of the triadic relationship. The extension of non-medical prescribing may offer a way out of this dead end.

As evidenced throughout this chapter, and its earlier complementary text (Page 2003), CMHN practice is influenced more and more by a new culture of dementia care and now the CMHN is being presented with a real opportunity to directly engage with the prescribing process and to change it for the better. The opportunity and framework are now before us and it is up to the profession to accept it.

Lessons for CMHN practice

- Appropriately qualified and registered nurses are legally permitted to practise as independent nurse prescribers.

- At present, supplementary prescribing remains the most appropriate mechanism for the CMHN and can be introduced to any number of areas of practice.

- Supplementary prescribing can only occur where a patient-specific clinical management plan has been written and agreed to by the patient.

- Directly involving the CMHN in the prescribing process is an opportunity to influence that process from a psychosocial perspective, which is known to offer benefit to the person with dementia.

- A collaborative style of consultation can do much to empower people with dementia and promote concordance with treatment regimes.

- The CMHN who assume a prescribing role is held legally and professionally accountable for his or her actions.

References

Bain, D.J.G. (1982) Patient knowledge and the content of the consultation in general practice, *Medical Education*, 11: 347–50.

Boyle, C.M. (1971) Differences between patients' and doctors' interpretation of common medical terms, *British Medical Journal*, 2: 286–9.

Brooks, N. et al. (2001) Nurse prescribing: what do patients think? *Nursing Standard*, 15(17): 33–8.

Caulfield, H. (2004) Responsibility, accountability and liability in nurse prescribing, *Prescribing Nurse*, Summer: 18–20.

Cumberledge, C. (2003) Keynote address: dicing with my mental health: medication management and supplementary prescribing in mental health, conference South Staffordshire Healthcare NHS Trust, November 2003.

Department of Health (1989) *Report of the Advisory Group on Nurse Prescribing*. London: The Stationery Office.

Department of Health (1998) *Review of Prescribing, Supply and Administration of Medicines: A Report on the Supply and Administration of Medicines under Group Protocol*. London: The Stationery Office.

Department of Health (1999) *Review of Prescribing, Supply and Administration of Medicines. Final report*. London: The Stationery Office.

Department of Health (2000a) *The NHS Plan: A Plan for Investment, A Plan for Reform*. London: The Stationery Office.

Department of Health (2000b) *Patient Group Directions (England Only)*. London: The Stationery Office.

Department of Health (2002) *Expanding Independent Nurse Prescribing within the NHS in England: A Guide for Implementation*. London: The Stationery Office.

Department of Health (2003) *Supplementary Prescribing by Nurses and Pharmacists with the NHS in England: A Guide for Implementation*. London: The Stationery Office.

Department of Health (2004) *Improving Mental Health Services by Extending the Role of Nurses in the Prescribing and Supplying of Medication: A Good Practice Guide*. London: The Stationery Office.

Department of Health (2006) Independent Nurse Prescribing: a guide for implementation, available at: www.dh.gov.uk

Department of Health and Social Security (1986) *Neighbourhood Nursing: A Focus for Care (The Cumberledge Report)*. London: HMSO.

Harrison, A. (2003) Mental health service users' views of nurse prescribing, *Nurse Prescribing*, 1(2): 78–83.

Helling, D., Lemke, J. and Semla, T. et al. (1987) Medication use characteristics in the elderly. *Journal of the American Geriatrics Society*, 35: 4–12.

Jones, M. (1999) Nurse prescribing: the history, the waiting, the battle, in M. Jones (ed.) *Nurse Prescribing: Politics to Practice*. London: Baillière Tindall.

Keady, J. and Nolan, M.R. (1994) Younger onset dementia: developing a longitudinal model as the basis for a research agenda and as a guide to interventions with sufferers and carers, *Journal of Advanced Nursing*, 19: 659–69.

Kitwood, T. and Benson, S. (1995) *The New Culture of Dementia Care*. London: Hawker.

Ley, P. (1988) *Communicating with Patients*. London: Croom Helm.

Ley, P. and Morris, L.A. (1984) Psychological aspects of written information for patients, in S. Rachman (ed.) *Contributions to Medical Psychology*. Oxford: Pergamon Press.

Luker, K., Austin, L. and Hogg, C. et al. (1997) *Evaluation of Nurse Prescribing: Final Report*. Liverpool: University of Liverpool and University of York.

MacNamara, L. (2000) Is prescribing really happening? *Primary Health Care*, 10(7): 32.

McCartney, W., Tyrer, S., Brazier, M. and Prayle, D. (1999) Nurse prescribing: radicalism or tokenism? *Journal of Advanced Nursing*, 29(2): 348–54.

Medicines Act (1968) *Medicines Act*. London: HMSO.

National Institute for Health and Clinical Excellence (2006) Donepezil, rivastigmine, galantamine and memantine for the treatment of Alzheimer's disease (including a review of existing guidance no. 19), available at: www.nice.org.uk

National Prescribing Centre (2001) *Maintaining Competency in Prescribing: An Outline Framework to Help Nurse Prescribers*. Liverpool: NPC.

Nolan, P., Carr, N. and Doran, M. (2004) Nurse prescribing: the experience of psychiatric nurses in the United States, *Nursing Standard*, 18(26): 33–8.

Nursing and Midwifery Council (2002a) *Code of Professional Conduct*. London: NMC.

Nursing and Midwifery Council (2002b) *Guidelines for the Administration of Medicines*. London: NMC.

Nursing and Midwifery Council (2002c) *Standards for Records and Record Keeping*. London: NMC.

Nursing and Midwifery Council (2006) *Nurse Prescribing and the Supply and Administration of Medication: Position Statement*. London: NMC.

Page, S. (2003) From screening to intervention: the community mental health nurse in the memory clinic setting, in J. Keady, C.L. Clarke and T. Adams (eds) *Community Mental Health Nursing and Dementia Care: Practice Perspectives*. Maidenhead: Open University Press.

Preece, S. (2002) Nurse prescribing: accountability and legal issues, in J.L. Humphries and J. Green (eds) *Nurse Prescribing*, 2nd edn. Bristol: Palgrave.

Rosenstock, I.M. (1990) The health beliefs model: explaining health behaviour through expectancies, in K. Glanz, F.M. Lewis and B.K. Rimer (eds) *Health Behaviour and Health Education: Theory, Research and Practice*. San Francisco: Jossey-Bass.

Seedhouse, D. (1991) *Liberating Medicine*. Chichester: John Wiley and Sons, Ltd.

Skidmore, D. (2002) Will you walk a little faster . . .? in J.L. Humphries and J. Green (eds) *Nurse Prescribing*, 2nd edn. Bristol: Palgrave.

10

Rural practice, dementia and CMHN activity

An Irish perspective

Aine Farrell, Suzanne Cahill and Shane Burke

Introduction

In 2002, there were 436,001 elderly people (aged over 65 years) living in Ireland of whom a slightly larger proportion (12.5 per cent) were older people living in rural rather than urban (10 per cent) communities (Central Statistics Office (CSO) 2003). Like other European countries, the Irish population is ageing (Connell and Pringle 2004). While currently there are some 436,001 people aged 65 years or over living in Ireland, 11 per cent of the total population, older people in 2021 will constitute about 15 per cent (O'Shea 2006). However, unlike the UK and other European countries, there is no Community Care Act in Ireland, which means that there is no legislation available that places a duty on Health Boards to provide statutory services to the frail elderly (Ruddle et al. 1997). A corollary of this is that community services for older people are not well resourced (Garavan et al. 2001) and, in particular, rural-based services remain under-developed (Convery 2001). The situation for older people diagnosed with dementia and living in rural areas until recently has been all the more challenging (O'Shea and O'Reilly 1999).

One of the paradoxes of our population ageing is that as we celebrate longevity, we also witness older people living with increased infirmity and being significantly at risk of developing age-related disabilities such as dementia (Gilleard 2000). Today there are approximately 34,000 people in Ireland known to have dementia. An additional 4000 new cases are expected to emerge annually (O'Shea and O'Reilly 1999; O'Shea 2006). In Ireland, people with dementia are located across 10 health board regions and around 26 counties (Figure 10.1). The Western and North Western Health Boards have the highest proportion of people with dementia in their populations and the Eastern Health Board has the lowest (O'Shea and O'Reilly 1999). Ironically, however, most of the new dementia-specific service initiatives such as case management, in home respite support, and the trial of enabling technologies have emerged in the Eastern Health Board area. Six counties have more than 1 per cent of the population experiencing dementia. The difference in prevalence rates reflects differences in age structure of the population across counties and regions (O'Shea and O'Reilly 1999).

The emergence in Ireland in more recent years of old age psychiatry teams and the advent and expansion of community mental health nursing (CMHN) services have been

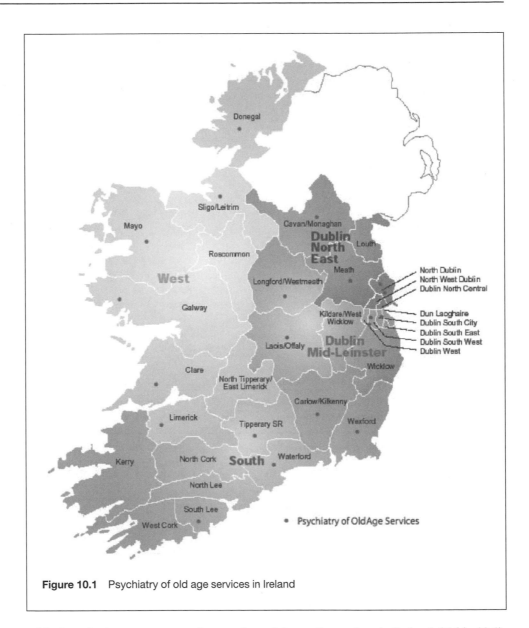

Figure 10.1 Psychiatry of old age services in Ireland

critical to the improvement and expansion of dementia services in Ireland (Table 10.1). This chapter aims to outline the way in which CMHN services evolved in Ireland, and to detail the role and unique challenges facing CMHNs working with people who have dementia living in rural Ireland. The specialist roles CMHNs have in attempting to provide care and support to persons with dementia and their family caregivers will also be outlined. The chapter is based on a review of available literature and on a small scale in-depth survey conducted with 19 CMHN practitioners employed in old age psychiatry teams around the country. Before proceeding to this more detailed analysis, some background information outlining the history behind the evolution of the CMHN service will first be provided.

Table 10.1 Psychiatry of Irish Old Age Resource data, 2005

Service	Date established	Population ≥ 65 yrs
NAHB Area 6 and 7	1989	30,500
SWAHB Area 3 and ½ 4	1991	20.228
ECAHB Area 1 and 2	1996	30,000
MWHB Limerick	1996	19,000
SWAHB Area 5½ 4	1998	15,600
MHB Laois/Offaly	1999	14,036
NEHB Cavan/Monaghan	2000	14,289
SEHB Waterford	2000	14,000
SEHB S. Tipperary	2000	10,200
MWHB Clare	2000	13,500
SEHB Wexford	2001	15,000
MHBLongford/Westmeath	2001	13,000
SHB South Lee	2001	18,000
NWHB Donegal	2002	17,300
NWHB Sligo/Leitrim	2002	14,600
NAHB Area 8	2002	18,600
SEHB Kilkenny	2002	14,000
WHB Mayo	2002	17,000
NEHB Meath	2003	13,000
Galway West	2004	25,500

Background

Community psychiatric nursing (CPN) first became a feature of the Irish health services in the 1960s (Commission on Nursing 1998). The development of this service arose largely in response to a local and worldwide move to shift the balance of care for those with mental health problems away from institutional to community care. During the 1950s and 1960s, civil rights groups were very critical of the standards and culture of psychiatric institutions (Hudson 1999). The development of new drugs to treat certain mental illnesses along with the excess disabilities created by maladapted institutional environments facilitated the return of patients to their homes. This transition was often difficult with many patients refusing to take their medication. Indeed, it was noted that the most significant reason for the return of psychotic symptoms was non-compliance with new medication together with poor preparation on the part of families to accept the recovered patient back home from the institution (Commission on Nursing 1998). In response to these and other needs, the establishment of the position of a new grade of CPN was deemed necessary to ensure that the patients' return to the community would be a successful one (Commission on Nursing 1998).

Since the position of CPN was first established in the 1960s there has been a significant growth in numbers employed across the country. However, until recently, the service focus has been generic rather than specific, and issues such as mental health promotion and high quality specialist nursing services to those at serious risk (including suicide prevention) have not been a priority (Commission on Nursing 1998).

The role of the CPN and community mental health nurse (CMHN)

The Commission on Nursing, established in 1997, was set up to review the evolving role of nurses including CPNs employed in the Irish health services and to examine their professional development. It recommended the development of a new position of Community Psychiatric Clinical Nurse Specialist. Appointees to this new position would be responsible for developing the role of the CPN and for psychiatric nursing services in the community. It was noted that promotion to this role would require application in accordance with procedures for the appointments of clinical nurse specialists (Commission on Nursing 1998). It was suggested that a specific grade for community psychiatric clinical nurse specialist should be developed and that their name would be changed to that of 'community mental health nurse' (CMHN).

Despite such recommendations, the reality was that no formal application was needed to advance to this new position. In fact, in 2000, the position of CPN was automatically upgraded to that of CMHN (Henry and Deady 2001) and no specialist training was required to make the transition. This upgrade, it was said, was largely due to recommendations made by the Commission on Nursing and the Post Strike National Nursing agreement (Kavanagh 2000). It was felt that these nurses should become more pro-active, working in crisis intervention so as to reduce the numbers going to outpatient clinics (Henry and Deady 2001). It was hoped that the upgrade would give CMHNs more status than staff nurses.

The diversification of community mental health nursing and the emergence of old age psychiatric teams in Ireland

The establishment of old age psychiatry services in Ireland in the 1990s greatly facilitated the further development and diversification of the role of CMHNs. In 1989, the first psychiatry of old age service was established in Ireland. It offered a comprehensive community-designated psychiatry service to elderly people within a specific catchment area. The service, located in North Dublin, was initially established as a pilot project. It was funded by the Eastern Health Board to provide assessment and management to patients with functional and organic disorders. A multi-disciplinary team approach characterized the service in which the role of the CMHN was considered central to this new model of service delivery.

Since the initial piloting of this new service, and over the past 17 years, a total of 20 old age psychiatry teams have been established across Ireland, four in the Dublin region (and its locale) and 16 across each of the other seven Health Boards. Each team employs at least one and in some cases two or more CMHNs. However, team composition varies considerably across the country, with some teams employing as few as four health service providers while others have a complement of 14 staff, including psychiatrists, CMHNs, psychologists, occupational therapists, social workers and registrars.

Unlike the UK, where some CMHNs may have a dementia-specific remit, in Ireland, CMHNs attached to old age psychiatry teams have a generic rather than disease-specific remit and even though dementia can sometimes account for a very significant component of the workload, there are no CMHNs in Ireland assigned specifically to the area of dementia. As a suitable planning recommendation for this evolving service, a norm of one

CMHN per 4500 people aged over 65 has been recommended. This would suggest a total of 90 nurses will ultimately be linked to the development of a comprehensive psychiatry of old age service (O'Shea 2004). To date, these benchmarks have not been reached.

Training

Training to become a CMHN in Ireland and to work on an old age psychiatry team is not mandatory, provided the individual has trained as a psychiatric nurse. It is argued therefore that because they do not need a specific qualification for their post, as a professional group, CMHNs are somewhat undervalued in comparison to public health nurses (Henry and Deady 2001). It is difficult, however, to compare the role of CMHN with that of a public health nurse, as they represent two very different fields. A public health nurse cannot become a CMHN, unless he/she first becomes a psychiatric nurse. Public health nurses have, however, been known to perform CMHN duties, which, according to some experts (Henry and Deady 2001), further devalues the role of the CMHN and the treatment of mental illness in general in Ireland.

All CMHNs working on old age psychiatry teams have equal status and make decisions equally. This teamwork approach, where health service professions come together to obtain a holistic view of the person's problems, is considered critical to effective assessment. The team allows realistic measures to be taken and realistic objectives to be set. The range of services available to CMHNs working on old age psychiatry teams includes out-patient clinics, day hospitals, psychiatric inpatient beds, extended care beds, respite beds and patient follow-up post-discharge. The development of old age psychiatric services in recent years is said to have improved the status of CMHNs since professional support can be offered and CMHNs are helped to set and attain goals in community services. Multi-disciplinary teams combine expertise from various health-care areas to provide better care for older people.

Community mental health nursing and dementia

As stated earlier, in Ireland no CMHN has a dementia-specific remit, however, the CMHNs attached to old age psychiatry teams have several roles to play in dementia care. These include that of assessor, consultant, clinician, therapist, educator and manager. In the context of dementia, initial referrals to CMHNs are made by GPs or other medical doctors such as geriatricians. After referral, the CMHN visits the person with dementia at home and using standardized assessment scales, undertakes a holistic assessment. In Ireland, standardized instruments used in initial dementia assessment include: the Hamilton Depression Scale, the Geriatric Depression Scale, the Mini Mental State Examination, the Clock Drawing Test, the Delayed Word Recall, OARS and the CAMCOG.[1] The CMHN will also take a physical, psychiatric and social history from the person and from family members or carers if available or necessary. For a more detailed medical/ psychiatric assessment, the CMHN refers the person to an outpatient clinic to be seen by a medical team. In situations where this is not possible, the CMHN will be accompanied by a doctor on a domiciliary visit.

After initial assessment and pending the nature of the problem, more specialist services may be recommended. If, for example, the presenting problem relates to a diagnosis of dementia or the need for a more differential diagnosis, or if it is of an acute medical nature, referral to a memory clinic or admission to a hospital under the specialist care of a geriatrician or old age psychiatrist may be recommended. If, on the other hand, the presenting problem relates more to the individual's psycho-social needs, referral to day care, social work, or psychiatry of old age day hospitals may be appropriate. Follow-up home visits can be arranged by CMHNs or at outpatient clinics.

Apart from assessment, behavioural and psychological symptoms associated with dementia are often common and problematic in community settings and represent a significant component of the day-to-day workload of CMHNs attached to old age psychiatry teams. Improving our recognition and management of challenging behaviours through observation, or through family members' education, medication, complementary therapies, or through admission to day hospitals can have a positive impact on the quality of life for people with dementia and their carers, and can potentially delay the transition from home to institutional care (Lawlor 2002).

There is a paucity of information available to older people in Ireland about local community support systems and the CMHN attached to an old age psychiatry team also has a key role to play in advising families about local community support services. The type of services available to people with dementia include: home helps, meals on wheels, day centres, mobile day centres, some care packages organized by the Alzheimer's Society of Ireland, respite care and day hospital admission, but many families have little knowledge of how to access these and other services and rely on the CMHN to help guide them.

Community mental health nurse and dementia in rural areas in Ireland

As stated earlier, there are marginally more older people living in rural rather than urban areas in Ireland and since most people with a dementia live at home (O'Shea and O'Reilly 1999), it is not surprising that some CMHNs spend much professional time in rural areas caring for people who have dementia. Several problems associated with providing health and social care to older people domiciled in rural areas have been highlighted in the literature and include long-distance travelling, professional burn-out, low personal accomplishment and the lack of access to trained personnel (Morgan et al. 2002; Innes et al. 2003). Similar problems also exist in rural Ireland where the CMHN spends a large part of his/her working day often in remote areas, away from colleagues, often driving alone from one client to another.

Apart from geographical issues such as these, there are also social barriers to community care for older people particularly those diagnosed with dementia. Lack of transport in rural Ireland constitutes a significant problem for older people (Convery 2001) including family caregivers of persons diagnosed with dementia (O'Shea and O'Reilly 1999). The lack of a driver's licence, or of an adequate public transport system, means that access to certain services such as day care are denied. Rural areas in Ireland are often close knit socially and as such those who live in them are very conscious about maintaining appearances (Morgan et al. 2002). This can sometimes mean that carers of people with dementia feel stigmatized and are unwilling to seek help or use community services, as this would expose the situation of those they are caring for. Families in Morgan et al.'s (2002) study suggested that better awareness of what dementia was would allow people to speak openly about it.

In general, there remains an absence of literature on Irish psychiatric nursing (Henry and Deady 2001) and in particular on the role CMHNs play in rural Ireland, especially in caring for persons diagnosed with dementia. This gap in the literature became apparent while researching materials for this chapter and it was for this reason that a small survey of CMHNs from across Ireland was undertaken. The following section reports on findings of this survey.

Survey of community mental health nurses

In June 2004, the Dementia Services, Information and Development Centre conducted a small survey of CMHNs who were attending a special study day in Kilkenny (Midlands of Ireland). A semi-structured questionnaire was developed which sought information from respondents about a variety of issues pertaining to service delivery to older people and their caregivers, living in rural areas. The aim of this survey was to gain a better understanding of the role of CMHNs and of the special problems faced by them, particularly when working in rural areas. The survey was also designed to investigate the extent to which CMHNs offered a service to families where a person had dementia, and to examine service needs and service usage. Questionnaires were distributed to 30 CMHNs, of whom 19 returned completed survey forms (thus yielding a response rate of 63 per cent). It therefore needs to be remembered that the sample is small and biased and consists of only those CMHNs attending a specialist study day. We do not know the experiences of other CMHNs. However, despite these limitations, our findings shed new light on the topic of how CMHNs perceive their role, and what their concerns are in the context of delivering care to people diagnosed with dementia.

Results demonstrated that most CMHNs saw their role as that of supporting and advocating on behalf of their clients, and coordinating services. Curiously, while no formal training is required to work as a CMHN on an old age psychiatry team in Ireland, almost half (41 per cent) had undergone specialist training. Most respondents had a caseload, of which 50 per cent of their clients had dementia. Some had as few as 25 per cent while others had as many as 75 per cent. In response to a question asked about which aspect of their work caused them most concern, two particular issues were highlighted. The first concerned CMHNs' concerns about leaving vulnerable and at risk people with dementia at home alone, particularly in the evenings and at weekends when the Health Boards offered no CMHN support. The second concern related to the nature of their workload, the possible long delays (up to one year) for non-urgent referrals and the fact that there was a general absence of relevant support services available to enable CMHNs carry out their work satisfactorily and provide back-up support to their clients.

Desirable additional resources identified by CMHNs through the survey included: respite facilities (some felt that nursing homes were not prepared to offer respite to persons with challenging behaviours), dementia-specific day care centres, more CMHNs, access to social workers and occupational therapists and more care workers. Other problems encountered by those employed in rural areas included a lack of transport, a lack of carers and day care, isolation, bad roads, and overall poor access to services. Fifteen out of nineteen respondents (79 per cent) claimed they had insufficient dementia-specific resources to do their job well. The large majority reported they could benefit from having additional specialist training.

Despite working in multi-disciplinary teams, the survey revealed that many of the rural-based CMHNs felt quite isolated. Issues highlighted by them included a feeling of being unsupported ('doing it alone') and the need for more policies and procedures to be developed for staff and for team building. Professional burn-out was often associated with the absence of services and inadequate training to do the job. One respondent highlighted the need in particular for specialist training in challenging behaviours.

Though findings from this work cannot be generalized, it seems that the workload of CMHNs in rural Ireland is particularly stressful when attempting to provide care to persons with dementia. A key problem highlighted by several CMHNs centred around the provision of respite services. This stems partly from the paucity of appropriate safe dementia-friendly environments in which clients can be offered respite care, along with inadequate transport in rural areas, which in turn creates problems in accessing services. Transport, however, is just one factor that creates a barrier to care services. The structure of the health system and the rules governing it may also be a factor.

Summary

This chapter has traced the history and development of the role of CMHNs in Ireland, from the 1960s, when the position of CPN was first instituted, to more recently when, with the advent of old age psychiatry teams, more CMHNs offering a designated service to older people have been employed across the country. The chapter has also shown that rural areas present difficulties to both service users and health service professionals as social services are grossly under-resourced, transport facilities are inadequate, and stigmatizing illnesses such as dementia may be neglected. Through a small-scale survey undertaken with a sample of CMHNs, the unique difficulties confronting CMHNs working with families living in rural areas have been outlined. In this study it was shown that while service provision to families where an older person has dementia constituted a significant proportion of the workload of CMHNs, overwhelmingly, most CMHNs reported that there were insufficient dementia-specific resources available to them to carry out their work adequately.

Lessons for CMHN practice

- In Ireland, the advent of old age psychiatry teams since 1989 means professional support can be offered to the CMHNs which helps them to set and reach goals in community services.

- Community mental health nurses are under-resourced and as such cannot do their job effectively.

- In rural areas, community mental health nurses suffer from professional isolation due to the solitary nature of their work.

- Rural areas present a real problem for both service users and service providers as transport facilities are inadequate in these areas and there is a paucity of social services.

● There is a need to invest more funding in community care services.

Note

1   CAMCOG: a concise neuropsychological test to assist dementia diagnosis: socio-demographic determinants in an elderly population sample.
OARS: Duke (Older American and Services) Multidimensional Assessment Questionnaire, see the Duke University Centre for the Study of Ageing and Human Development (1978) *Multidimensional Function Assessment: The OARS Methodology*, 2nd edn. Durham, NC: Duke University Press.

References

Central Statistics Office (2003) *Press Statement*. www.cso.ie.

Commission on Nursing (1998) *Commission on Nursing Report: Nursing in the Community*. Dublin: Stationery Office.

Connell, P. and Pringle, D. (2004) *Population Ageing in Ireland, Projections, 2002–2021*. Dublin: National Council on Ageing and Older Persons.

Convery, J. (2001) Social inclusion of older people in the health and social services in Ireland, in *Conference Proceedings: Towards a Society for all Ages*. Dublin: National Council on Ageing and Older People.

Garavan, R., Winder, R. and McGee, H. (2001) *Health and Social Services for Older People (HeSSOP). Consulting Older People on Health and Social Services: A Survey of Service Use, Experience and Needs*, Report No. 64. Dublin: National Council on Ageing and Older People.

Gilleard, C. (2000) Is Alzheimer's Disease preventable?: A review of two decades of epidemiological research, *Ageing and Mental Health*, 4(2): 101–18.

Henry, H.M. and Deady, R. (2001) *Mental Health Nursing in Ireland*. Kilkenny: Red Lion Press.

Hudson, M. (1999) Psychiatric hospitals and patients' councils in C. Newnes, G. Holmes and C. Dunn (eds) *This is Madness: A Critical look at Psychiatry and the Future of Mental Health Services*. Herefordshire: PCCS Books.

Huppert, F.A., Brayne, C., Gill, C., Paykel, E.S. and Beardsall, L. (1995) CAMCOG – A concise neuropsychological test to assist dementia diagnosis: Socio-demographic determinants in an elderly population sample. *British Journal of Clinical Psychology*, 34: 529–41.

Innes, A., Mason, A., Cox, S., Ribiero, P. and Smith, A. (2003) Dementia services in remote and rural areas, *Journal of Dementia Care*, July/August, pp 33–37.

Kavanagh, D. (2000) Community Psychiatric Nurses (CPNs), *Psychiatric Nursing*, 1(6): 9.

Lawlor, B. (2002) Managing behavioural and psychological symptoms in dementia, *British Journal of Psychiatry*, 181: 4063–5.

Morgan, D.G., Semchuk, K.M., Stewart, N.J. and D'Arcy, C. (2002) Rural families caring for a relative with dementia: barriers to use of formal services, *Social Science and Medicine*, 55: 1129–42.

O'Shea, E. (2004) *Policy and Practice for Dementia Care in Ireland*. Cardiff: The Edwin Mellen Press.

O'Shea, E. (2006) Public policy for dependent older people in Ireland: review and reform, in E. O'Dell (ed.) *Older People in Modern Ireland: Essay on Law and Policy*. Dublin: FirstLaw Limited.

O'Shea, E. and O'Reilly, S. (1999) *An Action Plan for Dementia*. Dublin: National Council on Ageing and Older People.

Ruddle, H., Donoghue, F. and Mulvihill, R. (1997) *The Years Ahead Report: A Review of the Implementation of its Recommendations*. Dublin: National Council on Ageing and Older Persons.

11

Younger people with dementia

Emerging needs, multi-disciplinarity and the CMHN

Jan Reed, Charlotte L. Clarke, Caroline Cantley and David Stanley

Introduction

This chapter is based on a study that was carried out to evaluate a community-based service for younger people with dementia, comprised of a community mental health nurse (CMHN), a social worker and an occupational therapist (Reed et al. 2000, 2002). For the team members, the challenge was for them to work together in mutually beneficial ways, sharing and extending their expertise, while maintaining a distinct field of practice. For the CMHN, there was a challenge to articulate and reflect on her expertise in a way that identified the distinct contribution of nursing knowledge. While this learning took place for all team members, this chapter will focus on the CMHN's experience, identifying ways in which CMHN contributions can add to multi-disciplinary teams for this particular client group.

The needs of younger people with dementia

The specific problems and service needs of younger people with dementia have been a national concern for some time. The Alzheimer's Disease Society (1996) claimed that many Health Authorities were failing to identify the number and care needs of younger people with dementia, a point reiterated by Williams (1995) and Daniel (2004). In the UK, the Alzheimer's Society (2003) estimate that 18,500 people aged between 45 and 65 have dementia. Jubb et al. (2003) argue that the NSF for Older People (Department of Health 2001) 'lacks clarity and detail on the specific and unique needs of younger people who have dementia, thus leaving them in danger of falling between service providers' (2001: 34).

These needs are identified by the Alzheimer's Disease Society (1996) as differing from the needs of older people (Jubb et al. 2003) in respect of greater need to understand and therefore greater frustration (Keady and Nolan 1997); greater physical fitness; different family and life circumstances; different employment status; and a more extensive range of disturbed behaviour (Keady and Nolan 1997).

In Newcastle a study undertaken in late 1993 identified 51 younger people with dementia (Joint Planning Group 1995). The study interviewed 35 carers and also utilized details about another 16 cases from professionals and medical notes. The findings can be summarized as follows:

- Most people accessed services via their GP.

- Many people were reluctant to seek help.

- Referrals on from GPs were to old age psychiatry, adult psychiatry or neurology.

- For many people the diagnosis came beyond the point at which the person with dementia was able to understand the implications.

- Carers criticized the methods of disclosure by some clinicians and the limited information available.

- The time taken to access support services varied; the old age psychiatry route was generally faster and clients felt better supported. Through the psychiatrist they accessed Social Work, Psychology, Occupational Therapy and Community Psychiatric Nursing; and, as a consequence of these introductions, they accessed day care, respite and residential care.

- Some people who were referred back to their GP by hospital consultants experienced a delay in accessing support services.

- Day care was the most valued service; relatives would have preferred centres specifically for younger people.

- Respite care was used reluctantly, despite carers needing a break; this reluctance was linked to carers' opinions that services were inappropriate, and that the person with dementia would deteriorate in a strange environment and that they might have problems in resettling at home.

- 14 people were placed in residential homes for older people; all carers would have preferred placement with younger people.

The report concludes with the following general principles, which should apply in developing services to meet the needs of this group:

- There should be psycho-educational support and information available throughout the illness for both the person with early onset dementia and their carer.

- There should be coherence between general practice, diagnostic and continuing care services.

- There should be flexible day care designed for and offered exclusively to people with early onset dementia.

- There should be flexible home care services available.

- There should be temporary and permanent residential care designed for and offered specifically to people with early onset dementia.

- Services should have trained and dedicated staff.

- There should be an identifiable service specifically to undertake multi-disciplinary diagnosis.

The service in Newcastle was subsequently initiated in response to this growing recognition of the needs of younger people with dementia. The service team included a full-time community psychiatric nurse, social worker and occupational therapist. A consultant psychiatrist was attached to the team but overall patient management remained with the referring consultant. People could only access the service after having received a diagnosis of dementia, from either psycho-geriatricians or neurologists, and could not self-refer or be GP-referred.

The original outcomes of the service were defined as:

1   To establish appropriate early diagnosis via effective active liaison by specialists in dementia services (old age psychiatry) with neurology and general medicine.

2   To develop more age-sensitive packages of care for people with dementia and intensive support for carers.

3   To establish existing resource use and develop appropriate future models for ongoing delivery and purchasing of services locally.

4   To raise awareness of the needs of this client group among service providers, increasing sensitive service delivery through publicity, education and training.

Aims and method of the evaluation

The aims of the evaluation study were, therefore:

1   To describe the nature of the work of the service team with clients and carers, specifically noting areas of age-specific care.

2   To describe the multi-disciplinary nature of the service and the process of developing the multi-disciplinary team.

3   To identify experiences of the service's functioning from three major perspectives: service users (clients and carers), team members and stakeholders.

4   To analyse the model of service delivery in relation to alternative models and in relation to its original and evolving aims.

The focus of the evaluation was therefore not the specific CMHN experience, but in the course of carrying out the evaluation it was possible to identify some particular issues for the development of CMHN work with this client group.

The evaluation involved collecting a range of data, including interviews with people with dementia and their family members; repeated focus group interviews with the practitioners in the team; interviews with a range of stakeholders who are concerned with the work of the service; case note analysis of the case-load of the service (see Reed et al. 2000, 2002). The results of the evaluation that are presented in this chapter draw only on the focus groups with team members.

Community mental health nursing in the multi-disciplinary team

The development of multi-disciplinary care is particularly complex, and one response to this has been to shift from thinking of individual practitioners as units of care delivery to teams. Such teams go through processes of learning about sharing skills, knowledge and experiences, where boundaries are crossed and perspectives integrated (Bond 1997). In the case of this team, providing a service for younger people with dementia, extensive learning and development had to take place because the client group were very different from those that they had met before – they had problems usually associated with an older group, but were younger. This meant that the skills, knowledge and expectations that the staff had built up with older people had to be re-evaluated when they worked with younger people.

In addition, the innovative structure of the team meant that professional working had to be negotiated. The team was non-hierachical, with members carrying a case-load of individual clients. The process of allocation was carried out by the team, based on their initial judgement of client needs, and 'best fit' with the team members' areas of expertise. This judgement could change over time, as the team found out more about the clients, or as different issues arose. The team therefore had developed a process of co-opting colleagues to work with clients when their expertise was needed. This informal working depended much on a good knowledge of each other's skills and knowledge, and a willingness to work flexibly.

The experiences of the team members reflected these themes and processes to some extent, although the data did not represent a longitudinal study. For the purposes of reporting and discussing this data, four broad areas or headings have been identified: (1) individual professional knowledge and skills; (2) team development and working; (3) multi-disciplinary working; and (4) age-specific care.

Individual professional knowledge and skills

Legacy of past experience and knowledge

The CMHN in the team was able to identify her core areas of experience and knowledge as being a holistic approach to understanding the issues facing the person with dementia and their families and carers. While her previous experiences had been with people with dementia, these experiences had largely been with older people, and so working with younger people was a challenge to some of the expectations developed in this experience.

> When I nursed people with dementia in the past, they had usually been on care of the elderly wards, and so they were generally written off as 'geriatric'. I hadn't realized how much this had coloured my approach until I found myself taken aback at how young the clients were.

In this sense, then, her past experience had not always been useful to the CMHN, and her previous training had also been restricted, with dementia care for all age groups having a minor part in the pre-registration curriculum, and post-registration training being limited. Development of specialized knowledge, therefore, had been very much 'on the job' for the CMHN, prompted by her own personal interest and commitment, and the stimulation of working with other professionals within the team. This development had, however, been founded on a nursing perspective, which had informed the focus of the developing expertise. As well as knowing her own individual skills, the CMHN recognized that her values of practice were located in her past professional practice, for example, in recognizing the special case of younger people with dementia before joining the team.

Skill development and use

The CMHN identified a range of skills she had developed since joining the team. In most cases, this was a matter of a changing emphasis in the range of skills used in previous posts, such that certain skills have become more important in her work with clients. This range of skills, however, was also refined and developed in the light of learning between the team members and as the result of the opportunity for altered work practices. In this way, the perception of the needs of clients change as the team learnt more about younger people with dementia, and consequently the skills they used to respond to the emerging needs developed. This is a process of reframing which builds on the individual frames of client perception that each team member held previously.

The following skills were identified as important for the care of younger people with dementia and their family:

- *Interpersonal skills.* Counselling, negotiation, gaining trust. One of the complexities of communication with clients and carers was that the CMHN had to communicate effectively with everyone, and this could include people with very different communication capacities and skills.

- *Building relationships with clients.* While nursing experience had provided the foundation for relationship building, incorporating empathy and trust, the relationship with clients were often complex. Clients could be very distressed by their dementia, and problems with recall meant that some conversations could be forgotten, although they seemed to have significant impact at the time. Issues of trust and confidentiality became problematic at times when discussions involved carers and the health and safety of the person with dementia or their carer.

- *Working at the client/carer's pace.* While CMHN work is flexible, a focus on goal-setting can impose expectations about how long it will take to achieve these goals. With these clients, these expectations would often have to be revised.

- *Identifying when to refer to others (within and outside the team).* Continuously assessing changing needs and being sensitive to emerging issues increased skills in identifying the potential contribution of other team members and other agencies. This also depended on knowledge and information about other inputs available, and the ability to identify the need for them.

- *Using specific therapeutic interventions.* These were varied and included areas such as memory skill acquisition through the use of client diaries, for example. These skills had been acquired through previous experience and through learning from other team members, rather than formal training.

Team development and working

The process of reframing their individual roles, and their understanding of the therapeutic nature of their work, was evident in the development of the team collectively as well as for the individuals within it.

Professional growth

There were two ways in which the CMHN enhanced her professional knowledge and role. First, this was through recognizing and learning about each other's skills in the team:

'It's acknowledging and recognizing people's expertise.' Second, professional growth was identified as taking place through an understanding of the boundaries of each other's work: 'You need to know how far you can go in a role.'

Reconfiguring professional support networks

As a result of this level of individual and collective professional growth, and their evolving reframing of the needs of younger people with dementia, the team members found that they needed to develop different support networks to those they had previously used. They found it increasingly difficult to identify other people with relevant clinical experience, and as they 'outgrew' previous support, they consolidated a new support framework, drawn from the internal strengths of the team. As one team member said: 'The team itself is the first port of call.'

However, they did strive to maintain their own professional links within the health-care organization and social services. This served two purposes: first, to maintain access to professional specific information and, second, the team members were mindful of the need to protect their future employment position outside of the team, and thus sought to retain a profile with their own professional group.

These very particular support needs of the members of the team reflected their need to feel professionally secure while working in an altered environment of colleagues and clients. Waterman et al. (1995) and Bell and Procter (1998) identify the importance of collegial professional support in complementing the individual's personal enthusiasm. This is seen to contribute to the individual's commitment to the change in client and service provision such that they accept the value of the change and have confidence in their ability to effect that change. Some 'key' characteristics of individuals who seek to develop, and reframe, practice can be identified from these two studies and are reflected in the process of adaptation to multi-disciplinary working with a new client group experienced by the team members:

• self-confidence and self-direction in personal development;

• participation in a supportive group who share similar clinical interests;

• access to staff with similar interests who are elsewhere in the organization;

• familiarity with the users of a service to identify practice development needs, and the organization to identify ways of responding to the needs.

Elements from the work of Waterman et al. (1995) and Bell and Procter (1998) which were less apparent in the work of the team were:

• academic skills and contact sufficient to utilize theoretical and research knowledge;

• participation in a culture that supports R&D activity.

The reframing of client need, the development of necessary professional knowledge and skills, and the development of appropriate support require a personal invest-ment by members of the team. This is more consistent with developmental models of change, emphasizing professional change and a challenging of professional assump-tions about care (Schön 1987), than project-orientated change that is task-specific and time-limited.

Structural issues in developing expertise and specialized practice

The structure and organizational location of the service impacted on the relationship of the team to other services, and strongly shaped their awareness of their contribution to care. They were an added extra to core service provision and therefore at times felt that they were outside of central lines of communication. However, in response to this, and other factors described earlier, the team developed a considerable degree of internal solidarity. This was an experience shared across the team, and not just by the CMHN, and affected the ways in which they all saw their roles and skills in relation to agencies and services outside the team. In relation to 'the outside world', then, identification with the team took precedence over identification with professional groups.

Multi-disciplinary working

Impact of working with other agencies

Working with other agencies was a key experience of the team members, and centred on the management of information. At times, the team perceived there to be unreliable channels of communication, which excluded their involvement in the care of the client: 'Unless the client or carer tells you they are going for a review appointment, you are not necessarily going to know.'

The team members also perceived there to be a need to prove themselves to other agencies as a necessary and valuable part of service delivery and client care. As one team member said: 'You have to prove yourself worthy of information.'

The team placed a high value on the relationship that they developed with clients and their carers, and perceived there to be a risk of fragmenting that relationship if the client were referred to another agency. However, the team members were also working to develop the interface between the team and other agencies, sometimes despite existing service systems: 'We're trying to work in conjunction with specialist care providers and it's somehow trying to work around those structures and how you actually do that.'

The team also worked closely with other agencies to develop and deliver the care which they recognized as necessary for younger people with dementia but which they themselves were unable to provide. For example, they worked with Dementia Care Initiative (now Dementia Care Partnership), a regional charity, to provide care by male carers for the male clients.

The team members also recognized that there were some aspects of care which were out of their control but which impacted on their practice. These included the diagnostic process and the involvement of medical staff with their case-load and in referring clients to the team. 'We've had to learn what we can change and what we can't change and I think initially we were quite depressed and frustrated by trying to change some of the things we actually can't change.'

One key concern of the team was to establish a base of support for younger people with dementia, and this centred on the position of the service within the health-care organization so that they moved from the position of being a project which was an add-on to mainstream care to being an integrated part of mainstream care.

They gave considerable thought, for example, to where the service could be located in the health-care organization, and where consultant support could be available. Integration into the mainstream activity of the organization was viewed by the team as being further enhanced by developing a single citywide referral point to facilitate a pathway of care 'from diagnosis to death', and a single citywide day hospital and inpatient resource within an Old Age Psychiatry Assessment Unit.

Development of an integrated service was perceived to have the advantages of creating further opportunity to 'promote and develop wider and more constructive networking, both locally and with specialist services developing nationally', and thus allowing the experiences of the team to be available as a resource.

Impact of working within the team

The experiences of the team members as they developed the nature of their work within the team is characteristic of Dechant et al.'s (1993) proposition that as teams learn together, their processes of learning increasingly revolve around collective thinking and action, such that ideas and information cross their individual professional boundaries, and their divergent views become synthesized to generate an integrated perspective about the reframed care need and the nature of the team's response to that need. However, the team also spoke of their initial anxiety because of unclear roles and responsibility.

Very visible indications of such an integrated perspective for the team included shared, comprehensive assessment documentation and shared client records, which were valued by the team members. They also identified a blurring of their roles, which allowed them to retain their specific professional roles and special knowledge.

> The skills we all share have increased and our expertise has become, it's not less, but it's become a smaller amount but more specific . . . our expertise has become extremely well defined in a way because we've shared so much and there's so much blurring.

In reaching this point of 'professional personhood' (Dombeck 1997), the team members recognized the process they had gone through in learning about each other's professional language, checking things out with each other, and developing things together. They also identified a number of positive outcomes of the way in which they worked together:

- The access to a range of disciplines within the service avoided the need to refer clients outside the team and consequently allowed the team members to respond quickly and efficiently to client need.
- Their wide professional networks allowed them to access, and be a resource to, other services.
- There were able to balance development work and direct care delivery.
- They acted as a key contact service.
- They provided support right the way through the experience of dementia for clients and carers.
- They saved time.
- They perceived the team to be providing a quality service.

As one team member put it: 'I do believe that by good multi-disciplinary working quality and effectiveness of service are enhanced.'

Age-specific care

There has been an increasingly strong voice calling for assessment of the service needs of younger people with dementia and the development of age-specific services for younger people with dementia (for example, Williams 1995; Alzheimer's Disease Society 1996; Robertson 1996; Barber 1997; Daniel 2004), and indeed this was one of the foundations for the development of the service.

The team members identified a number of ways in which the clients they were now working with differed from older people with dementia. One key area was in the relationship of the client to health and social care services. For example, the clients and carers of the team were perceived to have a different approach to health-care services and to reject traditional 'old-age' services such as day care and old age psychiatry. As one team member described it: 'Younger people don't put the medical profession on a pedestal – they challenge – they challenge the system through the team.' Consequently, the clients and carers were perceived to have different expectations of the outcomes of services: 'With this age group, you have to know you're going to get it more or less right first attempt because of their high expectations.'

Some of the very specific age-related need of the clients and carers which were identified by the team members stemmed from their different employment and financial situations, a factor also found in other services for younger people with dementia, for example, in London by Walton (1999), and discussed by Robertson (1996). As one team member said: 'People still have a strong need to fill their occupational role.'

In addition to these social and psychological imperatives, younger people with dementia were perceived to have also experienced a number of financial worries and problems. Usually they had not prepared for early retirement, and many had financial commitments. This required specific advice and support from the team, as clients tried to negotiate financial problems.

Generation-specific aspirations, for example, of retirement plans, and the lack of disengagement from society which is arguably expected of, and experienced by, older people (Reed et al. 2004), resulted in pressure for clients to remain at home for longer rather than move into a care facility and a pressure to develop different types of therapeutic intervention. For example, one team member described a particular challenge: 'Younger people need to have an occupational role and therefore we have needed to develop ways of meeting this outside the home.'

Additional issues were raised for the team by the physical activity of younger people with dementia, who would not necessarily experience the frailty encountered by older people. This activity, when coupled with frustration, anger, emotional liability and restlessness could threaten harm to people with dementia and carers, and they were also exposed to potential harm through wanting to continue with usual activities, such as driving. Giving up these activities may be advisable in terms of safety, but represented an unexpected and premature loss of activity for the person with dementia. Supporting people through these feelings, and developing strategies for managing them formed a large part of the team's work.

These perceived differences in the needs of younger people with dementia resulted in the team feeling that it is harder for professionals to engage with the younger client and family. Carers were described by the team members as having different problems from carers of older people with dementia, and again these were largely to do with the disruption of usual social roles and expectations. Carers were reported as experiencing financial and employment problems, and were not always able or ready to give up work – they had not anticipated or welcomed early retirement. The lack of provision which was felt by carers to be appropriate or acceptable made caring more difficult, and the untimeliness of developing dementia at a relatively young age meant that some carers felt that they had prematurely lost their relationship with the person with dementia, particularly if this was a spouse.

The team were able to identify gaps in service provision for younger people. This is certainly consistent with Tindall and Manthorpe's (1997) proposition that younger people have been required to 'fit' into services designed for older people although an alternative perspective would accept that services should be driven by need and not age. A team member echoed this idea: 'The person fits the age group but the services don't fit the need.'

As well as perceiving younger clients as having a high level of insight, perhaps because a relatively high proportion of them were in the early stages of dementia, the epidemiology of gender and age meant that the team's case-load had a much higher proportion of male clients than would be expected in a case-load of older people. This altered gender profile had a considerable impact on the appropriateness of existing services and triggered the need for the team members to develop some services with other agencies, as discussed previously. In particular, they identified the discomfort some clients felt about spending time with female staff, and their preference for male staff, particularly in public activities.

As the clients on the case-load of the service age, the team members were also concerned about their future care since the arbitrary cut-off point of 65 years (Cox and McLennan 1994; Tindall and Manthorpe 1997) has implications for continuity of care as people move out of the remit of care by the team.

Summary of the team's learning

The members of the team demonstrate the move from individual knowledge to mutual collaboration and sharing which is a classic feature of team learning as described by Dombeck (1997). Accordingly, their skills developed rapidly as they assimilated the knowledge base of each other. This learning took place in a context of conceptualizing the needs of a 'new' client group – younger people with dementia and their carers – and of being a 'project' rather than mainstream service providers. This context shaped the ways in which the team worked and the nature of their relationship with other professional groups and other agencies. The predominant impression is of the internal solidarity of the team but also of their having to make a special effort to overcome the disadvantages of not being mainstream service providers, such as in the areas of communication and service developments.

The need for the CMHN role

The need to improve services for young people with dementia is very widely recognized and supported (for example, Cox and McLennan 1994; Alzheimer's Disease Society 1996; Williams et al. 1997) and the role of the CMHN in this is critical. The development of a very broad range of services is advocated, providing:

- emotional support; early referral and diagnosis services; specialist day care; better information giving at diagnosis; support for carers (Sperlinger and Furst 1994);

- services for children (Dementia Relief Trust 1996; Robertson 1996). Robertson (1996) more specifically recommends a family systems approach to helping involve the children from the moment of diagnosis; information about dementia and practical advice on caring and behaviour management for all the family not just the main carer;

- opportunities for contact with others in a similar situation; befriending and advocacy for isolated people (Dementia Relief Trust 1996);

- 'work-assisted schemes' in normal or sheltered environments (Keady and Nolan 1997);

- mutual support for people in early stages plus a confidante from outside the family (Keady and Gilliard 1999).

Keady and Nolan (1997) more specifically advocate a central role for the CMHN in:

- promotion, support and facilitation of new coping skills for family members;

- dynamic assessment of individual, family and community support;

- preparation, information and empowerment in helping the family carer move from one stage of the process of dementia care to another;

- developing counselling approaches to address carers' feelings of loss and challenge;

- adopting the role of 'informed service networker' and liaison with other clinical and voluntary service personnel;

- responding to the need to 'be there' for the carer and the younger person with dementia, drawing on the nursing principle of presencing.

Comparing these recommendations to the data about the way in which the service described in this chapter developed, it can be seen that some aspects were being addressed and became a key feature of the way in which the service worked, for example, befriending and support services. Others, however, are not evident in the data, for example, support for children. This is to be expected in that existing clients at that time did not have young families, and these issues have not been in sharp focus. On the other hand, many older people will have grandchildren, and the finding that family systems have not been a focus of the service suggests that development may have been responsive rather than pro-active. In other words, the pressures of immediate care delivery may have hindered the development of broader or more strategic approaches.

Models of service provision

There is considerable debate about the model of service provision that will best meet the needs of younger people with dementia and their carers. Ferran et al. (1996) identified the following controversies and they remain issues that need to be tackled by any service seeking to develop provision for younger people with dementia: whether the extent of the problem warrants specialized service; who should provide the diagnostic service; and what the nature of the service should be. One aspect of these debates is consideration of the relative roles that neurologists and old age psychiatrists should play in the diagnosis of dementia in younger people. Allen and Baldwin (1995) argue for links between neurology and old age psychiatry services, with neurology providing the diagnostic service and old age psychiatry contributing to long-term management. Others argue that this model is flawed since it is often important for psychiatrists to have input to the diagnostic process particularly in distinguishing dementia from other psychiatric disorders. While the limitations of the current general practice input to services are widely recognized (DOH 2001), and a more central role is advocated, there is little clarity about how this should be effected. It is in this context that CMHNs must establish their own role in service provision for younger people with dementia.

There have been some notable attempts to outline the features of comprehensive service systems for younger people with dementia. The Alzheimer's Disease Society's (1996) Charter for Younger People with Dementia, for example, highlights the following areas which need to be addressed: early diagnosis, assessment and referral; access to specialist services; adequate financial support; good employment practice; and education, training and information for professionals.

One of the important features of the Charter (Alzheimer's Disease Society 1996) is that it identifies service needs that extend beyond the core responsibilities of health and social services. In order to fully address the Charter demands, wider issues relating to social security and employment policies and services will have to be tackled. The Dementia Relief Trust (1996) summarizes what is needed as follows: 'to provide a co-ordinated pathway from early diagnosis through to access to the range of services provided by health, social services, and the independent sector'. Williams et al. (1997) in a Health Advisory Service report focusing on health and social care, identify the following key features for effective inter-sector service provision:

- clinical leadership;

- comprehensive, expert and timely assessment, reassessment and treatment;

- multi-disciplinary working;

- good inter-agency communication and collaboration;

- use of the Care Programme Approach (soon to be replaced or augmented by the Single Assessment Process in the UK);

- a range of care options including continuing care;

- support and advocacy for service users;

- education, support and advice for carers;

- trained and experienced care managers and coordinators;

- staff training, development and support;

- effective needs-led service commissioning across statutory and non-statutory services.

Thus, the challenge for CMHNs is to develop their practices and services in a wide context that is inclusive of a range of professions, disciplines, agencies and policies.

Specialist and age-appropriate provision

Barber (1997) reports on a survey of NHS Trusts, which found that it is uncommon for Trusts to have specialist services for younger people with dementia. While only 12 Trusts had specialist services, many Trusts (101) reported that they thought specialist services to be necessary. This was reported particularly by those Trusts that had undertaken some investigation of needs. Barber also notes that the composition and function of established specialist services have varied with ad hoc development and no standard model of patient care.

Many people argue for the establishment of specialist services for younger people with dementia (Williams 1995; Alzheimer's Disease Society 1996; Walton 1999). Barber (1997) summarizes the potential advantages of specialist services as:

- improved coordination, effectiveness and age-appropriate services;
- clearer referral and care pathways and thereby improved access and continuity of care;
- provision of a framework to develop diagnostic, treatment and research clinics;
- closer links between statutory and voluntary services;
- the facilitation of staff training and supervision and development of expertise.

There is broad agreement that age-appropriate services are important for some people who are still aware of their surroundings and who may be anxious or upset by old age services. The need for age-appropriate services is highlighted particularly in relation to day care activity (Delaney and Rosenvinge 1995; Newens et al. 1995). There are also suggestions that as the condition progresses, the differences between younger and old people diminishes and consequently the need for specialist services diminishes from the perspective of the service user, although not necessarily from the perspective of their carer (Fosey and Barker 1995; Delaney and Rosenvinge 1995).

The age band which should apply to 'age-appropriate services' has not gone unquestioned. For example, Keady and Matthew (1997) cite Christi and Wood's (1988) argument that the boundary should be in the early 70s as symptoms are similar up to that age. Harvey (1998) argues that since dementia in people under 50 is very rare, and since this includes a wide variety of diagnoses, it is important that referral for these people is made to a specialist unit, at least for initial diagnosis. He argues that the number of cases is so low that local provision for this group is unlikely to be cost-effective or practical. Tindall and Manthorpe (1997) discuss the arguments for and against separate 'age-appropriate' services. They comment on the variety of arguments advanced for separate specialist provision:

- the inadequacy of services (but in many ways these arguments apply to services overall);
- criticism of 'fitting' younger people into a service designed for older people;
- perceptions of people and families about 'what fits'; it is seen as normal and ordinary to be with one's own age group and to be otherwise results in identity being further spoiled;
- the argument that specialist services are functional and enable need to be better met, e.g. by facilitating mutual support among relatives, and by professionals seeing enough cases to develop expertise.

Tindall and Manthorpe (1997) suggest arguments are often made in terms that mask underlying feelings about equity, justice and blame (including, for example, the 'tragedy' of early onset dementia; the 'unfairness' of early onset dementia as compared with older onset). They argue that behind many views are theories related to normalization with early onset dementia in many ways challenging normative images of adulthood. This theoretical understanding can help explain the emotional context of reactions to placing people with early onset dementia in service settings for older people. They also point to the need to link our understanding with theories of ageing and ageism. Services for older people are associated with negative attitudes and fears about old age. It is not surprising, therefore, that the people with early onset dementia, their relatives and professionals themselves perceive emotionally that this world is 'inappropriate' for younger people. They conclude that arguments for 'the potential utility of a separate service to deal with problems of employment or mid-life relationships' exist but only 'in the context of other social beliefs, emotions and structures' (Tindall and Manthorpe 1997).

Finally, it is important to note the methodological limitations of existing research, which provides little direct comparison of the experiences of younger and older people (cf. Sperlinger and Furst 1994).

For the service that was evaluated and reported in this chapter, these issues regarding organizational location and age-specific care had specific implications. While the service clearly provided a much-appreciated service for people with dementia and their carers, who had been unable to access equivalent levels of appropriate care elsewhere, the future of the service was connected to its structure and organization.

The data indicate that the service was thought by stakeholders to have two sets of aims. The first set of aims was about exploring and investigating the needs of younger people with dementia, and developing and facilitating services to meet these needs. The other set of aims was about providing a high quality service. While these sets of aims are not necessarily incompatible, some degree of prioritization is to be expected, and it would appear that providing a high quality service has taken priority. This is entirely understandable, given the immediate demands of service delivery. As staff meet daily with clients, and respond to the needs that they see, more strategic issues almost inevitably will receive less attention.

There were, however, some constraints on the provision of high quality care, which arose from the way the service sat in service structures. As a tertiary referral system that does not involve a consultant within the service for younger people taking over responsibility for patients, there were limits to the extent to which the team members could be involved in care. There were some disincentives to potential referrers, in that referral may lead to another layer of care added to a client's case, and moreover this is a layer of care that is not known to, or under the control of, the referrer. These disincentives limited the number and range of people referred to the team, which in turn limited their impact on care for younger people with dementia. The lack of an identified consultant made it difficult for the service to negotiate and communicate with other services and departments, particularly with other consultants. This meant, for example, that the team members were not necessarily informed of significant health problems or treatments that they could potentially support, or which might impact on dementia management. While such a structure may have promoted collegiate non-hierarchical working within the team, it made external relations more difficult.

One of the components of the investigative model of the service was described by one stakeholder as an 'action research' function. If this is taken to mean that the team should also be involved in changing or developing services, then this involvement could only extend to their own practice, as they did not have any commissioning, purchasing or monitoring role with other services. Gaps in provision, such as a lack of age-appropriate day care, which were identified in the original report and informally by the team, were beyond their remit. Furthermore, there did not appear to be any clear channels by which the team could influence or shape service development outside the project, nor was there any provision for research and development activity.

The focus on service provision within these constraints limited the extent to which the learning of the team was articulated or analysed. With a focus on responding to individual needs, it was not clear how the team members or the steering group had been able to build up a picture of potential strategies for the client group as a whole. This in part is traceable back to a lack of clearly articulated ideas of the specific problems presented by younger people with dementia, as opposed to older people. While the literature and some steering group members identify key features of being younger with dementia (such as rapid onset and progression, a lack of social acceptance, problems in maintaining age-appropriate roles, depression and hallucinations), it was not apparent that the service, the team members and the steering group had confirmed these differences, or developed a model of dementia in younger people.

It is possible to identify an implicit model from interviews with the team, stakeholders and service users. This model, however, is not based on distinct pathology, but on socio-cultural responses to untimely dementia. In a society that has certain expectations of people at certain ages, being younger with dementia, in the way that it prevents people meeting these expectations, has a number of social and personal implications. These implications include physical, social and psychological dimensions, and the corresponding model of response and care is similarly complex and broad. Looking at the needs identified as a basis for care by the team, stakeholders and users, these correspond to holistic approaches to care. In developing this implicit holistic model, the service sought to address and encompass a wide range of problems and issues at the individual level of care.

Developing such an approach may meet the needs of younger people with dementia, but there would appear to be no reason why it should be exclusive to this group. In other words, there is a question about whether this level of service should not be extended to older people with dementia too. There are arguments for assessing their financial situations and their family responsibilities as well.

Summary

This chapter has sought to articulate some of the needs of younger people with dementia as they are identified in the literature and explored through the evaluation of a service for younger people. It has also sought to identify and analyse the role of the CMHN in working with people with dementia. This has been analysed in relation to multi-disciplinary working and in relation to organizational arrangements of service provision. The CMHN's role ranges from the delivery of practice when working with people with dementia and their families through to identifying the needs of this group of service users and advocating further service provision to meet these needs. For a CMHN to be working with younger people is particularly challenging – services are underdeveloped as a result of long-term uncertainty about what needs younger people actually have and whether they even should constitute a distinct client group. These challenges are being played out throughout the country as CMHNs and their colleagues seek to respond to the unmet needs of younger people with dementia and their families. There is, however, no need for people to work in isolation and the failure to learn from each other's experiences makes it essential that CMHNs place policy, service and practice development as high on their agendas as they do the delivery of good quality care.

Lessons for CHMN practice

- Stereotypes of people with dementia need to be challenged.
- Younger people with dementia have different relationships and expectations than older people.
- Learning from colleagues in other disciplines begins with appreciation of their expertise.
- Maintaining a sense of nursing identity begins with valuing nursing skills and knowledge.

References

Allen, H. and Baldwin, B. (1995) The referral, investigation and diagnosis of presenile dementia: two services compared, *International Journal of Geriatric Psychiatry*, 10(3): 185–90.

Alzheimer's Disease Society (1996) *Younger People with Dementia: A Review and Strategy*. London: ADS.

Alzheimer's Society (2003) Numbers of younger people with dementia. Available at: www.alzheimers.org.uk/ypwd/Statistics.htm.

Barber, B. (1997) A survey of services for younger people with dementia, *International Journal of Geriatric Psychiatry*, 12: 951–4.

Bell, M. and Procter, S. (1998) Developing nurse practitioners to develop practice: the experiences of nurses working on a Nursing Development Unit, *Journal of Nursing Management*, 6(2): 61–9.

Bond, M. (1997) A learning team in the making, *Journal of Interprofessional Care*, 11: 89.

Cox, S.M. and McLennan, J.M. (1994) *A Guide to Early Onset Dementia*. Stirling: Dementia Services Development Centre.

Daniel, K. (2004) Dementia and younger people, *Community Practitioner*, 77(10): 369–70.

Dechant, K., Marsick, V.J. and Kasl, E. (1993) Towards a model of team learning, *Studies in Continuing Education*, 15: 1–14.

Delany, N. and Rosenvinge, H. (1995) Presenile dementia: sufferers, carers and services, *International Journal of Geriatric Psychiatry*, 10(7): 597–601.

Dementia Relief Trust (1996) *The Care Must Be There*. London: Dementia Relief Trust.

Department of Health (2001) *National Service Framework for Older People*. London: DOH.

Department of Health (2001) *National Services Framework for Older People*. London: DOH.

Dombeck, M.T. (1997) Professional personhood: training, territoriality and tolerance, *Journal of Interprofessional Care*, 11: 9–21.

Ferran, J., Wilson, K. and Doran, M. (1996) The early onset dementias: a study of clinical characteristics and service use, *International Journal of Geriatric Psychiatry* 11(10): 863–9.

Fosey, J. and Baker, M. (1995) Different needs demand tailored services, *Journal of Dementia Care*, 3(6): 22–3.

Harvey R.J. (1998) *Young Onset Dementia: Epidemiology, Clinical Symptoms, Family Burden, Support and Outcome*. London: NHS Executive (North Thames).

Joint Planning Working Group on Early Onset Dementia (1995) *Care Patterns of People with Early Onset Dementia in Newcastle and the Views of their Carers*. Newcastle: PCT internal report.

Jubb, D., Pollard, N. and Chaston, D. (2003) Developing services for younger people with dementia. *Nursing Times*, 99(22): 34–5.

Keady, J. and Gilliard, J. (1999) The early experience of Alzheimer's disease: implications for partnership and practice, in T. Adams and C. Clarke (eds) *Dementia Care: Developing Partnerships in Practice*. London: Baillière Tindall.

Keady, J. and Matthew, L. 1997 Younger people with dementia, *Elderly Care*, 9(4): 19–23.

Keady, J. and Nolan, M. (1997) Raising the profile of younger people with dementia, *Mental Health Nursing*, 17(2): 7–10.

Newens, A., Forster, D. and Kay, D. (1995) Dependency and community care in presenile Alzheimer's Disease, *British Journal of Psychiatry*, 166: 777–82.

Reed, J., Cantley, C., Clarke, C. and Stanley, D. (2002) Services for younger people with dementia: problems in differentiating need on the basis of age, *Dementia*, 1(1): 95–112

Reed, J., Cantley, C., Stanley, D. and Clarke, C. (2000) *An Evaluation of the Lewis Project: A Service for People with Early Onset Dementia*. Newcastle: Centre for Care of Older People, University of Northumbria, and Dementia North.

Reed, J., Stanley, D. and Clarke, C. (2004) *Health, Well-Being and Older People*. Bristol: The Policy Press.

Robertson, S. (1996) *Younger People with Dementia: The Impact on Their Children*. Stirling: University of Stirling.

Schön, D. (1987) *Educating the Reflective Practitioner*. San Francisco: Jossey-Bass.

Sperlinger, D. and Furst, M. (1994) The service experiences of people with presenile dementia: a study of carers in one London borough, *International Journal of Geriatric Psychiatry*, 9: 47–50.

Tindall, L. and Manthorpe, J. (1997) Early onset dementia: a case of ill-timing? *Journal of Mental Health*, 6: 237–47.

Walton, J. (1999) Young-onset dementia, in T. Adams and C.L. Clarke (eds) *Dementia Care: Developing Partnerships in Practice*. London: Baillière Tindall.

Waterman, H., Webb, C. et al. (1995) Changing nursing and nursing change: a dialectical analysis of an action research project, *Educational Action Research*, 3: 55–70.

Williams, D.D.R. (1995) Services for younger sufferers of Alzheimer's Disease, *British Journal of Psychiatry*, 166(6): 699–700.

Williams, R., Barrett, K. and Muth, Z. (eds) (1997) *Heading for Better Care: Commissioning and Providing Mental Health Services for People with Huntington's Disease, Acquired Brain Injury and Early Onset Dementia*. NHS Health Advisory Service Schematic Review. London: HMSO.

12

The CMHN: pathways for assessing vulnerability and abuse in dementia care

Simon T. O'Donovan

Introduction

The abuse of vulnerable adults has increasingly been under the spotlight in recent years, since the publication of the government policy documents *No Secrets* (England) (DOH, 2000) and *In Safe Hands* (Wales) (Welsh Assembly Government [WAG], 1999), which required Local Authorities to work in partnership with partner statutory agencies in preparing local policies and procedures to protect vulnerable adults from abuse and inappropriate care. More recently, the Health Select Committee of the House of Commons reported that as many as 500,000 older people may be subject to abuse, which is equivalent to 5–9 per cent of the older population in the United Kingdom (HC 111–1 2004). Furthermore, the Community and District Nurse Association found that 88 per cent of Community Nurses had encountered elder abuse in their case-loads (CDNA 2003), meaning that Community Mental Health Nurses (CMHNs) must be concerned about their own practice in response to suspected cases of abuse or inappropriate care.

This chapter aims to equip CMHNs with the essential information and guidance to inform their practice in order that they know how to respond to cases both by way of effective and timely referral to lead officers in their own and partner agencies, and by engagement in local multi-agency protection of vulnerable adult procedures. The chapter is underpinned by two anonymized case studies that highlight how the 'Protection of Vulnerable Adults Policy and Procedures (POVA)' are effectively implemented and the potential role of the CMHN in a variety of real-life scenarios. Each case study is presented with a series of key points in relation to assessment, intervention and reflective practice. For the purposes of this chapter, the definitions of 'vulnerable adult', 'abuse' and 'significant harm' are taken from *In Safe Hands* (WAG 1999).

Vulnerable adult
A person who is 18 years of age or over, and who is or may be in need of community care services by reason of mental or other disability, age or illness and who is or may be unable to take care of him/herself, or unable to protect him/herself against significant harm or serious exploitation.

Abuse
Abuse is a violation of an individual's human and civil rights by any other person or persons.

Indicators of abuse

- *Physical abuse*: Hitting; slapping; pushing; kicking; misuse of medication; undue restraint; any inappropriate sanctions.

- *Sexual abuse*: Rape; sexual assault; sexual acts to which the vulnerable adult has not consented/could not consent to/was pressured into.

- *Psychological abuse*: Threats of harm/abandonment; humiliation; verbal/racial abuse; isolation/withdrawal from services/support network.

- *Financial abuse*: Theft; fraud; pressure around wills, property or inheritance; misuse/misappropriation of benefits.

- *Neglect/acts of omission*: Failure to access medical care/services; negligence in the face of risk taking; failure to provide appropriate care.

- *Institutional abuse*: Several forms of abuse may occur within a care setting and affect several vulnerable adults.

Significant harm

Ill treatment (including sexual abuse and forms of ill treatment that are not physical); the impairment of or an avoidable deterioration in physical or mental health; and the impairment of physical, emotional, social or behavioural development.

Vulnerable adults: considering the issues

The primary responsibility for caring for a person with dementia usually falls upon one family member's shoulders, most often an elderly wife or adult daughter carer (Gilleard 1984), and this may engender considerable resentment if the carer perceives other family members as being unsupportive (Gilhooly 1986). The 'lone carer' who receives no assistance from informal supporters is more likely to seek institutional care than those who have contact with and support from family and friends and are satisfied with this help (Gilhooly 1986).

Aneshensel et al. (1993) found that carers who perceived they are captive in the caring role, i.e. the unwilling incumbents of caregiving through a lack of choices or by default, are most at risk of breakdown in their caregiving situation. Similarly, Hirschfield (1983) found carers who perceive that they are 'tied down' to caregiving; a lack of free time for carers and feelings of resentment, helplessness, hopelessness and guilt are major areas of tension for carers and important variables in predicting institutionalization. Annerstedt et al. (2000) found that carers with an impaired sense of self-identity resulting from caregiving and who perceive the needs of their dependant as overtaking their own, are most at risk of breakdown in their caregiving situation. Other key predictors for carers reaching 'breaking point' in this study were the amount of time spent in caregiving each week, the dependant misidentifying the carer, clinical fluctuations in the dependant's condition and nocturnal deterioration.

Austrom and Hendrie (1990) proposed that the quality of life of carers of people with dementia is invariably affected by caregiving, with 55 per cent reporting physical exhaustion and 75 per cent dissatisfaction with their current state of health. Intervening variables such as the strength of the existing relationship with the dependant and the presence of a social support network were found to be important mediating factors in quality of life impact. Interestingly, clinical depression in carers of people with dementia is recognized as being an important risk factor for breakdown in caregiving situations (Whitlach et al. 1999) and a major determinant of nursing home placement (Gilleard et al. 1984). Dura et al. (1990) found a depression prevalence level of 30 per cent in their study (carers meeting DSM III criteria), but levels as high as 77.8 per cent have been reported (Harper et al. 1993). Haley et al. (1987) found that carers of people with dementia report significantly higher levels of depression and negative affect towards their relatives than controls and have lower life satisfaction, significantly impaired social life and poorer physical health.

In considering the literature on carers of people with dementia as abusers, it is first necessary to highlight that not all highly burdened carers become abusers and that caregiving satisfactions may be evident even in the most complex and challenging situations (Nolan et al. 1996; Nolan and Keady 2001). McKee et al. (1997) found that most carers (74.5 per cent in their study) report that they are coping well with the demands of caregiving and that caregiving satisfactions, such as having an opportunity to repay past kindness, being closer to the person and trying to maintain the dependant's dignity and self-esteem, are important ways of coping. Moreover, Orbell and Gillies (1993) found that a lack of satisfaction gained from the caregiving role was the 'single most powerful determinant of carer preference not to continue providing care'. In this study, carers with a preference not to care saw themselves as being unable to satisfactorily meet the needs of their dependant. Nolan et al. (1996) suggested that there is a particular need to target carers who get no satisfaction from caregiving, as they may be more likely to be near to breaking point. They also found, based on the work of Hirschfield (1983) and Archbold et al. (1992), that caregiving situations in which there is 'low mutuality' in the relationship should be 'taken very seriously' in terms of risk for elder abuse.

Research by Sadler et al. (1995) confirmed the existence of a strong link between dementia and elder abuse. In this study, the co-existence of dementia with substance misuse or psychiatric illness on the part of the carer or pre-existing family conflict significantly increased the risk of abuse. Dementia in the dependant alone, even coupled with challenging behaviour, was not significantly associated with the risk of abuse, though carers themselves were more at risk of being abused by dependants in such situations. However, Homer and Gilleard (1990) did find such an association, with abuse perpetrated by carers being more likely as a response to violence or threat of violence towards them by the dependant. This finding, of the carer abusing in response to being abused, was also shown in a study by Coyne et al. (1993), who found that 26 per cent of carers who reported being abused by their dependant stated that they themselves had been abusive. An additional 4.8 per cent who did not report being abused stated that they had abused.

Quayhagen et al. (1997) found that behavioural deterioration and carer stress enhance the potential for burn-out and aggression in families coping with dementia. In this study, abusive behaviour was identified in 33 couples, with 17 carers and 16 dependants as perpetrators. The carer abusers scored higher for depression, anxiety and hostility and were more burnt out from mental, physical and emotional exhaustion. Cooney and Mortimer (1995) found that the duration of caregiving was also a significant risk factor, with those caring for the longest being most at risk of becoming abusers. In this study, 55 per cent of carers admitted to perpetrating at least one type of abuse, verbal being the most common. Social isolation and a pre-existing poor relationship with the person cared for were the main risk factors.

The above risk factors are a cause for concern for CMHNs' assessment and intervention practice. Carers who identify themselves as being highly burdened, clinically depressed, physically exhausted, socially isolated and unsupported may be in urgent need of increased support, to reduce the risk of them becoming 'end of tether' abusers. There is a vital role for CMHNs to play in assessing risk factors and intervening to achieve adequate risk reduction. For instance, by identifying caregiving problems that carers perceive as being the most stressful/difficult to manage, the CMHN as care manager can coordinate community service interventions to achieve maximum stress reduction, e.g. arranging home care support to relieve the carer of washing/dressing duties if these are times of high stress, conflict or aggression. Similarly, the CMHN is well placed to help educate and emotionally support the potentially abusive carer towards positive care, sensitively highlighting inappropriate coping/management strategies and pointing out alternative approaches.

Another important role for the CMHN is in identifying those caregiving situations which may be breaking down and where intensive CMHN/community services support is required. Two very different but equally valid outcomes may result following intervention. First, with access to intensive home care support, emergency respite care, emotional and educational support, etc., highly burdened carers may be enabled to continue in their caregiving role for longer, and until the dependant reaches a less active/disturbed and more passive/frail phase when caregiving may become somewhat less burdensome and more satisfying (O'Donovan 2004). Indeed, O'Donovan's (2004) research provides CMHNs with carers' assessment tools to both meet the requirements of the Carers (Recognition and Services) Act (DOH 1995) and determine those caregiving situations which are most at risk of breaking down. Second, through assessing the carer's subjective experience and their capability and willingness to continue in the caregiving role, it may become apparent that it would be in the best interests of both the dependant and carer to facilitate admission to permanent care at an earlier stage than might otherwise be achieved, i.e. before the caregiving relationship breaks down to the extent that it becomes abusive. Philp et al. (1997) state that in such cases institutionalization should be regarded as a positive outcome, especially if it improves the safety and comfort of the person with dementia, reduces carer stress and is achieved at a reasonable cost.

Vulnerable adult protection procedures – an outline

The POVA Policy developed in South Wales in response to *In Safe Hands* (WAG 1999) demands that all CMHNs be aware of the multi-agency approach to responding to cases of suspected abuse and inappropriate care, and undergo training in the identification and referral of potentially abusive caregiving situations, or when professional or stranger abuse is alleged. There is an absolute expectation that practitioners will make a referral (using the relevant 'VA1 Referral' document) whenever they have a professional concern or receive a disclosure from the vulnerable adult, their carer or any person on their behalf.

Within Wales, NHS Trusts have 'full partner agency' status within the POVA Policy, alongside the Police and Care Standards Inspectorate for Wales (CSIW). Social Services have the lead responsibility for coordination under the POVA Policy (the South Wales POVA Policy follows closely the *In Safe Hands* guidance, and thus the approach taken will be similar throughout Wales). In England, Health would appear to have less of a full partner status, although all agencies are required under *No Secrets* to designate a Lead Officer as a resource for operational staff.

Cardiff and Vale NHS Trust have responded to the POVA Policy and procedures by establishing a management structure of responsibility, developing a Trust POVA Operational Group and appointing a Named Nurse for Vulnerable Adult Protection who, with the Consultant Nurses for Older Vulnerable Adults, acts as Designated Lead Manager Health for the Policy.

The lead roles for POVA case coordination vary, according to where the abuse or inappropriate care is alleged to have taken place – Social Services have the Designated Lead Manager (DLM) role for all cases of abuse occurring within community settings, including residential and nursing homes; Health have the lead role for abuse or inappropriate care occurring within NHS Trust settings, whether perpetrated by visitors, strangers, other vulnerable adults or Trust staff. In all cases, there will be a collaborative, multi-agency approach involving, in every situation, the Social Services DLM together with:

- the Police DLM, if there is any potential criminal element to the concern, disclosure or allegation;

- the Health DLM, if there is a Health professional involved as an alleged perpetrator or if there are significant health issues to be addressed;

- the CSIW DLM, if there is any registered domiciliary care agency or care home involvement.

Once a VA1 Referral is received by the appropriate DLM (in most cases a senior Social Services officer), a Strategy Discussion is held with appropriate partner DLMs from Police, Health and CSIW, according to which agencies will need to be involved in investigating the concern or allegation of abuse or inappropriate care and in developing an intervention plan for protecting the vulnerable adult from further significant harm. (The VA1 referral should be sent via safe fax within 24 hours of the concern/disclosure being raised.)

The DLMs involved in the Strategy Discussion will between them decide whether a full Strategy Meeting should be called to plan for investigation and intervention and determine what information needs to be gathered in readiness for this meeting, e.g. outcome of medical assessment, medical photographs of bruising/injuries, collation of evidence from other professionals/records, a verbatim disclosure from the vulnerable adult, etc. A Strategy Meeting needs to be arranged with some urgency, i.e. within 48 hours of the referral, so that the earliest possible intervention can be planned to afford the highest level of risk management/safety possible. (In cases where a criminal offence appears to have been committed, more urgent Police intervention may be required, i.e. in cases of sexual or physical assault, where forensic or other evidence may need to be preserved.)

Possible outcomes from the Strategy Meeting may be that:

- no further action is required and the procedures are stood down, e.g. the preliminary information gathering exercise may secure an adequate explanation for the concern;

- a Police-led criminal investigation may be required, if there is sufficient evidence to suggest that an offence has taken place (a video interview with the vulnerable adult may need to be arranged to secure evidence to support prosecution of the perpetrator – under the new 'Achieving Best Evidence' guidance, video evidence can now be presented in court);

- an internal agency-led investigation may be required and an investigating officer may need to be appointed, in order to identify what has happened and what needs to happen to ensure the vulnerable adult's safety and well-being. (CSIW will lead any investigation relating to alleged registered care home or care agency abuse; Health will lead any investigation relating to abuse allegedly perpetrated by a Health professional or taking place within any NHS Trust setting);

- an interim Adult Protection Plan will need to be developed to ensure effective risk management/reduction and appropriate care management/community service intervention, and a Keyworker appointed to implement, monitor and feed back the effects of the Plan (this will often be a CMHN).

The final stage in the POVA strategic process is the Adult Protection Case Conference, which has to be held in all cases of sexual or physical assault, where there are serious and ongoing levels of risk present, or where there is more than one agency involved in coordin-ating the Adult Protection Plan. The Adult Protection Case Conference allows all inter-ested parties to come together to exchange information and share expert opinion (it will usually be a larger meeting than the Strategy Meeting, which would usually only involve DLMs and any individual holding first-hand information, e.g. the referrer), and should afford an opportunity for the vulnerable adult's voice to be heard – their presence should be facilitated wherever possible, and this may require advocacy and/or communication support. The main aims of the Adult Protection Case Conference are to hear the outcomes of the investigative process, ensure appropriate action is taken against perpetrators (which would include additional support for over-burdened carers) and further develop the Adult Protection Plan to ensure ongoing effective risk management/protection. Arrangements for urgently reconvening the Strategy Meeting/Adult Protection Case Conference should be in place if the nominated keyworker believes the plan has not achieved effective risk reduction or if further concerns/disclosures arise. Triggers for urgently reconvening should be built into the Adult Protection Plan.

Area Adult Protection Committees (AAPCs) are available in each Local Authority area to ensure that the POVA Policy and procedures are being effectively implemented and that consistent practice is being achieved. All agencies involved in the procedures are obliged to attend and to collect and present data on referrals received and outcomes of intervention. Importantly, the AAPCs provide a 'Learning the Lessons Forum' for DLMs and practitioners involved in adult protection to come together to share their experiences and learn lessons from practice.

Finally, a South Wales Adult Protection (SWAP) Forum is available to monitor and guide the work of the AAPCs, revise the Policy and procedures in light of outcomes from practice and new legislation and to ensure that appropriate levels of training are available for practitioners across South Wales. It can also undertake reviews of cases where the procedures have not been consistently implemented or where negative outcomes have resulted. (A Serious Case Review procedure is also in place for situations of abuse or inappropriate care which have resulted in serious injury to or the death of a vulnerable adult.)

Fundamental issues in vulnerable adult protection practice

Assessment of mental capacity

Fundamental to vulnerable adult protection work is the principle that vulnerable adults have the right to be involved to the fullest level possible in decision-making regarding their care, and that their wishes must be respected, within their mental capacity to anticipate and understand the risk. Vulnerable adults who are not mentally incapacitated are entitled, as are any members of society, to make their own choices, maintain their independence and refuse intervention, even if this means that they will continue to remain at risk. However, there may be occasions where it is unclear whether the vulnerable adult has sufficient mental capacity to decide. In such situations, making sound professional judgements may require a formal assessment of mental capacity in relation to consent.

In law, all adults are presumed to have legal mental capacity unless:

> The person is unable, by reason of mental disability, to make decisions for themselves on the matter in question or the person is unable to communicate their decision on that matter because they are unconscious or for any other reason.
>
> (Lord Chancellor's Department 1997)

As the legal starting point is the presumption that the vulnerable adult has mental capacity. Evidence to the contrary needs to be gathered to establish mental incapacity before decisions can be made and actions taken on the vulnerable adult's behalf in respect of vulnerable adult protection. (Many daily care interventions which are deemed as necessary to health and well-being can be undertaken without establishing mental incapacity under a duty of care in common law [doctrine of necessity].)

A GP or senior doctor in charge of the vulnerable adult's care may need to undertake an assessment of mental capacity, using the views of the multi-disciplinary team to inform their decision. In addition, specialist assessments from a Psychologist, Speech and Language Therapist or any professional trained in assessing mental capacity, can be sought in informing this opinion. Old Age Psychiatrists may be asked to provide a detailed second opinion assessment of mental capacity in complex cases, i.e. where there is a lack of consensus among the multi-disiplinary team; where the first assessment is a borderline one, or where litigation or court proceedings are possible.

Fundamental to good practice in assessing mental capacity is that the assessment should be single issue-specific, i.e. relating to one complex decision only. Blanket assessments of mental capacity cannot be undertaken, as mental capacity can fluctuate or improve/deteriorate over days or weeks. The test of mental capacity, as laid out in the Mental Capacity Act (2005), should be cogent and probative. Decisions must be evidence-based and made on a balance of probabilities assessment.

In assessing mental capacity, the vulnerable adult should be taken through the following four stages (they must pass on all four parts to be assessed as having mental capacity to decide). An individual must have the ability to do the following:

1   understand the information relevant to the decision (what is being proposed and why it is being suggested);

2   retain the information (for long enough to process the information and make an effective decision);

3   use or weigh that information as part of the process of making the decision (appreciate the principal benefits, risks and alternatives of pursuing/not pursuing the option/s suggested);

4   communicate their decision (whether by talking, using sign language or other means).

If *all* of the above are achieved, then the person must be regarded as having mental capacity to make their own decision and this is inviolate. If the person fails even one part of the test, then he/she must be regarded as mentally incapable of making his/her own decision and professionals can make decisions on his/her behalf, under a duty of care in common law. However, in making decisions, professionals *must* give full regard to what is in the person's best interests. This includes consideration by the professional making the determination of all the circumstances which appear to be relevant, and considering the following:

1   the person's past and present wishes and feelings;

2   the beliefs and values that would be likely to influence his/her decision if he/she had mental capacity; and

3   the other factors that he/she would be likely to consider if he/she were able to do so.

The professional must also take into account, if it is practicable and appropriate to consult them, the views of:

4   anyone named by the person as someone to be consulted on the matter in question, or on matters of that kind;

5   anyone engaged in caring for the person or interested in his/her welfare;

6   any donee of a Lasting Power of Attorney granted by the person (this will be a future role when the Mental Capacity Act (2005) is fully implemented, which will extend to personal welfare and health care related decisions in addition to financial matters); and

7   any Deputy appointed for the person by the Court of Protection.

The above best interests factors also require professionals making decisions on behalf of vulnerable adults to ensure that the person is involved to the fullest extent possible; any action taken or decision made is the least restrictive of the person's rights and freedom of action possible, to effectively achieve risk reduction/management, and to act always in a manner which respects the vulnerable adult, minimizes distress to him/her and supports him/her throughout any actions which need to be taken.

The CMHN has an important role to play in gathering and documenting evidence to inform assessments of mental capacity, e.g. in assessing cognitive functioning; in ascertaining what the vulnerable adult's wishes are (or were); in contributing to decision-making regarding risk prevention/management and, most importantly, in supporting the vulnerable adult through the process and outcomes of the assessment of mental capacity.

Case example 1

Mrs A. has suffered with Alzheimer's disease for five years. She has been cared for by her husband at home and is supported by an extensive community care package coordinated by a CMHN, which includes three days a week day hospital care. Mr A. is felt by the CMHN to be devoted to his wife and there have been no previous concerns regarding abuse or inappropriate care. He is, however, felt to be significantly depressed and overburdened in his caregiving role.

VA1 referral. On her most recent attendance at day hospital, Mrs A. was using sexually disinhibited language and told a member of staff that she was 'going to have a baby'. During a bath, she was noted to have some bruising around her vulva and concerns were raised about possible sexual abuse. In response to a potentially very serious concern, a Strategy Meeting was urgently convened for later that day (the identifying day hospital nurse and CMHN were invited to attend). The Social Services Community Mental Health Services for Older People Team Manager was identified as being the Lead DLM and the Police DLM and Health DLM agreed during Strategy Discussion that their input was required. The Consultant in Old Age Psychiatry was also invited to attend the Strategy Meeting.

Strategy Meeting outcomes

Plan for protection. It was decided that Mrs A. should be admitted to hospital for emergency respite care pending a POVA investigation. Assessments of her physical condition and mental state would be undertaken during her stay, including a full medical examination and, if necessary, medical photography of her injuries. It was also decided that an assessment of her mental capacity to consent would be urgently required as this would be fundamental to decision-making and intervention.

Plan for investigation. It was decided that as Mrs A.'s bruising was probably sustained during sexual intercourse between husband and wife. Police involvement to lead a criminal investigation was not required and would be inappropriate at this stage (assuming no third party was involved). It was therefore agreed that Mr A. would be interviewed by the Lead DLM with the Consultant in Old Age Psychiatry in order that his account of how his wife's bruising was sustained could be heard. The interview would also aim to identify any unmet mental health or service needs that Mr A. perceived as Mrs A.'s main caregiver.

An Adult Protection Case Conference was planned to hear the outcomes of the investigation/ interim Adult Protection Plan.

Adult protection case conference outcomes

Mrs A. settled onto the ward well and showed no signs of distress when her husband visited her and spent time with her. Mr A.'s contact with his wife on the ward was reported to be gentle and affectionate. Mr A. stated to ward staff that he was happy to have the break from his caregiving role.

An assessment of Mrs A.'s mental capacity by her Consultant in Old Age Psychiatry found that she was no longer capable of giving valid consent to continued sexual intercourse with her husband. Ward staff observed that Mrs A. sometimes misidentified her husband as being her grandfather. In respect of her physical condition, no further bruising or other injuries were noted. Mrs A.'s dementing illness was assessed as having progressed significantly since her last admission for assessment one year ago – her MMSE score had reduced to 10/30 from 20 previously and she was noticeably more confused and disorientated. An especial difficulty was her night-time waking and walking.

As planned, Mr A. was sensitively interviewed for his perspective regarding his wife's bruising and the changes in her behaviour noted at day hospital. He disclosed that he had continued to have a sexual relationship with his wife and that in the past this had provided her with great comfort. However, he stated that this aspect of their marriage had become less frequent over the last few months and on one recent occasion his wife had not recognized him and had become afraid and pushed him away. He was very tearful during the interview and agreed that continued sexual activity with his wife was no longer appropriate or legal. With support, Mr A. decided to sleep separately from his wife and accepted that he may benefit from treatment for his depressive illness.

During the above interview, Mr A. expressed a strong desire to continue caring for his wife at home. The remainder of the meeting was spent in developing a plan for increased support to Mr A. This was to include frequent rotational respite care, continued day hospital care, home care support for washing/dressing in the morning and putting to bed at night and a carer's support group for husband carers for Mr A. to access increased social and emotional support. Mrs A. was also to be tried on some night sedation to aid her sleep and lessen her husband's fatigue.

Outcome

Based on the findings of the investigation and the agreed modifications to the community services intervention/treatment plan, it was decided to stand down the POVA procedures. The CMHN would remain closely involved and report back on the success or otherwise of the agreed plan or if any further concerns were forthcoming.

Mrs A continues to be monitored at day hospital/during respite and Mr A. has accepted counselling support from his CMHN, which has enabled him to grieve for the loss of this aspect of his relationship with his wife.

Notes for CMHN practice

- The POVA Policy states that families should be helped to remain together wherever possible. To remove Mrs A. from the family caregiving situation without assessing the significance of the risk/s to her and trying alternative measures first would be contrary to her best interests. The POVA Policy states that the least restrictive intervention should be used before escalation.

- To criminalize this sort of behaviour would be inappropriate, based on the information provided, and would more than likely result in worse outcomes for both Mr and Mrs A. However, if Mrs A. was subject to continued sexual intercourse in the absence of mental capacity to consent, this would be illegal in the eyes of the law and Police intervention or measures to remove her to a place of safety might become necessary.

- This case study highlights how the CMHN can play an important role in supporting the alleged perpetrators of abuse or inappropriate care. It also shows how the POVA procedures need to be applied with care and sensitivity to result in positive outcomes.

- The multi-agency and consensus approach the POVA procedures afford results in improved decision-making and the CMHN as lone practitioner can share the responsibility of such cases with a team of lead professionals. However, their role as care manager/key worker is also strengthened by the POVA procedures.

Question for practice development reflection

How would this case have been managed prior to *No Secrets/In Safe Hands*, and has the new multi-agency/collaborative approach made a real difference to your work with vulnerable adult protection cases?

Discuss this question with colleagues from your own team and other agencies, and share your ideas for further improved practice with your AAPC or equivalent vulnerable adult protection forum.

Safe discharge planning

If the vulnerable adult, as part of clinical or care management, needs to enter hospital care for medical or mental health assessment and/or treatment, or is receiving health-provided respite care, there may be occasions where the risk of harm may be considered as being so great as to require an assessment of whether discharge home would be contrary to their best interests. The hospital Consultant in charge of the patient's care can refuse discharge and retain the person in hospital under a duty of care in common law (doctrine of necessity),[1] if there is clear evidence that their care needs cannot be safely met at home *and* they have been assessed as lacking mental capacity to make their own decision regarding discharge planning. (If the vulnerable adult was assessed as having mental capacity to make their own decision, and they wished to return home to the vulnerable situation, then they could not be retained in hospital against their wishes and there would be a duty of care to work with partner agencies to effect as safe a discharge as could possibly be afforded.)

The CMHN, or any member of the community or hospital-based team, should be able to call a Safe Discharge Planning Case Conference if they have a significant concern about a patient returning home either to live alone or with a family member. It could be that the person may be at risk of self-harm/neglect if they returned home, that a family member may be judged to be incapable of providing appropriate care, or that there is an ongoing risk of abuse (this should have been previously addressed under the POVA procedures).

Prior to the Case Conference, the following evidence should be gathered:

* the views (and records) of the care manager and professionals involved in community care, including evidence of previous concerns;

* the mental capacity and wishes of the vulnerable adult, following the above guidance;

* the capability and willingness of the main carer/family members to provide appropriate care (contact with alleged perpetrators of abuse or inappropriate care must be coordinated by the POVA DLM);

* an assessment of the suitability of the home environment in which care will take place;

* a review of the patient's requirements for community care services and specialist aids and equipment.

During the Case Conference, based on this evidence, a consensus decision should be reached by the multi-disciplinary team as to whether or not the vulnerable adult would be safe to return home, with or without intensive monitoring and support; if they should be allowed home for a defined period, with a planned re-admission for formal review, or if they should be retained in hospital pending further assessments and consideration of legal powers. These could include the main carer/family members being invited to participate in the delivery of personal care in hospital under supervision, perhaps accompanied by some skills training, e.g. in how to administer PEG feeds or use a hoist; a second opinion by a psychiatrist of the vulnerable adult's mental capacity to make decisions regarding their future care, or an exploration of alternative placements for post-hospital discharge care. If the person is assessed as being unsafe to return home and he/she does not require ongoing hospital care, an assessment of their NHS Continuing Care status may be required to determine the funding arrangements for residential or nursing home care. If the nearest relative refuses to support placement, legal powers to secure transfer of care may need to be explored, e.g. Mental Health Act (1983) or Declaratory Relief. In some situations displacement of the nearest relative via a Section 29 Court hearing as part of a Guardianship Order may need to be considered to ensure the vulnerable adult's continued placement in a residential or nursing home setting and to prevent their relative from taking their discharge.

Obviously, how decisions are documented and communicated in these cases is crucial.

If there is a decision to retain the vulnerable adult in hospital pending consideration of legal powers, the nearest relative should be informed and given an opportunity to discuss the decision with the Consultant in charge of care. A formal entry regarding the decision should be made in the vulnerable adult's multi-disciplinary notes and staff involved in care should be informed that the patient's nearest relative/family members must not be allowed to take their discharge against medical advice. Security and/or the Police will need to be involved in cases of attempted removal from the hospital setting to prevent abduction of the 'at risk' vulnerable adult, and all cases of actual abduction should result in a POVA VA1 Referral (this also applies to unplanned removal from residential/nursing homes).

If the vulnerable adult is to leave hospital and is felt to be at significant risk, e.g. if they are assessed as having the mental capacity to make their own decision regarding future care and choose to take their own discharge against medical advice, then formal alerts to the CMHN as community care manager and other key professionals involved in care management must be issued at the earliest opportunity so that effective risk management can recommence.

Case example 2

Mrs B. has moderate vascular dementia and was cared for at home by her middle-aged nephew, who had always lived with her. He works full time and has consistently refused to allow his aunt to undergo a Social Services assessment for home care services. He has also refused access to the family home for assessment for aids and equipment. The only service Mr B. has accepted, facilitated by a CMHN (who has only recently become involved following an urgent GP referral), is hospital-based respite care (this was in a non-psychiatric hospital setting).

VA1 Referral. On Mrs B.'s admission to hospital, concerns were raised by nursing staff about the unkempt state in which she arrived (she was wet and heavily soiled with dried faeces and not wearing an incontinence pad), the damage to her pressure areas – she had a grade 3 pressure ulcer to her sacrum, and her poor physical state – she was chairbound and assessed as being at high risk of falling from her bed/chair. They completed a VA1 Referral form and this led to a Strategy Discussion between the DLM Social Services (despite there being no previous Social Services involvement) and the DLM Health. It was decided that a Strategy Meeting was required, and the GP and CMHN were invited to attend.

Strategy meeting outcomes

Plan for protection. It was decided that Mrs B. would be retained in hospital under a duty of care in common law (doctrine of necessity) until further assessments could be made, including a Mental Health Act (1983) assessment if Mr B. demanded his aunt's discharge home, and until such time as Mr B. accepted support from community care services to meet his aunt's high level of frailty/care need.

Plan for investigation. Mr B. was informed (by the DLM Health) that there were concerns about the state in which his aunt arrived in hospital. Mr B. refused to acknowledge that his aunt was incontinent or had a pressure ulcer when at home. However, he did accept an invitation to attend a family meeting with the Consultant and Social Services DLM and Health DLM. This took place a few days later, at his convenience, with the family GP in attendance. The CMHN was not invited to attend this meeting, as it was felt that attendance could damage her future relationship with Mr B.

The meeting took place as planned, but Mr B. continued to refuse to accept that his aunt had a dementing illness or had high-level care needs. However, the following initial plan was developed, with Mr B.'s stated agreement:

- Mr B. agreed to allow the CMHN to undertake a home visit to assess suitability of the home environment for care and what aids and equipment would be required to support discharge planning.

- Mr B. agreed to meet with a voluntary sector care provider to discuss the provision of some limited home care support for washing/dressing, etc., which he said he would prefer to pay for himself. However, he refused to engage with Social Services regarding financial assessment towards the provision of a community care package or for a carer's assessment to be undertaken.

- Mr B. refused to agree for a Consultant in Old Age Psychiatry to assess his aunt's mental state and mental capacity to make her own decisions regarding future care. This was recorded, but Mr B. was told that this was required to inform decision-making and would be requested in his aunt's best interests.

Adult Protection Case Conference outcomes

Following her home visit (with a male colleague), the CMHN reported that the room in which Mrs B. had lived was badly soiled and that the furniture provided was inappropriate to meet her mobility needs. The Consultant in Old Age Psychiatry reported that he had assessed Mrs B. as having moderate to severe dementia and lacking mental capacity to make her own decisions regarding future care – she thought she was a young girl and living at home with her brother in mid-Wales.

Mrs B. was reported to have improved during her two weeks stay in hospital – she had put some weight on, her pressure ulcers had improved somewhat and she was enjoying the company of fellow patients. Further assessments were made regarding Mrs. B.'s mobility and she was assessed as having contractures in her knees and requiring hoist transfers. Due to her risk of falling from bed/chair, she was reassessed as having a 24-hour nursing need.

Mr B., who attended for part of the meeting, adamantly refused to allow care workers into the family home, despite his initial indication that he would allow voluntary sector workers in to provide some limited care. He remained of the belief that his aunt was not severely confused; could wash, dress and toilet herself, and would be safe left at home alone while he was at work.

On the basis of the above assessments, and especially the view of the multi-disciplinary team that Mrs B. required 24-hour nursing care and would be unsafe left alone for any period, it was decided that Mrs B. would continue to be retained in hospital until such time as Mr B. accepted a full care package and could ensure that his aunt would not be left alone for significant periods. Mr B. was informed that if he refused to accept that his aunt required ongoing hospital care, or later placement in a nursing home setting if it was assessed that she did not meet the eligibility criteria for NHS Continuing Health Care, legal powers would need to be considered to ensure her discharge home was prevented.

Outcome

After several months in hospital, Mr B. continued to demand his aunt's discharge home. Mrs B. was reassessed as needing 24-hour nursing care but not requiring ongoing hospital care – her condition was stable and it was felt that she could be managed in an EMI Nursing Home environment. Her nephew appealed against this assessment and the dispute over her NHS Continuing Health Care eligibility was referred to the Local Health Board's appeals procedure.

Notes for CMHN practice

- Carers who fail to provide appropriate care may have their own physical/mental health needs and vulnerabilities. They may even be considered as being a vulnerable adult in their own right.

- Carers and family members should be engaged with throughout the above procedures, unless this is judged by the Consultant/multi-disciplinary team as being contrary to the best interests of the vulnerable adult.

- In some situations, the implementation of the Mental Health Act (1983) may be required, e.g. to displace the nearest relative as part of Guardianship procedures.

- Even in such cases of retention/detention in hospital, continued relationships between vulnerable adults and their carers/relatives should be supported, again unless this is considered contrary to their best interests, in which case supervised or restricted visiting may be required.

- The POVA procedures ensure that decision-making is coordinated at a service manager (DLM) level, meaning that the CMHN can be perceived as not being directly involved in such difficult and challenging decisions and practitioner/client/carer relationships can be maintained.

Question for practice development reflection

How could communication/collaboration between hospital-based services and community services (CMHNs, in particular) be further improved to effect safer discharge from hospital and prevent vulnerable adults being subjected to inappropriate care or rapid readmission?

Discuss this question with colleagues from your own team and with hospital-based colleagues, and share your ideas for further improved practice with your Health DLM or equivalent lead manager.

Cases of self-neglect/harm

Cases of self-neglect/harm may also need to be considered under the POVA Policy, as often these situations require an urgent, multi-agency response, often involving the Police. For example, the person who is failing to care for him/herself and refusing community services involvement may suddenly come to the attention of emergency services because they are becoming a nuisance (or a concern) to neighbours or members of the public. Among the older vulnerable adult client group this is often a result of a chronic cognitive impairment which inhibits self-care functioning and/or appropriate social behaviour, or an acute delirium or psychotic episode which leads to sudden and often dramatic changes in behaviour and/or risk of significant harm. Common risks may include malnutrition and/or dehydration resulting from inability to provide meals and drinks; infection/pressure area damage as a result of soiled clothing/furniture/bedding arising from inability to toilet/ cleanse self; hypothermia due to leaving windows/doors open or dressing in inappropriate clothing, or road traffic accident from disorientated wandering in the street. This group may also be particularly vulnerable to opportunistic abuse by strangers, as doors may be left unlocked, money may be poorly handled and the individual may be less able to call for help or to report abuse.

With an estimated 154,000 people with dementia living alone (Alzheimer's Society 1994), the role of the CMHN is these cases is essential, both for risk assessment and ongoing risk management intervention, e.g. by monitoring diet and hydration, ensuring medication compliance, facilitating the highest level of home safety possible and assessing self-care, continence and skin care needs. If situations continue to deteriorate, to a level at which the vulnerable adult's health and safety are severely compromised, the CMHN also has a vital role to play in facilitating a referral to the Consultant in Old Age Psychiatry for assessment under the Mental Health Act (1983) (Section 2). This may require forced entry to the client's premises to remove him/her to a place of safety by the Police under Section 135 of the Act, if there is:

> reasonable cause to suspect that a person believed to be suffering from mental disorder has been or is being ill-treated, neglected or kept otherwise than under proper control, in any place within the jurisdiction of the justice . . . or is unable to care for him/herself and is living alone in any such place.

If the client is assessed as not being sufficiently mentally disordered to fall under the Mental Health Act (1983) (there may be instances where the CMHN is involved for initial assessment when dementia/late onset mental illness is suspected but not yet clinically diagnosed), then the Public Health Doctor may be required to undertake an assessment under the National Assistance Act (1948). Section 47 of this Act allows for an application to the Magistrates' Court for an order authorizing the removal of a person from their place of residence to a hospital or care home, if the Public Health Doctor and Magistrate are satisfied that the person is:

- suffering from grave chronic disease;
- aged, infirm or physically incapacitated (the person does not need to be mentally incapacitated to use this measure);
- living in insanitary conditions;
- unable to devote to (look after) themselves;
- not receiving proper care and attention from other persons;
- in need of being removed from their home, either in their own interests or for preventing injury to the health of or serious nuisance to other persons.

Usually, seven days' notice must be given to any person involved in caring for the client before they are removed to a place of safety, which provides an opportunity for the application to be contested. Initially, the order will last for three months with a further three months on renewal by the Court. However, if removal is considered urgent by the Public Health Doctor and another doctor, then under an emergency procedure (provided by the National Assistance [Amendment] Act 1951), the person can be removed to a place of safety without delay. This order is only for three weeks and any application for an extension must comply with the full procedure.

Future developments

It is important for the CMHN to be aware of several key developments in the field of vulnerable adult protection that have either recently occurred or are expected.

The first and perhaps most significant of these is the establishment of a new criminal offence (in the Mental Capacity Act 2005) of 'ill-treatment or wilful neglect of a person lacking capacity by anyone responsible for that person's care', which will be punishable by up to five years custodial sentence. This measure will give vulnerable adult protection procedures some real 'teeth', but also means that the gathering of evidence in support of prosecutions will be of critical importance. The CMHN will undoubtedly play an important role in this respect.

The Safeguarding Vulnerable Adults Bill (2006), when enacted (anticipated 2008), will extend the existing POVA List to the NHS. Proven perpetrators of vulnerable adult (or child) abuse-working in NHS Trusts and other Health settings will, when accepted onto the POVA List, be barred from working with vulnerable groups again. This measure, together with enhanced CRB checking, will help prevent staff abusers from moving geographically or between care sectors and continuing their abuse. CMHNs need to be aware of this development as being a possible disciplinary outcome, alongside NMC referral. However, an important point is that NHS staff without a professional qualification, or indeed those previously qualified staff who have been struck off their professional register, can be barred from working with vulnerable groups via the POVA List whereas NMC deregistration only prevents the person working in a qualified nurse capacity.

Another new measure for the CMHN to be aware of is Declaratory Relief (Schwehr 2003).[2] This is an alternative to using the Mental Health Act 1983, i.e. it can be used in situations where the person is not mentally disordered under the Act, and the National Assistance Act 1948, i.e. it can be used in situations where the person is not gravely ill. However, in order for it to be used, the person must be assessed as being mentally incapacitated. The Local Authority or NHS Trust solicitor makes an application to a High Court Judge for him/her to make a Declaration as to what planned care, including place of residence, would be in the vulnerable adult's best interests (initially a Declaration can be made over the 'phone, but a full High Court hearing needs to follow to secure a lasting provision). In making their application, the Local Authority/NHS Trust would have to demonstrate that:

- Mental incapacity was established.
- There was a serious issue relating to welfare and that an adjudication was required.
- Alternative risk management approaches had been explored and failed.
- Professional opinion, including that of a Consultant Psychiatrist and independent Social Worker, was in support of the application.

It seems that Declaratory Relief will become an important additional power in the armoury of measures available to Local Authorities and NHS Trusts in their vulnerable adult protection work and could be useful in many situations, including those where a carer is incapable of providing appropriate care and refuses to accept community services intervention or placement.

Summary

The duty to protect vulnerable adults from abuse and inappropriate care has always been implicit in the CMHN role and is explicit in the NMC Code of Professional Conduct (NMC 2002): 'As a registered nurse, midwife or health visitor, you must act to identify and minimise the risk to patients and clients.' Therefore, it is imperative that CMHNs familiarize themselves with their local POVA Policy and receive training to ensure its effective implementation. This chapter intends to demonstrate that the CMHN has a key role to play in vulnerable adult protection work and they need to strengthen their role in this respect, especially in relation to the section concerning professional practice.

In the past, there has been a tendency to view abuse intervention work as often being negative and punitive. It is hoped that this chapter goes some way to demonstrating that the new POVA policies and procedures are sensitive to the uniqueness of each individual situation; respectful of the vulnerable adult's wishes, which are of paramount importance throughout, and are supportive of family carers as the perpetrators of unintentional abuse. The multi-agency approach and the collaborative decision-making that the POVA policies and procedures afford result in better decision-making and increased support for practitioners, who previously often carried these most difficult cases on their own. In this respect, the CMHN can view the new POVA policies and procedures as an additional supportive and protective measure.

As a result of *No Secrets/In Safe Hands*, vulnerable adult protection is a growing area of concern within health and social care and this is long overdue. The new POVA policies and procedures will help us all to continue to improve our practice and the care that vulnerable adults receive. The hope for all of us must be that the anticipated Mental Capacity Act (2005) and future primary legislation will bring this vital area of practice further to the fore, with the same status that child protection currently holds. Only then will the most vulnerable members of our society begin to be adequately protected.

Lessons for CMHN practice

- The CMHN must discuss their concerns with their professional line manager at the earliest possible opportunity and he/she is responsible for communicating with the relevant DLM and ensuring the VA1 Referral form is completed (part 1 by the CMHN as identifier; part 2 by the professional line manager as referrer) and submitted to the identified Lead DLM via safe fax.

- Unilateral decision-making must be avoided; the multi-agency approach in taking cases forward that is assured by consistent implementation of the POVA strategic process leads to better outcomes for the vulnerable adult and in increased support for practitioners.

- The CMHN must never promise to keep information received from the vulnerable adult or carer alleging abuse a secret. There is a moral and legal duty to act to prevent further abuse from occurring by making a referral under the POVA Policy.

- It is important not to contaminate evidence, therefore the CMHN should not engage in a formal interview with the vulnerable adult/witnesses but simply clarify what is being said and ensure verbatim records are kept and communicated to the Lead DLM. (Formal interview will be undertaken by a nominated Police officer or practitioner trained in vulnerable adult interview techniques.)

- The Police will advise on how forensic evidence should be preserved and may need to intervene more urgently, i.e. sooner than Strategy Meeting, if a criminal offence is thought to have been committed.

- The CMHN as referrer will be expected to attend the Strategy Meeting and give a first-hand account of their concerns/their reason for making the VA1 Referral. He/she may also be involved in the development of an Adult Protection Plan and may be nominated as Keyworker for the implementation of this plan.

- Advice and support for the CMHN in their POVA-related work will be available from their professional line manager and Health DLM throughout the procedures.

Notes

1   Following the recent European Court of Human Rights judgment on the informal detention of H.L. at Bournewood Hospital being a violation of his human rights (5 1 'right to liberty and security' and 5 4 'right to have legality of detention reviewed by a court'), this power over discharge has been diminished and prolonged informal retention could be challenged as being a 'deprivation of liberty'. Thus, the Consultant may only retain the person in hospital in their best interests for their treatment rather than to prevent discharge. Formal legal powers such as the Mental Health Act (1983) or Declaratory Relief would need to be considered to enable longer-term retention in hospital.

2   It should be noted that when the Mental Capacity Act (2005) is fully implemented, this function will be taken over by the new Courts of Protection, which will make Declarations as to what care would be in the mentally incapacitated adults' best interests and involve 'Court Appointed Deputies' to make ongoing decisions for them.

References

Alzheimer's Society (1994) *Right from the Start: Primary Health Care and Dementia*. London: Alzheimer's Society.

Aneshensel, C.S., Pearlin, L.J. and Schuler, R.H. (1993) Stress, role captivity, and the cessation of caregiving, *Journal of Health and Social Behaviour*, 34: 54–70.

Annersdedt, L., Elmstahl, S., Ingvad, B. and Samuelson, S.M. (2000) Family caregiving in dementia – an analysis of the caregiver's burden and the 'breaking point' when home care becomes inadequate, *Scandinavian Journal of Public Health*, 28(1): 23–31.

Archbold, P., Stewart, B., Greenlick, M. and Harvath, T. (1992) The clinical assessment of mutuality and preparedness in family caregivers of frail older people, in S. Funk, E. Tornquist, S. Champagne and R. Wiese (eds) *Key Aspects of Elder Care: Managing Falls, Incontinence and Cognitive Impairment*. New York: Springer Publishers.

Austrom, M.G. and Hendrie, H.C. (1990) The grief response of the Alzheimer's disease family caregiver, *The American Journal of Alzheimer's Care and Related Disorders and Research*, 5(2): 16–27.

Community and District Nurses Association (2003) *Responding to Elder Abuse*. London: CDNA.

Cooney, C. and Mortimer, A. (1995) Elder abuse and dementia, *International Journal of Social Psychiatry*, 41: 276–83.

Coyne, A., Reichman, W.E. and Berbig, L. (1993) The relationship between dementia and elder abuse, *American Journal of Psychiatry*, 150: 643–46.

Department of Health (2000) *No Secrets: Guidance on Developing and Implementing Multi-agency Policies and Procedures to Protect Vulnerable Adults from Abuse*. London: Department of Health.

Dura, J., Stukenberg, K. and Kiecolt-Glaser, J. (1990) Chronic stress and depressive disorders in older adults, *Journal of Abnormal Psychology*, 99(3): 284–90.

Gilhooly, M.L.M. (1986) Senile dementia: factors associated with caregivers' preferences for institutional care, *British Journal of Medical Psychology*, 59: 165–71.

Gilleard, C.J. (1984) *Living with Dementia: Community Care of the Elderly Mentally Infirm*. London: Croom Helm.

Gilleard, C.J., Belford, H., Gilleard, E., Whittick, J.E. and McKee, K. (1984) Emotional distress among the supporters of the elderly mentally infirm, *British Journal of Psychiatry*, 145: 172–7.

Haley, W.E., Levine, E.G., Brown, S.L. and Bartolucci, A.A. (1987) Stress, appraisal, coping and social support as predictors of adaptational outcome among dementia caregivers, *Psychology and Aging*, 2: 323–30.

Harper, D., Manasse, P., James, O. and Newton, J. (1993) Intervening to reduce distress in caregivers of impaired elderly people: a preliminary evaluation, *International Journal of Geriatric Psychiatry*, 8: 139–45.

HC 111–1 House of Commons Health Committee (2004) *Elder Abuse: Second Report of Session 2003–4*, Vol. 1. London: The Stationery Office.

Hirschfield, M. (1983) Homecare versus institutionalization: family caregiving and senile brain disease, *International Journal of Nursing Studies*, 20(1): 23–32.

Homer, A. and Gilleard, C. (1990) Abuse of elderly people by their carers, *British Medical Journal*, 301: 1359–62.

Lord Chancellor's Department (1997) *Who Decides? Making Decisions on Behalf of Mentally Incapacitated Adults*. London: Lord Chancellor's Department.

McKee, K.J., Whittick, J.E., Ballinger, B.B., Gilhooly, M.M.L., Gordon, D.S., Mutch, W.J. and Philp, I. (1997) Coping in family supporters of elderly people with dementia, *British Journal of Clinical Psychology*, 36: 323–40.

Nolan, M., Grant, G. and Keady, J. (1996) *Understanding Family Care: A Multidimensional Model of Caring and Coping*. Buckinghamshire: Open University Press.

Nolan, M. and Keady, J. (2001) Working with carers, in C. Cantley (ed.) *A Handbook of Dementia Care*. Buckinghamshire: Open University Press, pp. 160–72.

O'Donovan, S.T. (2004) Dementia caregiving burden and breakdown, unpublished doctoral thesis, University of Glamorgan.

Orbell, S. and Gillies, B. (1993) Factors associated with informal carers' preference not to be involved in caring, *The Irish Journal of Psychology*, 14(1): 99–109.

Philp, I., McKee, K.J., Armstrong, G.K., Ballinger, B.R., Gilhooly, M.L.M., Gordon, D.S., Mutch, W.J. and Whittick, J.E. (1997) Institutionalization risk among people with dementia supported by family carers in a Scottish city, *Aging and Mental Health*, 1(4): 339–45.

Quayhagen, M., Quayhagen, M.P., Patterson, T.L., Irwin, M., Hauger, R.L. and Grant, I. (1997) Coping with dementia: family caregiver burnout and abuse, *Journal of Mental Health and Aging*, 3(3): 357–64.

Sadler, P., Kurrle, S. and Cameron, I. (1995) Dementia and elder abuse, *Australian Journal on Aging*, 14: 36–40.

Schwehr, B. (2003) Declaratory Relief: legal breakthrough for adult protection, *Signpost to Older People and Mental Health Matters Journal*, 8(1): 10–12.

Welsh Assembly Government (1999) *In Safe Hands: The Implementation of Adult Protection Procedures in Wales*. Cardiff: Welsh Assembly Government.

Whitlach, C.J., Feinberg, L.F. and Stevens, E.J. (1999) Predictors of institutionalisation for persons with Alzheimer's disease and the impact on family caregivers, *Journal of Mental Health and Aging*, 5(3): 275–88.

13

Supporting people with a learning disability and dementia
The role of the community learning disability nurse

Fiona Wilkie, Catherine Brannan, Kenneth Day and Heather Wilkinson

Introduction

In comparison to other areas of practice development within nursing, there has been little research into the role of the community learning disability nurse (CLD nurse) (Jenkins and Johnson 1991; Barr and Parahoo 1994; Parahoo and Barr 1996). In this chapter we use the experiences of the CLD nurses within the Lothian Community Learning Disability Team (CLDT), and a series of four case studies,[1] to explore the development of practice, identity and roles of the CLD nurse in the field of learning disability and ageing. In particular, we will illustrate their journey from hospital-based practice to providing a wide-ranging and specialist service within the community. The exploration will highlight just how far the role of the CLD nurse has changed in light of UK government legislation (Department of Health 1990) and how far the role has to progress in order to meet recent concerns over its 'identity crisis' (Mitchell 2004).

The development of CLD nursing has taken place against the background of, and indeed has been partly driven by, demographic shifts in the population of people with a learning disability. As people with a learning disability experience increased longevity, they encounter illnesses of older age, including dementia. Service providers have had to address a number of practice and philosophical issues in providing good care and support for people with a learning disability as they live with dementia (Watchman 2003). The work developed in Lothian illustrates the centrality of the CLD nurse role, their increasingly specialized position and their expertise in the area of learning disability and dementia.

Learning disability

The term 'learning disability' applies to the developmental condition also known as intellectual impairment and is classified as a 'condition of arrested or incomplete development of the mind' (ICD-10 1994), the impairment being present during the developmental phase (pre-adulthood). The assessment of learning disability is typically conducted through the use of psychometric tests and through examining the individual's level of adaptive functioning.

Incidence of dementia in people with a learning disability

Recent UK reviews give some indication of relevant demographic statistics, with estimates of about 210,000 individuals with severe and profound learning disability in England, 25,000 of whom are over the age of 60 (Department of Health 2001). It is estimated that, in Scotland, around 12,000 people have a learning disability (Scottish Executive Health Department 2000a). It is anticipated that the number of people with a learning disability will continue to grow by over 1 per cent a year over the next 10 years (Scottish Executive Health Department 2000a; Department of Health 2001).

Life expectancy of people with a learning disability has also increased significantly. The average life expectancy of a person with Down's syndrome has increased from only nine years in the early twentieth century (Baird and Sadovnik 1987; Holland and Moss 1997) to 70 per cent of people with Down's syndrome now living over 30 years and 44 per cent reaching 60 years (Marler and Cunningham 1994). A consequence of this increase in longevity is the increased likelihood that people will experience illnesses of older age, in particular, dementia (Janicki and Dalton 2000).

Analysis of studies investigating the prevalence of dementia among people with a learning disability shows that there is wide variance in the reported rates (Zigman et al. 1996). The prevalence of dementia among people with a learning disability can be four times higher than found in the general population (Cooper 1997b) and risk factors can relate to medical factors such as chromosomal differences, head traumas and the high use of medication to control psychiatric and neuroleptic disorders (Popovitch et al. 1990; Durkin et al. 1994). By contrast, other studies have examined the prevalence of dementia in people with a learning disability (where the learning disability is not Down's syndrome) and have found there to be little difference between this group and the general population (Evenhuis 1997; Zigman et al. 1997). Accordingly, it would appear that, apart from age, the major risk factor for developing dementia in people with a learning disability would appear to be Down's syndrome (Carr 2003).

The link between Down's syndrome and dementia, specifically dementia of the Alzheimer's type, is well documented (Lai and Williams 1989; Prasher 1995; Visser et al. 1997; Zigman et al. 1997; Janicki and Dalton 2000). Prasher (1995) reports prevalence rates of 9.4 per cent at age 40, rising to 54.4 per cent at age 60. Coupled with this is the presence of the neuropathology of Alzheimer's disease in almost all individuals with Down's syndrome at post-mortem (Wisniewski and Rabe 1985).

In the past 30 years, the profession of learning disability nursing has undergone major changes in role, approach and position. These changes, from a hospital to community context, partly reflect the major shifts in philosophical underpinnings to supporting people with a learning disability illustrated by the move to community care, and are partly due to the contested nature of their role within the wider nursing profession (Mobbs et al. 2002; Mitchell 2004).

The National Health and Community Care Act (1990), a major piece of legislation which sets out the basis for the provision of health and social care in community settings, provided the impetus required to speed up the process of deinstitutionalization started in the 1950s (Bradley and Knoll 1990). Specifically, the Act imposed upon local authority social services departments overall responsibility for community care and the obligation to arrange the provision of care. This forced health and social care providers to discuss provision in more joint ways. As the work of the Lothian CLD nurses has developed against this background, we will look at the background in more detail by examining three key aspects of the work: position, approach and role of the CLD nurse, before moving to look specifically at the work of CLD nurses in Lothian.

The CLD nursing context

Drawing on a literature review focusing on the position of the CLD nurse within the wider nursing profession, Mitchell (2004) comments on their 'ambiguous professional location' and 'anomalous position'. In the recent past they have been viewed as 'a small grouping on the margins of the nursing profession' (Mitchell 2004). Such a marginalized position could be considered to be a result of their approach to their work where they failed 'to be part of the sickness model of care that has been at the centre of the values of nursing' (Mitchell 2004). Again, this is perhaps a reflection of the wider context of learning disability provision where the stigma attached to living with a learning disability has been increasingly challenged in Western societies and where the role of the CLD nurse relates more to supporting a socially integrated lifestyle rather than taking a very narrow approach to 'curing ill health'.

While their location within the wider nursing field remains contested, the role and working practices of the CLD nurse have become much clearer and specialized. Previously, one of the key difficulties in defining the role of the CLD nurse was in distinguishing between the 'nursing' and 'social' aspects of their work with people with a learning disability (Mobbs et al. 2002). Following the shift to community-based services for people with a learning disability, the need for joint working between health and social work providers was highlighted (Department of Health 1990). Since this time, an ongoing debate has taken place with the CLD nurse role increasingly being defined and redefined in terms of specialist health provision (Carlisle 1997). As part of the wider policy and practice context, the Kay Report (Kay et al. 1995) on CLD practice recommended that the role of CLD nurses be defined with an emphasis on health and promoting the autonomy of people with a learning disability. This corresponded with the *Health of the Nation* report (DOH 1995) which presented key principles for improving the health of people with learning disabilities, a role for which CLD nurses appear well prepared (Mobbs et al. 2002).

A further indication of role development is illustrated by descriptions of CLD nurse working practices, gathered from managers in 136/170 NHS Trusts in England and Wales by postal questionnaire (Mobbs et al. 2002). The results demonstrated wide variations in CLD nurse practice, but what was consistent across the responses was that CLD nurses worked not as autonomous individuals but as part of a Community Learning Disability Team (CLDT). The majority of the CLDTs included a psychologist, a psychiatrist, a speech and language therapist, an occupational therapist, a physiotherapist, a social worker and a CLD nurse (Mobbs et al. 2002).

With the increased emphasis on 'joint working', from a policy perspective the role of the CLD nurse in supporting the health and social care needs of people with a learning disability has become a clearer and more central part of the CLDTs. This positioning of CLD nurses is grounded strongly in wider philosophical approaches to supporting people with a learning disability. Gates (2002) describes the potential for CLD nurses as 'agents of inclusion' through their contribution to current health-care and social care reforms and their central role in developing services for people with learning disability. Despite practice being open to variation on a geographical basis, increasingly, CLD nurses have specialist roles such as in epilepsy and health promotion (Mobbs et al. 2002: 13). Such developments have been due to the characteristics of continuity and flexibility inherent in the CLD approach (Salvage 1985) and have led to CLD nurses having a strong sense of identity, essential to being able to develop effective practice.

This position of strength based on a clear role, central team position and strong identity is now illustrated from the perspectives of the Lothian CLD nurses through a description of their specialist working practices with people with learning disability and dementia.

The Lothian experience

The relocation of service provision from hospital to the community, arising out of the closure of long-stay hospitals, necessitated a reassessment by health-care and social care providers of the numbers and needs of the population of people with a learning disability in Lothian. An attempt was also made to identify the number of individuals with Down's syndrome in Lothian, hitherto undocumented, with a view to, *inter alia*, extrapolating the number of people with Down's syndrome who would go on to develop dementia.

As outlined above, the wider policy context was influential in the local development of services. In Scotland, people with a learning disability still experience high levels of unmet and unrecognized health needs (Cooper 1997a; NHS Health Scotland 2004). However, recent years are witness to policy drives to improve the access to health services for people with a learning disability (Scottish Executive 2000b). Within this wider context, the role of the CLD nurse was highlighted in *Caring for Scotland*, the nursing strategy document supporting the policy focus on improving quality of life for people with a learning disability; and the results of a national review of the contribution of all nurses and midwives to the care and support of people with a learning disability (Scottish Executive 2002b). A more recent report, *Shaping the Future: A Vision for Learning Disability Nursing* (Northway et al. 2006), reinforces the ideal of improving quality of life, community integration and equity of access to mainstream services. While in support of these ideals, a note of caution has to be added, that mainstream services have to be 'ready' and capable before they totally replace specialist services and even then it is possible that some specialist services would still be beneficial.

One significant outcome of the deinstitutionalization process was the transfer of the expertise and skills of nurses based in the long-stay hospitals (including particular expertise in nursing individuals admitted for end-stage care), to their work in community settings. Supporting this process of knowledge transfer in Lothian was the creation of the Older Adults with Learning Disabilities Working Group (OALD) in 1999. This multi-disciplinary group of psychologists, nurses, social workers and allied health professionals examined the perceived difficulties involved in the provision of a high level of care to individuals growing older in a community setting, and explored aspects of good practice that could be implemented. Sub-groups were also formed to develop good practice tools for an assessment diagnostic care pathway for Lothian which covers screening, assessment, diagnosis and management, training resources and health promotion material. In terms of improving assessment and diagnosis of dementia for people with a learning disability, the care pathway has been a key development in the effective provision of services, especially for individuals with Down's syndrome (who, as previously referred to, have a significantly higher likelihood of developing dementia than the rest of the population).

The implementation of the care pathway illustrates the key position of the CLD nurse both within the CLDT and for the care of the person with dementia in partnership with their other formal and informal carers. In the next section we explore the context of the role of the CLD nurse in more depth before developing this context through the experience of the CLD nurses in Lothian.

A key issue for CLD nurses is the ageing population of people with a learning disability and the increased health-care and social care needs associated with ageing. The Lothian CLD nurses have developed their practice in this area to provide a wide-ranging and specialist service within the community. In particular, they have undertaken an essential role in raising basic awareness of issues relating to ageing, including indications of dementia, among other professionals, care staff and family members of people with a learning disability. Working in partnership has been essential to the success of this process and their work in establishing the care pathway has provided the basis for a system of assessment, diagnosis and management where all participants, including family and carers, have a route to follow in supporting someone with a learning disability and dementia. We now look at the implementation of the pathway, including the central role of the CLD nurse and, in particular, highlight how problems around effective management and service provision have been addressed, beginning with the issues of diagnosing dementia.

Diagnosis of dementia in people with a learning disability

The process of diagnosing dementia is based on a 'ruling out' of alternative causes of symptoms and no definite diagnosis can be given until post-mortem. Diagnosing dementia is problematic in any individual but, for an individual with a learning disability, there are additional barriers to reaching a clear diagnosis (Burt and Aylward 2000). Neither ICD-10 nor DSM-IV refers to dementia in people with a learning disability specifically (Cosgrove et al. 1999), and diagnosis tends to be based on the symptoms observed in mainstream populations and not specifically people with learning disability. This may result in misdiagnosis as some symptoms are only found in some people with a learning disability, for example, an increase in seizures in people with Down's syndrome in early/middle stages of dementia (Kerr and Wilson 2001).

Methods of diagnosis also vary between the mainstream population and those with a learning disability. Mainstream diagnosis centres around a change from 'normal' functioning. However, people with a learning disability are already cognitively impaired and instruments used to objectively assess the presence of dementia may only evidence the presence of an already established cognitive impairment.

Diagnostic overshadowing is also a problem. Carers and professionals may attribute aspects of cognitive decline to the presence of the learning disability rather than any process of decline associated with the dementia. Allied with this is the possibility that individuals with a learning disability may already be assisted in a number of aspects of daily living and therefore not have had the opportunity to display loss of skill.

Communication difficulties may also mean that the individual is unable to inform staff or professionals of any changes. This can lead to an over-reliance on second-hand information. This in itself causes further problems in that staff turnover and level of ability of experienced and qualified staff can affect the quality of the information provided. The Royal College of Speech and Language Therapists (2003) highlight the need for maintaining effective communication for people with a learning disability and dementia, particularly as a way of supporting relationships and for addressing the challenges of including the client in the assessment, despite high levels of communication difficulties.

In order to combat these difficulties, a number of techniques and assessments have been advocated (Gedeye 1995; Evenhuis 1997) although there is no gold standard assessment approach or tool. To address the difficulties in differentiating between an already present cognitive impairment and the onset of dementia, the establishment of a baseline level of cognitive functioning is widely regarded as the key factor in providing a tool for diagnosis of dementia. It is this baseline and ongoing monitoring that is the starting point for the care pathway.

Lothian's dementia care pathway

The pathway, throughout which the nurse plays a central coordinating role, is outlined in Figure 13.1. The following areas in which CLD nurses play a key role have been identified and will now be examined using case studies to illustrate practice: diagnosis; support and training for staff and carers; challenging behaviour; environmental issues; eating and drinking; maintaining skills; sleep; mobility and epilepsy. This spectrum of expertise illustrates the blurring of boundaries between nursing and social care.

Diagnosis

The key point throughout the implementation of the pathway is that the role of the CLD nurse is central. In achieving a diagnosis of dementia, the need is for the CLD nurse to coordinate the steps of the pathway, starting with the first step of excluding other conditions from consideration, and use is made of what is called a 'differential diagnosis'. The purpose of this is to check that conditions that can mimic dementia, for example, bereavement depression, underactive thyroid gland and sensory impairment, are ruled out (Prasher 1995; Thorpe 1999). Figure 13.1 is used to assist staff and carers in ruling out

Under-active thyroid	Hearing loss	Eyesight	Depression	Loss and bereavement
Blood test	Audiology referral	Optician referral	Psychiatry	CLD nurse psychology
↓	↓	↓	↓	↓
Medication	Hearing aid	Check for cataract or glaucoma Spectacles or hospital referral	Medication – support	Bereavement support Stress management Cognitive behaviour therapy

Figure 13.1 Differential diagnosis chart

Source: Adapted from Kerr and Wilson (2001)

certain conditions and was used in Lily's case in case example 1 to rule out other possible causes before she went through the full assessment process for dementia.

Case example 1

Lily was a 54-year-old lady with Down's syndrome. She lived in a group home with three flatmates. The house was supported by a minimal staff group with sleepover night staff. Lily was reported by her care staff to have been experiencing difficulty visuo-spatially when entering the bathroom, sitting on the toilet, walking around the house, and had started to refuse to get out of a taxi/bus/car. She was becoming disorientated to time and space, although she still recognized familiar faces. She was also beginning to experience episodes of urinary incontinence. Following the first visit assessment by the CLD nurse, history taking and health screening were carried out by members of the CLDT and it became evident that there were changes occurring for Lily that made the CLD nurse suspicious that dementia was occurring. Following recommendations from the OALD working group, a flowchart assessment pathway was implemented for Lily and she is now receiving additional support for her dementia from the CLDT.

The results of the early assessments recommended in the pathway will then inform the treatment of the client. If the client has a historical baseline, then a comparison is made. If significant changes are noted, and all confounding factors are ruled out, then a diagnosis of dementia can be made. However, if the client has no baseline information, then the current assessment would be viewed as baseline and a follow-up assessment would be conducted in six months. This process allows for a comparison of the individual's ability over time.

In the event that a diagnosis of dementia is made, then at a CLDT case conference the client is allocated a coordinator, who begins the process of formulating a dementia pathway. This means that the team's involvement with the client will be reviewed every quarter and the progression of the disease will be monitored with the team phasing in support when required.

The role of the nurse through the care pathway

The implementation of the care pathway is reliant on a team approach and all clients referred to the CLDT for possible cognitive decline or behavioural problems that may be indicative of a dementia are discussed as a team. The multi-disciplinary nature of the CLDT allows for a full investigation into the possible contributory factors to the client's presentation. A decision is then made regarding whether or not further investigation is required. If further investigation is viewed as necessary, then the various disciplines will begin their work.

Within Lothian CLDTs, it has been good practice for many years to offer health assessment. The community nurse will conduct basic recordings, such as weight, BMI, BP, etc., as well as assessment of epilepsy, mental health, sexual health and lifestyle risks. It is well documented that individuals with a learning disability have a high level of unmet health needs (Scottish Executive 2000a, 2002b) and CLD nurse practice can address this. Following the assessment, the nurse will either refer the individual to mainstream services or refer within the CLDT.

In keeping with national policy, health promotion is seen as a high priority within the Lothian CLDT. Nurses from Lothian recognized the need for health promotion material that is accessible for people with a learning disability themselves, and worked alongside the Family Advice Information Resource (FAIR) to produce health promotion leaflets covering topics that ranged from dental care to testicular cancer. The OALD health promotion subgroup produced a leaflet for carers called *Older People with a Learning Disability – Keeping Healthy Checklist* and the Scottish Down's Syndrome Association produced the checklist in a user-friendly format.[2]

Although the CLDT is integral to the assessment and treatment of the client with dementia, the role of the community nurse becomes more pertinent following diagnosis. Usually the coordinator of the care pathway will be a community nurse. This requires the nurse to instigate a planned pathway that allows for the CLDT and the care provider to assess the future needs of the individual and to provide for these accordingly. The skills required to facilitate this are based on the ability to communicate accurate and realistic information to people who may be emotionally involved in the process. Good judgement and a desire to provide the best model of care for the individual are essential to the role. The community nurse will also act as a link between the service provider, family carers and the CLDT as well as providing the necessary support and reassurance for the staff teams who are involved in the day-to-day care of the person with dementia. In short, the community nurse provides a link between all the disparate agencies and services, with a view to providing a service that best suits the individual's needs.

The nurse has a central role in responding to the person's changing needs and supporting care staff throughout their experience of living with dementia. Initially the main focus will be on adapting the environment, keeping up day activities, responding to changes in daily living skills and communication. The structure and routines in the person's day should remain, although day centres may need to adapt activities or make activities achievable. People with Down's syndrome and Alzheimer's disease may develop epilepsy in the early stages and require treatment and carers will need training on the management of epilepsy.

As the dementia progresses, and particularly for people with Down's syndrome, physical deterioration becomes more evident (Kerr and Wilson 2001; McCarron 2002; McCarron et al. 2002). The person's mobility decreases, swallowing difficulties occur, daily living skills are lost and incontinence can develop. Again, carers need to adapt the environment, take on more of a physical care role. People with dementia can develop severe mental health problems characterized by depression, hallucinations, delusions, fears and anxieties. The CLDT has a crucial role, particularly the psychiatrist, to diagnose and offer medication and the clinical psychologist who can offer advice on behavioural issues, such as aggression. The CLD nurse, as the person who has probably been monitoring the person, has a central role in asking other professionals for help and ensuring family and paid carers are well supported.

Later, towards the end stages of dementia, the person will experience further deterioration of cognitive and physical abilities. They will probably have decreased mobility progressing to wheelchair use and eventually become bed-bound. The nurse will liaise with the physiotherapist and occupational therapist, in order to assist with the provision of equipment such as wheelchair and hoists. Care staff need to be trained in manual handling and use of equipment. Immobility brings its own problems such as risk of fracture, joint contractures, breathing difficulties and pressure sores. Maintaining a person's skin in good condition is vital to prevent pressure sore development. The person with dementia's skin is compromised due to loss of muscle and fat, incontinence of urine and faeces and poor nutrition. The nurse can advise on pressure sore prevention and the provision of specialist pressure relieving mattresses. Crucially the CLDN may now have to involve the wider health team calling on a tissue viability nurse and a district nurse to prevent pressure sores developing. At the end stages of dementia, carers need to concentrate on keeping the person comfortable and safe. In particular, the person's ability to recognize and communicate pain may be further compromised by the dementia. Staff must be alert to the signs of pain and be wary of interpreting signs of pain as challenging behaviour (Kerr et al. 2006).

Often carers don't get an opportunity to carry out end-stage care as the person with dementia may be hospitalized due to pneumonia or infection. If a person is required to go into hospital, the CLDT have access to Lothian Acute Liaison Nursing who work jointly within the community and the hospital. The liaison nurse will coordinate the inpatient stay and liaise with others regarding a discharge package. However, if the person does remain at home, it can be very difficult for staff, but also be very rewarding, in that they have managed to care well for somebody and the person has died with family, friends and carers around them. The community nurse is central to the care planning and providing support for carers and family when caring for the dying person. The recent report, *Home for Good* (Wilkinson et al. 2004) advocates keeping the person at home with good support and clear advanced planning as a preferable model of care.

The central role of the nurse is evident throughout the care pathway and we suggest that the nurse's involvement follows a circular model of assessment, implementation, monitoring and assessment. The dynamic nature of the model is evidenced across the following areas of specific practice including training which cuts across the areas of: challenging behaviour, environmental issues, eating and drinking, maintaining skills, sleep, mobility and epilepsy.

Training

Staff training is vital to ensure the person is looked after by people who understand the condition, what it means and how it will progress. It is extremely important that staff can respond to and understand the changing needs of the person. If staff are well trained and supported by the Community Learning Disabilities Team, it can mean the difference between somebody staying at home or moving to another establishment (Kerr and Wilson 2001). A key part of the CLD nurse work is ensuring that information, training and support are offered to everyone involved in the care of the person with dementia.

Another aspect of training is to consider the needs of the person's peer group and friends (Wilkinson et al. 2003). They may not understand what is happening to the person and may need appropriate levels of information and support, for example, the Down's Syndrome Scotland leaflet (Kerr and Innes, no date) or the materials produced by and for people with a learning disability by the Norah Fry Institute (see Wilkinson and Kerr 2004). In addition, the CLD nurse can adapt information and often offer materials and key points in pictorial form.

Challenging behaviour

The behavioural aspect of the training for dementia aims to address the possible misattribution by carers of particular aspects of an individual's behaviour. The progression of dementia can result in a number of behavioural changes, which can cause a great deal of confusion and stress among staff members and other residents. Increases in violence, defiance and agitation are often seen and the ability to properly assess the triggers for these behaviours can result in greater staff efficacy and client satisfaction. The role of the nurse is to ensure that staff and carers have the information needed to understand what is causing these behavioural changes and how to modify care, interactions or the environment in order to reduce the overall occurrence. The CLDN draws on a behavioural approach to educate staff and act as the main link between the care group and the clinical psychologist.

The initial approach is to try and help staff understand the difficulties being experienced by the individual with dementia. Through the use of role plays, staff are often asked to describe their own reactions to situations that are experienced by people with dementia. For example, how would they respond if they were awoken and taken through to the bathroom and undressed? By using this technique the CLD nurse is able to support carers to view the situation from the perspective of the person with dementia.

Possible triggers and motivations can then addressed using the ABC (Antecedents, Behaviour and Consequences) of behavioural analysis with staff/carers as a means of finding the explanations for a behaviour. By accurately recording situations involving difficult behaviour, staff are better able to understand the reasons for the behaviour. For example, the idea of behaviour as a communication tool is often used and staff are asked to consider how they would react if they consistently were presented with things they did not like at dinnertime and had no ability to communicate that this was not what they wanted. A person with LD may react very differently to situations so the ability to analyse the causal aspects from their point of view is important. The identification of the triggers can allow for manipulation of the environment to lessen the likelihood of the behaviour occurring.

The communication with the client with LD and dementia is an extremely important aspect of care. Working in partnership with a speech and language therapist in the training gives carers the chance to explore augmentative and alternative communication devices, which may facilitate understanding and increase the quality of care. Ongoing behavioural analysis and support is provided by the CLDT with specialist input from clinical psychology.

Environmental issues

Staff need to know how the environment will affect a person with dementia and there are increasing amounts of evidence regarding environmental modifications (Cohen and Day 1993; Bawley 1997; Hutchings et al. 2000; Wilkinson et al. 2004). Many problems identified can be directly related to how the person with dementia is interpreting their environment due to declining cognitive functioning and sensory problems.

It is important that the nurse assists carers to examine their environment and look at triggers that may cause anxiety and confusion such as noise. It can be a difficult balance to ensure that the needs of other residents are still met but often planning and negotiation will help. Generally, it is important to keep the environment calm and try to plan where a person will be if, for example, lots of visitors are expected.

People with Down's syndrome and dementia can also have visuo-spatial problems – this means seeing things in 3D is difficult. Again, looking carefully at the home and work environments can be important and often quite simple strategies can be very effective as illustrated in the case study of Evelyn.

Case example 2

Although previously very mobile and active, Evelyn was finding it difficult moving from one room to another within her house. Staff described her as trying to step up between the living room and hallway where no step existed. The carpets were highly patterned and different patterns in both areas and Evelyn was finding it difficult to distinguish between the two areas. This was solved by putting yellow tape across the threshold so she could clearly see the threshold. Better lighting could also have been used and avoiding patterned carpets, furnishing and décor are also recommended.

Most importantly, staff need to consider safety and finding a balance regarding issues of risk (Alaszewski et al. 1999; Clarke et al. 2003). For example, strategies such as access to a pathway in a safe garden to allow for walking/wandering can provide a supportive environment in which people with dementia can remain active. In addition, it is important for staff to know a person's routines so they can be consistent in giving the person with dementia a structure and guide to their day. In this way their lifestyle can be maintained as long as possible rather than activities being curtailed through over-protective risk management strategies.

Eating and drinking

The community nurse and the wider community team have a vital part to play in maintaining good nutrition and helping care staff understand the importance of the difficulties for the person with eating, drinking and swallowing. In a recent survey of speech and language therapists, feeding was regarded as 'a multi professional process, which required different professionals implementing individual strategies' (Lillywhite and Atwal 2003: 134). The speech and language therapists would assess for swallowing, the dietician for content, the physiotherapist for posture and the nurse role would be to liaise between the carers/staff and to manage medical aspects of feeding.

In Lothian, the health screening by the CLD nurse will include establishing weight, body mass index and asking about any swallowing difficulties. Taking eating and drinking into account is fundamental as the person with dementia is likely to have problems with eating and drinking throughout the course of their illness and the risks associated with poor food and drink intake are weight loss, dehydration, constipation, increased risk of infection and pressure sores (Bucht and Sandman 1990). Collectively, eating, drinking and swallowing problems are known as dysphagia. In the early stages of dementia loss of memory affects the person's ability to remember to eat and loss of physical skills affects the person's ability to coordinate the process of eating. Therefore, carers require to monitor food and drink, to prompt food and to assist in feeding. The occupational therapist can assist with modified cutlery, plates and non-slip matting. Carers can help by having structured mealtimes, supervising and assisting at meals, regular dental checks, and anticipating hunger and thirst if the person cannot communicate their needs.

Case example 3

Billy was having difficulty eating and the nurse came to assess his needs during mealtimes. He seemed to eat when he got the food to his mouth, but had difficulty locating it. Working with the staff it was suggested that the flowery plastic cover on the table and the highly patterned plate used for his food made it difficult for Billy to see and find his food. These were changed to a plain tablecloth and a plain plate with a bold coloured rim and he managed much better.

As dementia progresses, eating, drinking and swallowing difficulties become common and can be potentially fatal due to the risk of aspiration. The most common signs of aspiration are coughing, choking, weight loss, repeated chest infections and pneumonia. The CLD nurse, along with care staff, need to be constantly monitoring for dysphagia and if there are any signs, they must immediately refer to speech and language therapist. The speech and language therapist will assess for dysphagia and advise care staff about modifying the texture of food and possibly using thickener in drinks. This assessment will be carried out jointly with the dietician who will work with care staff to advise on how to achieve a modified diet. Within Lothian there is a Rapid Response team for dysphagia consisting of speech and language therapist, dietician, occupational therapist and physiotherapist to advise on all aspects of the management of dysphagia. An interim treatment plan will be put in place within 48 hours until the fuller assessment is complete. There is also training given to carers on safe feeding techniques, positioning the person and providing a nutritionally balanced diet.

Over time, further deterioration of eating, drinking and swallowing can take place, and this may lead to the need to consider enteral feeding. Enteral feeding is a method of providing nutrition to people who cannot sufficiently obtain food by eating, or those who cannot eat because they have swallowing difficulties. A tube is inserted, either down the nose or if the feeding is considered to be long term, the tube will be placed endoscopically into the stomach. Making a decision to enterally feed is complex and requires full assessment and discussion with the family, carers and the multi-disciplinary health team. As with any treatment, the benefits verses the burdens need to be carefully weighed up. This can be very emotive for families and carers and the health team can help with all necessary information and supports to help come to an informed decision. Experience within the team would suggest that enteral feeding be used to improve quality of life, but not to extend life in the terminal stages where physical deterioration has generalized (Pennington 2002).

Maintaining skills

It is important that ways are thought about of maintaining skills, especially if the carers are new to the person with dementia. Crucially, to be able to help a person maintain skills, carers need to know which skills and abilities were previously held, so an important role of the CLDT when involved with a person in the early stages of dementia would be to help staff prepare a life story/communication passport. This would then be regularly updated and travel with the person through any transitions that may occur in later life. If this has not been developed, then carers would need to be able to find this information. Due to the individual's particular difficulties with communication or memory, it may be impossible to elicit this directly from the client. Therefore carers would need to seek help from relatives or key people who have known the person for a long time.

In maintaining preserved skills, the person can achieve positive results, thereby increasing self-esteem. These skills can be maintained by carers through highlighting social cues and providing environmental cues to trigger behaviours, e.g. bedtime routines, table setting at mealtimes. The CLD nurse role is then to help carers to prepare action plans and goal plans to enable them to focus on the person's abilities, without feeling overwhelmed. It also allows for baseline and ongoing recording of levels of functioning, which will help the carers to review the person's abilities, to acknowledge changes/declines and to adapt their practice as needed.

It is important that carers develop each plan to meet the needs of the individual. This will be achieved by negotiating with the person and all members of care staff. In doing so, this should provide continuity and consistency of care for the person with a learning disability and dementia.

Sleep

People with Down's syndrome are prone to sleep apnoea. This may be more noticeable once dementia is established, e.g. sleeping during the day and disturbed sleep pattern. The CLD nurse will work with carers/staff to support them to effectively assess the problem, using sleep diaries to implement solutions. This usually entails keeping a diary for two weeks to give a clear picture of events, then analysing the results and producing guidelines to manage behaviour. Cooperation and communication between agencies are essential for giving accurate information.

Again an assessment of the environment is always helpful, checking for factors such as light curtains or blackout blind, night light, safety gate or pressure-sensitive alarm pad, temperature of room, width of bed, appropriate bedlinen/night clothes, and so on.

Communication between agencies, i.e. day service and house care, is paramount, if the person is lethargic, sleeping and dozing while at day-care, but returns home and is left to catnap in the chair; staff thinking they have had a busy day, then day/night reversal may occur. The person with dementia may not know that it is time for bed, and they may have forgotten their usual bedtime routine. Often towards the end of the day, they may become confused, uncooperative and disorientated, known as 'sundowning'.

In these circumstances the use of visual/physical cues becomes crucial. Staff need to be aware of how to re-establish good night-time routine, seeing the need for continuity of this routine to create familiarity for the client to ease manageability of this time. Generally in consultation with the GP, Melatonin, a natural sedative, could be prescribed to enable establishment of good sleep routine.

Case example 4

On the initial assessment by the CLD nurse, sleep was identified as an issue for Mike after his diagnosis of dementia as he appeared tired when he arrived at his Adult Training Centre (ATC) and sometimes was found to be asleep, which was not like him. On closer investigation, his sleep pattern was found to be totally erratic. He liked watching videos and would watch them until 2–3 a.m., sometimes falling asleep on the sofa. He would need to be awake at 7 a.m. to be ready for his ATC. On return from work, he often fell asleep for 3–4 hours and woke at about 8 p.m. A timer was tried to switch off the TV at 12 midnight with Mike's agreement, however, he soon decided to plug the timer into a light instead. It was agreed that Mike had real difficulty setting his own bedtime and needed a physical presence of care staff to prompt him to go to bed.

Mobility

One of the queries most often made to the CLD nurses in the CLDT was how to help a person who has 'gone off their feet', or stopped walking. Similar to the initial assessment where the CLD nurse will look at differential diagnosis, when people are reported to have 'gone off their feet', it is important not to assume that the person has simply forgotten how to walk. There is a need to do a general health check to rule out alternative reasons for the person's change in mobility, i.e. urinary tract infection, poor foot care, pneumonia, fractured neck of femur.

As discussed earlier in modifying a person's environment, flooring within the home needs to be assessed to reduce mobility problems and in particular things such as shiny or self-coloured flooring avoided. The person needs well-fitting shoes, regular chiropody and easy access to all areas – level surfaces.

By enabling carers to discuss different aspects of changing needs with regards to mobility for the person with learning disability and probable diagnosis of dementia, we would hope that they would access the CLDT physiotherapist who will be able to assess the person at each stage of their disease and provide equipment as required. Having enhanced the carers' understanding of why people 'go off their feet', the ultimate aim of this section would be that carers are able to keep the person with dementia fit and mobile for as long as possible, enhancing the person's quality of life.

Epilepsy

The onset of epilepsy, a neurological condition caused by electrical activity in the brain, in a person with no history of seizures should always be investigated. If carers inform the CLDT of possible seizure activity, they would be asked to keep a seizure diary to determine the type, severity and frequency of seizures. Within Lothian there is an epilepsy specialist nurse who will offer advice and training to carers and will monitor medication. A referral would also be made to the CLDT psychiatrist/specialist epilepsy liaison service to provide further assessment/diagnosis, prescribing of appropriate medication and regular monitoring of blood levels.

Diagnosis once again needs to be made in order to exclude other causes, particularly as epilepsy is rare in the early stages of dementia, but is seen to occur in excess of 40 per cent of people with Down's syndrome towards the end of mid-stage dementia (Kerr 1997).

This can be a very stressful time for carers, as the person's decline is becoming more apparent. As well as offering emotional support, the CLD nurse would offer training and education to help the carers understand the changes happening to the person and how best to meet their needs with regards to epilepsy.

Discussion

The development of the work of the CLD nurse in Lothian is indicative of a number of important practice developments for the CLD nurse within the CLD team context. The case studies reflected upon in this chapter in particular highlight the centrality of the CLD nurse in coordinating the screening and monitoring activities essential to informing a diagnosis and management of dementia in someone with a learning disability. Early diagnosis is fundamental to ensuring that all the elements of an effective health-care and social care package can be put in place for the person with dementia.

In the case examples of Lily, Evelyn, Billy and Mike, it is the CLD nurse's skills and knowledge that can lead to the implementation of quite simple measures that can support their inclusion and quality of life. It is often these very simple changes that can prevent the escalation of difficult situations that may lead to the person being moved to another care setting.

Summary

The increased life expectancy of people with a learning disability and the associated increased incidence of dementia are creating a relatively new phenomenon. Service providers are receiving increased demands to support older people with a learning disability and dementia and their families. Issues for service providers include the lack of effective and accurate assessment and diagnostic tools and pathways; the need for accessible and supportive housing, health and care services; the lack of training and support for staff; and the need to develop effective models of care to support people with a learning disability and dementia, and their carers, during illness and until death (Watchman 2003). Central to negotiating a pathway through these concerns for older people with learning disability and dementia and their carers is the role of the LD nurse.

The example provided by the Lothian CLDT is only one of many possibilities. The format and implementation of the pathway are considered to be a 'work in progress' and there are certain areas of practice that require further consideration as they become more of a common concern to the CLDT practice and experience. In particular, these concerns relate to being more person-centred; being more effective in diagnosis sharing; and improving the experience for the person when dying.

It is exactly through the highlighting of areas of practice which are becoming increasingly part of the requirements of health care and social care of older people with a learning disability that the imperative is created to have effective policies and practices to ensure a good quality of life for the individual. Such philosophy and practice bases are indicative of how the CLD nurse's role and position have changed in the past ten years. The example of the work of the CLDT and the CLD nurse in Lothian highlighted the strong position, role and identity now occupied by the CLD nurses and their key position in shaping future services. The report *Shaping Futures* (Northway et al. 2006) acknowledges the CLD nurse's unique role in being the only professional exclusively trained to work with people with a learning disability and emphasizes the impact they can make on the quality of care for someone with dementia.

Lessons for CMHN practice

- Life expectancy for people with a learning disability has increased significantly and, as a result, nursing staff in Learning Disability Services will be required to work more and more with people with dementia.

- There is a high prevalence of Alzheimer's disease in people with Down's syndrome, with approximately 50 per cent developing dementia at age 60.

- Accurate diagnosis is difficult but vital. This is complicated by the already global intellectual impairment.

- The nurse has a central role within the multi-disciplinary team, as they provide coordination, support and education to carers and other professionals.
- The progression of the condition will place more responsibility on the nurse as they become more involved in the maintenance of the person's living situation.

Notes

1   This chapter has been written collaboratively by members of a CLDT team in Lothian and Heather Wilkinson, a researcher with a special interest in learning disability and dementia.
2   Scottish Down's Syndrome Association 2004 – available from Down's Syndrome Scotland, 158–60 Balgreen Road, Edinburgh EH11, 0131–313–4225 or www.sdsa. org.uk. See also Wilkinson and Kerr (2004).

References

Alaszewski, A., Alaszewski, H. and Parker, A. (1999) *Empowerment and Protection: The Development of Policies and Practices in Risk Assessment and Management in Services for Adults with Learning Disabilities*. London: Mental Health Foundation.

Baird, P. and Sadovnik, A.D. (1987) Life expectancy in Down syndrome, *Journal of Paediatrics*, 110: 849–54.

Barr, O. and Parahoo, K. (1994) A profile of learning disability nurses, *Nursing Standard*, 8(42): 35–9.

Bawley, E. (1997) *Designing for Alzheimer's Disease: Strategies for Creating Better Environments*. Chichester: John Wiley and Sons, Ltd.

Bradley, V.J. and Knoll, J. (1990) *Shifting Paradigms in Services to People with Developmental Disabilities*. Cambridge MA: Human Services Research Institute.

Bucht, G. and Sandman, P. (1990) Nutritional aspects of dementia, *Age and Aging*, 19: 832–36.

Burt, D.B. and Aylward, E.H. (2000) On behalf of the Members of the Working Group Establishment for criteria for the diagnosis of dementia in individuals with intellectual disability, *Journal of Intellectual Disability Research*, 44: 175–80.

Carlisle, D. (1997) Triumphant return in a new role, *Nursing Times*, 93: 77–9.

Carr, J. (2003) Patterns of aging in 30–35 year olds with Down's syndrome, *Journal of Applied Research in Intellectual Disabilities*, 16: 29–40.

Clarke, C., Wilkinson, H. and Keady, J. (2003) Risk construction and management in dementia care: a research report, *Journal of Dementia Care*, 11(2): 36.

Cohen, U. and Day, K. (1993) *Contemporary Environments for People with Dementia*. Baltimore, MD: Johns Hopkins University Press.

Cooper, S.A. (1997a) Deficient health and social services for elderly people with learning disabilities, *Journal of Intellectual Disability Research*, 41(4): 331–8.

Cooper, S.A. (1997b) High prevalence of dementia among people with learning disabilities not attributed to Down's Syndrome, *Psychological Medicine*, 27: 609–16.

Cosgrove, M.P., Tyrrell, J., McCarron, M., Gill, M. and Lawlor, B.A. (1999) Age at onset of dementia and age of menopause in women with Down's syndrome, *Journal of Intellectual Disability Research*, 43: 461–5.

Deb, S. and Braganza, J. (1999) Comparison of rating scales for the diagnosis of dementia in adults with Down's syndrome, *Journal of Intellectual Disability Research*, 43(5): 400–7.

Dewing, J. (2002) From ritual to relationship: a person-centred approach to consent in qualitative research with older people who have a dementia, *Dementia*, 1(2): 157–71.

Department of Health (1990) *National Health Service and Community Care Act*. London: HMSO.

Department of Health (1995) *Health of the Nation: A Strategy for People with Learning Disability*. Wetherby: Department of Health.

Department of Health (2001) *Valuing People: A New Strategy for Learning Disability for the 21st Century*. London: HMSO.

Durkin, M.S., Schupf, N., Stein, Z.A. and Susser, M.W. (1994) Epidemiology of mental retardation, in M. Levine and R. Lifford (eds) *Fetal and Neonatal Neurology and Neurosurgery*, 2nd edn. London: Churchill Livingston.

Evenhuis, H.M. (1997) The natural history of dementia in ageing people with intellectual disability, *Journal of Intellectual Disability Research*, 41: 92–6.

Gates, B. (2002) The new learning disability nursing. Agents of inclusion for people with a learning disability in the 21st century. Guest editorial, *Learning Disability Bulletin, British Institute of Learning Disabilities*, Autumn 2002, review.

Gedeye, A. (1995) *Dementia for Down Syndrome: Manual*. Vancouver, BC: Gedeye Research and Consultancy.

Holland, A.J. and Moss, S. (1997) The mental health needs of older people with learning disabilities, in R. Jacoby and C. Oppenheimer (eds) *Psychiatry in the Elderly*. Oxford: Oxford University Press, pp. 494–506.

Hutchings, B.L., Olsen, R.V. and Ehrenkrantz, E.D. (2000) Modifying home environments, in M.P. Janicki and E.F. Ansello (eds) *Community Supports for Aging Adults with Lifelong Disabilities*, Baltimore, MD. Paul H. Brookes Publishing.

ICD-10 (1994) *International Statistical Classification of Diseases*. Geneva: World Health Organization.

Janicki, M.P. and Dalton, A.J. (2000) Prevalence of dementia and impact on intellectual disability services, *Mental Retardation*, 38(3): 276–88.

Jenkins, J. and Johnson, B. (1991) *Community Nursing Learning Disabilities Survey 1991*. Penarth: Mental Handicap Nurses Association.

Kay, B., Rose, S. and Turnbull, J. (1995) *Continuing the Commitment: The Report of the Learning Disability Nurse Project*. London. Department of Health.

Kerr, D. (1997) *Down's Syndrome and Dementia: Practitioner's Guide*. Birmingham: Venture Press.

Kerr, D., Cunningham, C. and Wilkinson, H. (2006) *Responding to the Pain Experiences of People with a Learning Difficulty and Dementia*. York: Joseph Rowntree Foundation.

Kerr, D. and Innes, M. (no date) *What is Dementia?* Edinburgh: Scottish Down's Syndrome Association.

Kerr, D. and Wilson, C. (eds) (2001) *Learning Disability and Dementia: A Training Guide for Staff*. Stirling: DSDC.

Lai, F. and Williams, R.S. (1989) A prospective study of Alzheimer disease in Down syndrome, *Arch Neurol*, 46: 849–53.

Lillywhite, A. and Atwal, A. (2003) Occupational therapists' perceptions of the role of community learning disability teams, *British Journal of Learning Disabilities*, 31: 130–5.

Marler, R. and Cunnningham, C. (1994) *Down's Syndrome and Alzheimer's Disease: A Guide for Carers*. London: Down's Syndrome Association.

McCarron, M. (2002) The influence of Alzheimer's dementia on time spent caregiving for persons with Down syndrome, unpublished thesis, Trinity College, Dublin.

McCarron, M., Gill, M., Lawlor, B. and Begley, C. (2002) Time spent caregiving for persons with the dual disability of Down syndrome and Alzheimer's dementia: preliminary findings, *Journal of Learning Disabilities*, 6(3): 263–79.

Mitchell, D. (2004) Learning disability nursing, *British Journal of Learning Disability*, 32: 115–18.

Mobbs, C., Hadley, S., Wittering, R. and Bailey, N.M. (2002) An exploration of the role of the community nurse, learning disability, in England, *British Journal of Learning Disability*, 30: 13–18.

NHS Health Scotland (2004) *People with Learning Disabilities in Scotland: The Health Needs Assessment Report*. Glasgow: Health Scotland.

Northway, R., Hutchinson, C. and Kingdom, A. (2006) *Shaping the Future: A Vision for Learning Disability Nursing*. London: UK Learning Disability Consultant Nurse network.

Parahoo, K. and Barr, O. (1996) Community mental handicap nursing services in Northern Ireland: a profile of clients and selected working practices, *Journal of Clinical Nursing*, 5: 221–8.

Pennington, C. (2002) To peg or not to peg? *Clin-Med*, May–June, 2(3): 250–5.

Popovitch, E.R., Wisniewski, H.M., Barcikowska, M., Silverman, M., Bancher, C., Sersen, E. and Wen, G.Y. (1990) Alzheimer neuropathology in non-Down's mentally retarded adults, *Acta Neuropathologica*, 80. 362–7.

Prasher, P. (1995) Age-specific prevalence: thyroid dysfunction and depressive symptomology in adults with Down's syndrome, *International Journal of Geriatric Psychiatry*, 10: 25–31.

Royal College of Speech and Language Therapists (2003) *Position Paper: Speech and Language Therapy Provision for Adults with Learning Disabilities*. London: RCSALT.

Salvage, J. (1985) *The Politics of Nursing*. London: Butterworth-Heinemann.

Scottish Executive (2000a) *The Same as You? A Review of Services for People with Learning Disabilities*. Edinburgh: HMSO.

Scottish Executive (2000b) *Caring for Scotland: The Strategy for Nursing and Midwifery in Scotland*. Edinburgh: HMSO.

Scottish Executive (2002a) *Research Governance Framework for Health and Community Care*. Edinburgh: Scottish Executive.

Scottish Executive (2002b) *Promoting Health, Supporting Inclusion*. Edinburgh: The Stationery Office.

Thorpe, L.U. (1999) Psychiatric disorders, in M. Janicki and A. Dalton (eds) *Dementia Aging and Intellectual Disabilities*. Philadelphia: Brunner/Mazell.

Visser, F.E., Aldenkamp, A.P., van Huffelen, A.C., Kuilman, M., Overweg, J. and van Wijk, J. (1997) Prospective study of the prevalence of Alzheimer-type dementia in institutionalised individuals with Down syndrome, *American Journal on Mental Retardation*, 101: 400–12.

Watchman, K. (2003) Critical issues for service planners and providers of care for people with Down's syndrome and dementia, *British Journal of Learning Disabilities*, 31: 1–4.

Wilkinson, H. and Kerr, D. (2004) *Dementia and Learning Disability*. Plain Facts materials. Bristol: Norah Fry Institute. Available from University of Bristol, 3 Priory Road, Bristol BS8 ITX.

Wilkinson, H., Kerr, D., Cunningham, C. and Rae, C. (2004) *Home for Good? Preparing to Support People with Learning Difficulties in Residential Settings When They Develop Dementia*. York: Joseph Rowntree Foundation.

Wilkinson, H., Kerr, D. and Rae, C. (2003) Might it happen to me or not? What do people with a learning disability understand about dementia? *Journal of Dementia Care*, 11(1): 27–32.

Wisniewski, H.M. and Rabe, A. (1985) Discrepancy between Alzheimer-type neuropathology and dementia in persons with Down's syndrome, *Annals of the New York Academy of Sciences*, 477: 247–60.

Zigman, W., Schupf, N., Haveman, M., et al. (1997) The epidemiology of Alzheimer disease in mental retardation: results and recommendations from an international conference, *Journal of Intellectual Disability Research*, 41(1): 76–80.

Zigman, W., Silverman, W. and Wisniewski, H.M. (1996) Aging and Alzheimer's disease in Down syndrome: clinical and pathological changes, *Mental Retardation and Developmental Disabilities Research Reviews*, 2(2): 73–9.

14

The role of the community mental health nurse and the creative arts

Kevin G. Wood

Introduction

While there is a substantial quantity of information and evidence-based research on the impact and effectiveness of the use of the arts in dementia care, there is little that focuses on the community mental health nurse (CMHN) and their role in this process. Drawing on my personal experience as a manager of a CMHN team in dementia care and team manager of many years standing, the arts offer an alternative means of assessment and intervention that complement existing and more traditional approaches of care delivery, such as individual psychotherapy, carer stress-reduction and cognitive rehabilitation. This alternative approach to assessment and intervention was discussed by Benham (2003) in a paper that explored the importance of 'improvisational drama' which was used and integrated into a clinical tool that helped transform the lives of people with dementia who attended a day hospital in North Dorset. To highlight the impact that the arts and creativity are having in the field of dementia care, it is noteworthy that the first two awards given by The Queen's Nursing Institute and Alzheimer's Society for innovation in dementia care nursing included arts-based projects.

The aim of this chapter is twofold. First, to outline and demonstrate how the CMHN can integrate the use of the arts in their practice. Second, to explore the achievements of the community mental health team based at Ysbyty'r Tri Chwm, Blaenau Gwent, South Wales, who were awarded in 2002 one of The Queen's Nursing Institute's innovations in practice awards for the development of a social dancing support group in the community. The chapter will, however, start with a literature review of the arts and how such practices have been operationalized within the context of CMHN practice.

What are the arts?

Whatever our age, the arts has the ability to energize and motivate, to take human experience to a different level of being and improve quality of life. Being creative gives us the opportunity to succeed and gain a sense of achievement, whether this involves getting up for a dance to a favourite song, writing a poem or creating a collage. Through the variety of arts, we can relax and enjoy the moment and link past memories to present circumstances. This biographical and expressively creative context can make the arts the ideal medium to help people with dementia express their sense of self and personal identity. Indeed, 'art' and 'the arts' can mean many things to many people so, for the purpose of this chapter, the arts will be addressed by exploring the following five descriptors:

1   *The performing arts.* This includes music, drama, theatre and dance and is the most popular forms of arts for enjoyment and participation. Most people, whatever their age, enjoy listening to music and it can be a powerful tool for expression and relaxation alike. Drama offers an opportunity to explore feelings and has the potential for therapeutic benefits as well as being an enjoyable and social activity of its own. Dance also has many proven benefits, and when used in conjunction with music and drama, provides real alternatives to managing some of the challenges and issues faced by people with dementia in their day-to-day life. For example, social dancing is an ideal way to support spontaneous activity and stimulate people to communicate with others. Humans are essentially social beings and dancing is a social activity that contributes towards improved self-esteem and a more positive outlook on life. Unlike many forms of exercise, dance doesn't consist of continuous repetitive movements, and it can improve concentration as people focus on the dance steps and movement. Moreover, dancing is a weight-bearing exercise and will help strengthen bones (tibia, fibula and femur); this can help prevent, or a least slow down, loss of bone mass (osteoporosis). Social dancing has also been observed to increase physical activity as it is possible for people to move freely while dancing. Muscular tone and basic movement styles have been seen to improve, resulting in individuals gaining more confidence to engage in everyday activities.

2   *The language arts.* This explores the use of literature, creative writing and poetry as a means of expression. Reading has always been seen as an enjoyable way to 'escape' and, when used in a group setting, it can be a good way of supporting people who have become withdrawn and socially isolated. Another way to use these art forms is through the medium of storytelling. This can stretch the imagination and help create a focus for group participation.

3   *The tactile and visual arts.* This includes the use of textiles, clay and paints to create and display individual artwork. It can be a very powerful way of promoting a sense of achievement, leading to an increase in personal confidence.

4   *The broadcast and media arts.* This medium explores the use of film, radio and computer-based technology and their utility in the arts. Film and radio in particular can be forceful tools for use with reminiscence material, while the 'new technology' of computer-based arts can incorporate photographic and video diaries. For people with dementia, this medium can be a valuable way of capturing, storing and retrieving memories, using them to connect to a biographical sense of self.

5   *The participatory arts.* This is a term used for collaborative approaches between artists and other people, although the terminology may be interchangeable, depending upon where you live. For example, the approach may be called the 'community arts', 'arts in the community' or 'outreach arts'. Indeed, participatory arts are a movement that began in the late 1960s and aimed to stimulate involvement in the arts among people in disadvantaged conditions (Frances 1999). It also sought to empower individuals and communities. The Arts Development Team (as is the case in the author's work area of Blaenau Gwent, South Wales) works with local communities and encourages

them to identify and address issues of personal importance. They have employed artists in the field of drama, dance and the visual arts who are able to work with and support disadvantaged groups in the community and help develop skills, improve equality of opportunities, combat social exclusion and promote the effective working together of community agencies.

The benefits of participatory arts programmes are shown to be:

For people with dementia

- complements general health care provided by the community mental health team;
- addresses social needs;
- improves the self-esteem of people by creating opportunities to make a contribution;
- balances an otherwise illness-orientated experience;
- instils feelings of wellness;
- combats isolation through increased social contact;
- empowers;
- offers new opportunities and skills;
- provides choices.

For staff

- increases staff morale by recognizing their personal effort and commitment to quality person-centred care;
- improves communication;
- presents the patient as a whole person – not solely as an ill body;
- offers new opportunities and skills;
- allows staff to demonstrate their appreciation of a patient's circumstances.

For the wider team

- reduces dependency on valuable resources;
- publicly communicates a positive image of the team's commitment and concern for patients as people, and shows pride in the quality of service;
- strengthens partnerships between hospitals and communities.

Why choose the arts?

As these five descriptors illustrate, use of the arts has enormous potential when working with people who have mental health problems, especially those living with dementia. Creative activities can help people express themselves in many different ways and for those with cognitive impairment, this could make a significant difference to their voice being heard. To ensure success, it is vital to adopt a person-centred approach and ensure that the subject matter is understood fully – this will facilitate real engagement rather than superficial conversation and token communication.

The arts can also offer people with dementia opportunity for self-expression and enhanced communication both during and after the activity. Killick (2000) observed that when people with dementia are offered opportunities in this area, some surprising outcomes could often be observed, this includes: spontaneous creativity; sustained concentration; and satisfying collaboration which helps break down isolation. This observation also suggests that creativity through the arts can facilitate enjoyment and help stimulate the imagination. To enable this to occur, as much biographical knowledge about each person is essential. An ideal way of capturing this information is through the use of memory diaries that can be completed with families. Indeed, collecting oral histories and sharing with family member's past experiences can become a vital way for siblings and others to gain an in-depth knowledge of the person with dementia as an individual, and also have the opportunity to engage in a number of creative activities.

The *Strategy for Older People in Wales* (Welsh Assembly Government 2003) highlights the need for a health promotion framework for older people. The use of the arts would support this as an area for heath, social care and well-being. In England, the National Service Framework for Older People (Department of Health 2001) aims to ensure fair, high quality, integrated health and social care services for older people. Two of the main themes of this policy are to respect the individual and promote an active healthy lifestyle. Therefore, use of alternative therapies that include the arts may contribute to an increase in the quality of life of people with dementia and facilitate dignity in old age. This premise was explored by Landy (1993) who stated that 'healing' can occur when people are involved in a creative process and that this will eventually support positive change, growth and health. Further, Reisberg et al. (1999) found that storytelling stimulated patients to express and communicate feelings and to reactivate memories. Music has also been used as a nursing intervention to help people with dementia who are seen to be 'agitated'. In a quasi-experimental study using one of group repeated measures, Ragneskog et al. (1996) compared three different types of background music: relaxation, popular and pop and rock, played at dinnertime during three periods of two weeks. The sequence of the three types of music chosen for the study was randomly assigned and the aim of the study was to assess the effect that music had on food intake, irritability, restlessness and uninhibited behaviour. The results demonstrated that people with dementia were affected by music, particularly relaxing music, and a conclusion was reached that indicated that playing relaxing music could beneficially affect restless and agitated behaviour.

Research and practice experience have also demonstrated that people with dementia can continue to sing songs and dance to past tunes when given the opportunity to do so (Aldridge 1998). Indeed, singing and dancing is often used in the management of older people and it has been found that dancing has recreational, therapeutic and caring potential (Palo-Bengtsson and Ekman 2002). Dance and movement in a group may help people with dementia to develop outlets for positive and negative emotions, social interactions, physical activity and relaxation, assisting them to establish a meaningful relationship with others. Dancing has also been seen as a therapy for people with dementia. In a study by Palo-Bengtsson et al. (1998), the aim was to find out how people with dementia living in a nursing home functioned in social dance sessions. Six people with dementia were videotaped during four dance sessions. The findings revealed that retained abilities were prominent in dancing and it was evident that social dancing was supportive and seemed to have meaning to both patients and their carers. Indeed, social dancing seems to be a nursing intervention that supports patients' positive feelings, communication and behaviour.

Dance, as a mode of creative expression and therapeutic engagement, will be discussed later in the chapter.

Another alternative approach to working with people with dementia and their families is through drama. This includes group activity in fictional role-play situations, for example, where participants learn to explore issues, events and relationships in a safe and supportive manner. It is important to involve the carers in any programme to provide an example of how people with dementia can be stimulated by drama. Furthermore, by keeping people with dementia active, cognitive functioning can also be exercised in a manner that helps to obtain the person's maximum possible functioning abilities (Sterritt and Pokorny 1994). Similar findings were also expressed by Miller et al. (2000) who suggested that people who had demonstrated exceptional visual and musical abilities before the onset of their dementia maintained their creativity, even though difficulties with other skills may begin to manifest themselves. For example, in one of the study sample (N = 12), a patient who had been linguistically talented began to lose this ability while a new musical ability began to emerge; indeed, of the study sample, 7 reportedly developed new skills during the progression of their dementia (5 visual and 2 musical). Miller's team concluded that the functioning of people with dementia in this sample 'offer[ed] an unexpected window into the neurological mediation of visual and musical talents'.

Using different mediums in the arts can therefore have an important function of providing biographical and external cues in aiding reminiscence. This is based on access to long-term memories and provides a means for older people with dementia to present their lives to themselves, and to others, in a way that sheds light on present-day experiences.

An interesting project that demonstrates the importance of creativity using reminiscence is the 'Elderflowers programme' for older people with dementia in hospital care; this programme is run in the United Kingdom by the registered charity 'Hearts and Minds'. The aim of the 'Elderflowers programme' is to improve the quality of life for people with advanced dementia and is based on a belief that creativity, communication and humour will benefit people with dementia and increase their feelings of well-being and quality of life. As their *modus operandi* suggests, the team use the arts including drama, improvisation, music, song, 'clowning' and storytelling and tailor what they do to meet individual needs and wants. This personalizing of the programme will take into consideration the age, abilities and interests of people with whom they work. With a little adaptation, this project work could be implemented in a community setting offering an ideal opportunity for supportive intervention.

Putting theory into practice: the case of 'Walking Mrs Jones'

An example of how the arts can be incorporated into a community health-care setting was seen during a project that was developed to celebrate the new millennium as part of an 'arts festival', developed in conjunction with the Blaenau Gwent Community Arts Development Team in South Wales.

With the involvement of CMHNs and other members of the primary care team, the project involved the use of reminiscence, theatre, music and dance and the performance consisted of a staged production in the local theatre. This performance used the memories and stories of people with dementia and associated mental health issues from a day hospital in the local area. Through a sequence of group meetings a local theatre director worked with service users and through the arts devised a play that catalogued their lives through the twentieth century. What started out as a creative writing opportunity quickly became a staged production and led to a significant sense of achievement for all those taking part.

The success of this project and the partnership developed by both teams were the catalyst in exploring how the creative arts could enhance the lives of people with dementia Several themes were then discussed to consolidate the partnership, one in particular involved using dance and movement with people with dementia attending our day hospital, while combining it with the visual arts as a medium to assist with communication. The visual arts component involved the use of a professional artist to help people with dementia express themselves through this medium. The aim of the project was twofold. First, to provide stimulation and interest to assist with cognitive functioning and maintain ability so people with dementia could continue to live in the community for as long as possible. Second, to increase the self-esteem of people with dementia who attended the day hospital, while creating an opportunity for enjoyment.

The community arts development team also arranged for a dance therapist, who was a trained choreographer, to visit the day hospital and discuss with staff the type of activity that could be introduced. A local artist, known to the team, was contacted and he immediately saw potential in the project and followed this up with a visit. He agreed to start in conjunction with the dance therapist. The Arts Council for Wales, via the Blaenau Gwent Arts Development Team, agreed financial support for the project that oiled the wheels of operationalization.

The project was later named 'Walking Mrs Jones' and demonstrated that through effective partnerships and person-centred values, much can be achieved to support and help people with dementia to live a more fulfilled life while also expressing creativity. In our experience, we found the CMHN to be ideally placed to liaise with organizations in the community to help establish opportunities for these types of activities to take place and this level of engagement will be explored later in the chapter.

Social dancing: developing a support group

In our clinical experience we have found many people with dementia who are ready for discharge from the inpatient or day care unit, are apprehensive about this process and require some additional support to help in the transition from institutional to community living. In many areas of the UK there is a lack of support networks within the community and people with dementia can find themselves isolated and in need of companionship – this is also the case in residential homes where there can be a need for social stimulation and community integration. From our project activities we have found social dancing to be one way of bridging this gap and developing strategies for support (Jenkins 2003).

The specific aims of the community-focused project has become known affectionately as the 'tea dance support group', and from the time of its setting up we have found a number of benefits for people with dementia, such as building confidence in social situations, increasing physical activity and improving muscular tone, and promoting communication with others. The wider implications, however, have promoted self-help and support in an innovative and creative way. The main success of this development has been the increased focus on joint activity across agencies and the promotion of collaborative working. This has proved successful in what has now become a joint initiative between health and social services. Another key issue was the importance of responding to the previously identified need for social inclusion of a vulnerable client group.

The current project involves a weekly tea dance, which takes place in a local senior citizens' hall, which we rent, for an hour and a half. The Community Team including CMHNs, social workers and occupational therapists, assist attendance of people with dementia and take part in the activities. Through a variety of psychosocial skills they enable the people who attend opportunities to get out and re-establish contact within the community. They can also assess any difficulties that people may be experiencing. For some individuals it is the first time they have had contact with the wider community for a number of years. A dancing instructor attends weekly and provides skilled tuition. Some interesting patterns of behaviour and social etiquette can be observed during the tea dance, including the way men feel confident when they recognize the dance being played and they walk across the dance floor to ask a lady to dance. Especially when the offer is taken up!

There are other examples of working creativity with people with dementia such as using music, art and ceramics, all with similar effects. Positive engagement and finding out as much as possible about the person are the key to helping people with dementia cope with the changing world in which they live. Creativity gives nurses and other staff a real opportunity to facilitate communication and involve both the person with dementia and their family in a range of enjoyable activities. In essence, promoting creativity has substantial benefits and can ultimately open up new horizons and assist with the delivery of person-centred care. An example of the value and importance of creativity and the arts, to support the person with dementia in the community is now presented.

Case example 1

It was during October 1995 that a problem first became evident. Bob Fay, who was the local general practitioner (GP), went to visit a lady whom he had been seeing regularly. He didn't recognize her. Also, he was becoming more and more tired and was having to write longer notes to compensate for his failing memory. This and other worrying incidents caused Bob to realize there was something wrong.

The Fays felt isolated, however, with the help of their own GP, and through their network of friends and medical colleagues, they eventually found their way to the National Hospital for Neurology and Neurosurgery. While there Bob had extensive neurological testing and, almost two years after its onset, was diagnosed with Fronto-Temporal dementia, or Pick's Disease. Bob's wife Ginty discovered the existence of the Pick's Disease support group and through this was able to network to find out more about the progression of the illness and what could be done to help.

In the early stages of Bob's illness, a variety of his previous skills became impaired, for example, driving, dinghy sailing and playing the piano. These involve doing several things at once which he no longer found easy to do. A skill acquired in his early life was carpentry; Bob has been able to enjoy this once more by attending 'The Bont', a local mental health day hospital.

Both Bob and Ginty realized the need for a focus during the winter months as these months can lead to frustration and aimlessness. In the support group several ideas were discussed. Jigsaws were considered but Bob found them boring.

Another winter was fast approaching and by pure chance Ginty came across an advert in *Country Living Magazine*. Rug making . . . Ginty contacted a lady who was passionate about the process and lived in Kent. She was convinced this would be a good idea. They eventually went to her rug-making workshop. They learned a method called continuous rug hooking and they both enjoyed this, with Bob really taking to it.

It was going to be quite a challenge. Purchasing the equipment was the first hurdle to overcome.

The specialist wool required needed to be bought from America. There seemed to be a problem around every corner, but that seemed to make the challenge more exciting and Bob's first rug was soon completed. It really was teamwork with Ginty designing the pattern and Bob filling in, and enormously rewarding in the process.

While the project was both enjoyable and therapeutic for Bob, it was becoming expensive and difficult to maintain, so the next option was for Ginty to spin her own wool. The local adult education group had a spinning and weaving class. They went to see the course tutor, agreed it would be a good idea and both joined. While the spinning was not a success for Bob, Ginty enjoyed this activity and spun the wool which Bob would use to weave. He continued to enjoy this enormously and a real partnership arrangement developed. 'Jacob's fleece' was used to create textures and patterns, and Bob created cushion covers using basic weaving techniques.

For the couple, another project has been the creation of a wall hanging. Ginty has spun and plied the fleece in three tones and Bob undertook the weaving on a loom he made in one of his carpentry classes and the end result is stunning. Bob also created a scarf on a four-shaft loom using another weaving technique. They have also developed a form of finger weaving on tiny looms and this has become a helpful diversion for Bob's agitation on distance travelling.

The motivation shown by Ginty has been remarkable. Her objective has always been to ensure that Bob has a meaningful quality of life and occupation. The way she has used the arts has created a person-centred means of support, arguably the assimilation of the arts into everyday living could be adopted by CMHNs and other carers/professionals as a means of supporting people with dementia at home. The commitment in time and energy for Ginty has been enormous and, though at times lonely, there is no doubt that the result for both Bob and Ginty has been an absorbing way to spend time, especially during the winter months. There has been a huge sense of achievement for Bob and they have met new friends and contacts. Social inclusion and mixing with others have resulted in real satisfaction, relaxation and less stress and confirms the place of the arts in the management of dementia as a real therapeutic intervention (Wood 2003).

The arts: evaluating success

An evaluation tool has been designed by the Blaenau Gwent community mental health team to assess and monitor the effectiveness of any group activity or arts involvement. This chart is shown in Appendix 1. As a brief explanation, however, in the evaluation of arts activities we have found that a number of sections are important and these are summarized below.

First, the interest of individuals and their willingness to take part in the session need to be ascertained. The next section reviewed awareness and looked at how much was understood about the activity. Section 3 concentrated on levels of interaction and how much prompting was required and also assessed whether patients were able to volunteer information. Section 4 assessed concentration levels and for how long concentration could be achieved. Section 5 monitored whether there were any beneficial visual aspects during the session, for example, how much enjoyment was shown and whether any patients found the group distressing. Section 6 looked at how able the person was to comprehend and understand the content of the session and finally, the last section looked at ability to use voice, which could indicate confidence. Two staff monitor and observe the interactions/communication and support one another during each session. The evaluation chart is completed immediately after the session. In the case of the social dancing group the evaluation tool was used to monitor the progress of the activity.

The results indicated that the sessions held were beneficial and nearly all people with dementia participated by getting up out of their chairs and dancing or moving with the trained choreographer. They also showed that, out of a possible score of 24, most scored between 12–18, which indicated that they had certainly enjoyed the session and there would have been actual benefits from this form of activity. Although memory was a major challenge for most of the participants, they would leave the day hospital smiling, singing and with an obvious feeling of well-being.

Discussion

While reviewing the literature, there is clear evidence that 'arts in the community' work is an ideal medium to complement more traditional ways of supporting the person with dementia. Through the variety of arts there is something for everyone, whether it is culture, religion, gender or age, there are no boundaries and the scope for inclusion is broad. The participatory arts offer an ideal mechanism for partnership working and collaboration, enabling new and innovative projects for people with dementia and their carers.

Health promotion initiatives are supported by government strategy with the National Service Framework for Older People (in England) devoting a standard to the subject (Department of Health 2001). It looks at identifying barriers to healthy living and encourages working together with other agencies to develop healthy communities that support older people to live lives that are as fulfilling as possible. Using arts-related work offers a real opportunity to enable people with dementia to regain confidence in a social setting by using skills from their past. Indeed, many of the arts have a definite link to the promotion of health and well-being, which figures very strongly in the strategy for older people in Wales.

Community mental health nursing also offers an ideal opportunity to help people who have developed a mental health problem move on and find ways of integrating their life back into mainstream activities; ideas about how to set up and start arts programmes is shown in the resource section on p. 215, whether it is through the establishment of self-help groups with a theme approach or through becoming involved with established groups already available. Health promotion initiatives are fundamental to successful care in the community, as explored by Diane Beavis in Chapter 8, and the arts can also provide an excellent way to promote this idea.

We have seen that music can help agitation, restlessness and uninhibited behaviour and looked at how social dancing supports patients' positive feelings, communication and behaviour. Through the development of two innovative projects, and Bob and Ginty's illustrative case history, the use of the arts has been shown to be instrumental in supporting people with dementia and their carers adapt to the next phase of their life.

Reminiscence has been used for many years in the support of people with dementia and by using the arts can complement the effect through a range of enjoyable activities and events. For example, the arts offer a definite opportunity to promote person-centred care in a creative way, providing carers of people with dementia with new avenues for managing some of the problems that might have led to early institutional care. This is a direct challenge to staff to develop new skills to work alongside people with dementia and lose inhibitions that may inhibit participation in community arts projects.

Another indicator for using the arts in mental health care can be to support, train and develop care workers in a person-centred approach to care. This is a role often undertaken by the CMHN and, as already mentioned, affords an ideal opportunity for improving standards of care in nursing and residential homes.

Summary

In this chapter, I have looked at how, by using the arts as an alternative approach to care, the community mental health nurse is able to offer a wider range of strategies in supporting the person with dementia in the community. The main aim of the CMHN is to maintain individuals with dementia in the community while supporting the carer in that role.

The Audit Commission (2000) briefing paper *Forget Me Not* highlighted that most older people prefer to be supported in their own homes, if they are given the choice. To enable this to happen, older people need to be given the opportunity to make decisions for themselves and experience empowerment. This further consolidates the role of the CMHN in supporting carers, and as carers are integral to the support of people with dementia, the partnership development is essential. The arts also afford excellent opportunities for diversion and meaningful occupation.

Health promotion and education in nursing and residential care homes are also an important liaison and in-reach role. This can prevent unnecessary admission to already stretched NHS inpatient facilities. Offering a variety of alternatives for intervention gives both informal and formal carers new hope for an improved quality of life for people with dementia.

Lessons for CMHN practice

- The importance of partnership working to make things happen cannot be underestimated, working in isolation can be frustrating and time-consuming.

- Don't be put off by the many barriers that occur, there is always a way around them, be patient and don't get disheartened if things don't happen as you planned.

- Sometimes the answer is on your doorstep, you just need to ask the right people the right questions.

- Be realistic in your expectations and you will always be surprised.

- Support from the wider team and especially your manager is important during the early process.

References

Aldridge, D. (1998) Music therapy and the treatment of Alzheimer's disease, *Journal of Clinical Geropsychology*, 4(1): 17–30.

Audit Commission (2000) *Forget Me Not*. London: Audit Commission.

Benham, L. (2003) Acting out a serious purpose, *Journal of Dementia Care*, Sept/Oct: 8.

Department of Health (2001) *National Service Framework for Older People*. London: The Stationery Office.

Frances, F. (1999) *The Arts and Older People*. London: Age Concern.

Jenkins, S. (2003) 'Just your cuppa tea', *Working with Older People*, 7(4): 21–4.

Killick, J. (2000) 'Holding a rainbow in our hands': arts activities with people with dementia, *Signpost*, 6(3): 20–1.

Landy, R.J. (1993) Introduction: a research agenda for creative arts therapies, *The Arts in Psychotherapy*, 20: 1–2.

Miller, B.L., Boone, K., Cummings, J.L., Read, S.L. and Mishkin, F. (2000) Functional correlates of musical and visual ability in fronto-temporal dementia, *British Journal of Psychiatry*, 176: 458–63.

Palo-Bengtsson, L. and Ekman, S.L. (2002) Emotional response to social dancing and walks in persons with dementia, *American Journal of Alzheimer's Disease and Other Dementias*, 17: 1–5.

Palo-Bengtsson, L. Winblad, B. and Ekman, S. (1998) Social dancing: a way to support intellectual, emotional and motor functions in persons with dementia, *Journal of Psychiatric and Mental Health Nursing*, 5(6): 545–54.

Ragneskog, H., Brane, G., Karlsson, I. and Kihlgren, M. (1996) Influence of dinner music on food intake and symptoms common in dementia, *Scandinavian Journal of Caring Science*, 10: 11–17.

Reisberg, B., Kenowsky, S., Franssen, E.H., Auer, S.R. and Souren, L.E.M. (1999) Towards a science of Alzheimer's disease management: a model based upon current knowledge of retrogenesis, *International Psychogeriatrics*, 11: 7–23.

Sterritt, P.F. and Pokorny, M.E. (1994) Art activities for patients with Alzheimer's and related disorders, *Geriatric Nursing*, 15: 155–9.

Welsh Assembly Government (2003) *The Strategy for Older People in Wales*. Cardiff: Welsh Assembly Government.

Wood, K.G. (2003) Spinning a yarn to weave the arts into care, *Journal of Dementia Care*, 11(3): 19–21.

Resources

Alzheimer's Society

Arts access e.mail@artsaccess.com.au

Arts Council of England www.artscouncil.org.uk

Arts Council of Scotland www.scottishscreen.com

Arts Council of Wales www.ccc-acw.org.uk

Association of Voluntary Organisations: these are situated throughout the country and offer opportunity for good partnership projects.

The Dementia Services Development Centre for your region can be accessed through their website and have a page for the creative arts.

Local Authority Community Arts development teams as part of participatory arts programmes.

Voluntary Arts Network (VAN) aims to promote participation in arts and crafts, recognizing that they are a key part of our culture and that they are vital to our health, social and economic development. www.voluntaryarts.org

www.heartsminds.org.uk

Appendix 1 Evaluation tool to assess effectiveness of group activity or arts involvement

Level of change in cognitive ability	Date											
	Activity code											
1 Interest, willingness to join in and participate in group	Refuses to attend	0										
	Attends but shows little interest	1										
	Shows some interest	2										
	Interested	3										
	Interested, participates and appreciates	4										
2 Awareness	Unaware of group activity	0										
	Distracted by illness/other	1										
	Sometimes aware of activity	2										
	Usually aware of activity	3										
	Always aware of activity	4										
3 Participation/interaction	Does not talk	0										
	Sometimes asks direct questions	1										
	Talks too much and can dominate	2										
	Sometimes volunteers comments and answers	3										
	Usually volunteers comments and answers	4										
4 Concentration	None	0										
	Some of the session but patchy	1										
	Most of the session	2										
	All of the session	3										
5 Beneficial aspects	Found group distressing	0										
	Showed no signs of enjoyment	1										
	Occasionally showed pleasure	2										
	Enjoyed the majority of the session	3										
	Thoroughly enjoyed the session	4										
6 Comprehension	Unable to comprehend	0										
	Usually comprehends	1										
	Always comprehends	2										
7 Voice	Does not speak	0										
	Speaks in a low voice	1										
	Speaks in a medium voice	2										
	Speaks in a loud voice	3										
Total Score												

15

The community mental health nurse in the care home sector

Issues of assessment and intervention

Caroline Baker and Dawn Brooker

Introduction

The overall aim of this chapter is to increase the practitioner's awareness of how dementia care can be improved within the independent sector, primarily through the application of Dementia Care Mapping (DCM) (Kitwood and Bredin 1992; Bradford Dementia Group 2005) and its associated interventions. Drawing on real-life practice (anonymized) examples, this chapter will outline the role of the community mental health nurse (CMHN) in working in partnership with staff teams in care homes. The authors will draw on their extensive experience of DCM as a tool to help practitioners in their understanding of the experience of people with dementia living in care homes and to foster a person-centred approach to finding solutions in difficult situations. Furthermore, the chapter will illustrate how interventions using positive person work (Kitwood 1997) and a person-centred approach can enhance the care for people with dementia who have previously been labelled as 'difficult' or 'challenging'. We will consider the challenges for people with dementia living in care homes and how working in a person-centred way can help meet some of these challenges. We will then illustrate this by describing the work of a specialist dementia team using DCM and provide case examples from this work.

People with dementia in care homes: the challenges

The numbers of people affected by dementia-type disorders requiring specialist care continues to rise (Knapp et al. 1998). Five per cent of people over 65 and 20 per cent of those aged over 80 have dementia, equating to approximately 700,000 in the UK alone. Residential and nursing homes form an integral part of the care network for these individuals, particularly during the later stages of the disease process (Bowman et al. 2004) or when concurrent psychiatric morbidity or behavioural problems arise (Steele et al. 1990).

The majority of people with dementia in long-term care experience additional psychiatric disturbances or behavioural problems (Margallo-Lana et al. 2001) and providing good quality care for this group is particularly difficult (Wilcocks et al. 1997). A large audit (Ballard et al. 2003) identified that the quality of care was poor or very poor in all 17 care facilities surveyed (both NHS and private sector) across three regions of the UK. It is therefore not surprising that the quality of care within residential and nursing home facilities has been a matter of serious concern to the government (Department of Health 1999).

The negative impacts of poor quality care are also associated with behavioural disturbances and falls. These are associated with serious cost implications, as both frequently lead to hospitalization and often increase the subsequent level of care needs. In particular, many people with intractable behavioural and psychiatric symptoms require ongoing treatment within expensive specialist NHS continuing care facilities.

As dementia progresses, it becomes increasingly difficult for most family members, staff and volunteers to go beyond care that is purely physical. True engagement with people with dementia is difficult to achieve and daunting to many. A cycle of avoidance of social contact often results with the person with dementia finding it even more difficult to initiate and respond to human contact.

In many areas of the UK there is a shortage of specialist provision for people with dementia. Those requiring full-time care are placed either in Elderly Mentally Ill (EMI) residential care homes or integrated within Elderly Frail (EF) Nursing Homes. Although placing people with dementia into non-specialist facilities has some advantages, many care teams find it difficult at times to provide the extra care that people with dementia require. Added to this, residents who do not have dementia and their families can find it difficult to share their living environment with those who have dementia, particularly those showing high levels of distress. Care teams can find themselves torn between balancing the rights of the few against the many.

Taking a person-centred perspective

Person-centred care emphasizes the importance of seeing the whole person rather than just focusing on the disease deficits (Kitwood 1997; Woods 2001; Brooker 2004). Dementia is understood as a bio-psychosocial condition. It recognizes that quality of life and well-being are determined by a multiplicity of factors including neurological impairment, physical health, sensory ability, the individual's biography and personality and the social environment and context in which they live. It rests on a value base that promotes the rights of people with dementia, regardless of age or cognitive impairment. People are treated as individuals, recognizing that all people with dementia have a unique history and personality. The perspective of the individual with dementia is seen as the starting point for care and that empathy with this perspective has its own therapeutic potential. Care is provided that recognizes that all human life, including that of people with dementia, is grounded in relationships and that people with dementia need an enriched social environment which both compensates for their impairment and fosters opportunities for personal growth.

The person-centred approach has been applied to understanding behavioural aspects of dementia (Kitwood 1997; Stokes 2000). Rather than accepting behavioural aspects as an inevitable feature of neurological impairment, a person-centred approach argues that much of what is described as 'challenging behaviour' is a misunderstood response to an altered reality. Taken from an understanding of, and empathy with, the perspective of the person with dementia, behaviour is viewed as a way of attempting to meet needs arising from an impoverished or unsupportive social environment. For example, people with dementia are often presented with little stimulation or opportunities for engagement in long-term care settings (Ballard et al. 2001). It is perhaps unsurprising that people seek their own stimulation by way of what is commonly labelled 'wandering' or 'disruptive vocalizations'. Common cognitive impairments in dementia such as poor learning of new information, dysphasias, dyspraxias and visuo-perceptual deficits mean that people with dementia will interpret their social and physical environments in a unique way. If these interpretations of the environment are not understood and compensated for, then the person with dementia will experience excess disability. All too often, however, challenging behaviour is attributed to neurological impairment rather than as a function of an unsupportive care environment.

Looking to our own experience

Before we begin to look at antecedents for behaviour that is deemed challenging by care teams, it may be useful for us to take a view within our own world and think about some of the experiences that we encounter, our own behaviour, and the possible consequences of that behaviour.

Imagine you are experiencing terrible pain, you think you may have a tooth abscess. It's Friday evening and you cannot get to your dentist until Monday morning, what would you do? You may take analgesia to try to relieve your pain but imagine that the pain is becoming unbearable. Your mouth feels very sore. It is uncomfortable to eat anything and besides, you feel nauseous because of the infection so you don't want to eat. How would you feel? How would you act?

Your friend comes to visit. She does not acknowledge that you are in pain at all, although you feel that it is quite obvious. Your friend is very happy, chattering away and trying to encourage you to come out for a meal. You tell her then about your tooth abscess. Your friend, who has never experienced a tooth abscess, laughs at you and states that a curry will do you the power of good. You become angry and you shout at her. Your friend is visibly shocked by your behaviour. How do you feel? What would be the consequences of your behaviour for her, and for you?

Imagine a similar scenario but that you also have dementia. You are unable to communicate to anybody the pain that you are feeling or indeed, where the pain is. You did not want to get up that morning. You felt unwell. The only way to communicate your desire to remain in bed was to take hold of the duvet tightly. The carers, however, did not recognize this need and proceeded to get you out of bed, commenting about the dementia getting worse. They washed you, and brushed your teeth. You push the brush away and shout. You become frightened as they are obviously cross with you. One carer takes hold of your hands so that the other can brush your teeth. The pain is immense, you struggle, you shout, but your determination to communicate is viewed as further resistance and aggression. You are 'tossed' into a wheelchair and taken to the lounge. You hear the carer talking to another nurse telling her that you were 'awful' and that you needed some medication to calm you down. You feel completely powerless and upset. What is likely to happen now?

Challenging behaviour?

Despite a plethora of information being delivered via articles, conferences, videos and included within training days it is overwhelming how many people continue to maintain the view that anything 'out of the ordinary' is deemed to be 'challenging behaviour'. How can we begin to lose this dreadful term? How can we help practitioners recognize that an expression of need is not necessarily a behaviour that needs management interventions? How can we help staff to see this behaviour as a trigger point to begin the process of clarifying the individuals' needs and establishing a care plan to support those needs? In Table 15.1 we list some of the questions that should be triggered when common 'Behaviour Problems' occur.

Clinical Nurse Specialists and a Dementia Care Team: a possible way forward

One response to help care homes work in a more person-centred way with people with dementia is the development of a specialist nursing team to work with the independent sector. The work of the first author is described here by means of an illustration.

The role of a liaison nurse working between the NHS, the independent sector and social services in the Borough of Walsall originated in 2001 as a joint project between health and social services to improve the level of knowledge about dementia and person-centred care of staff working within these sectors.

Nursing homes, both EMI and EF were referring a lot of people with perceived 'challenging behaviour' with an expectation that the person would be moved on as the home felt unable to cope. Providing support and education enabled homes to continue to care for the person experiencing difficulties. This meant that the person with dementia did not need to be moved and therefore avoided the likelihood of further confusion and or disorientation. As the role developed further, it was recognized that there was a need for a clinical specialist in dementia care with a focus on introducing and improving person-centred care across the catchment area.

The Dementia Care Team was established in 2003 in recognition of the need for increased training and interventions within both the independent sector and the acute general health sector. The team comprises a clinical nurse specialist in dementia care, three full-time F grade specialist nurses and a full-time secretary who has also been trained in person-centred care and DCM. The team's primary focus is to provide training to enable practitioners and carers to be able to continue to care for the person within their home environment in an attempt to prevent admission to residential or nursing home care.

In primary care, the Dementia Care Team provide 10-week training courses for family carers to enable them to feel confident about continuing to provide care at home. In secondary care, the team work alongside the staff to improve the person's well-being and provide support and supervision to enable staff to continue to provide person-centred care. The Dementia Care Team also works within the acute hospitals. Their remit here is to work alongside the staff to enable people with dementia to maintain or improve their psychological well-being and continue to receive the physical care required to facilitate discharge to their previous environment.

Members of the Dementia Care Team have been highly commended for both the Nursing Times 2003 Awards and the Community Care Awards 2004. Similar projects that have been developed include the CHESS project (Whyte 2003), the EQUAL project (Smyth 2000) and the EDGE project (Ronch et al. 2004).

Table 15.1 Re-thinking behaviour problems: questions to ask to identify unmet need

Perceived behaviour problem	Label	Questions to be asked
Shouting out Grabbing at others	Verbally and physically aggressive	Are you in pain? Is there a problem with sight and hearing? Is there something that you need? Are you worried?
'Inappropriate' urination Incontinence	Awkwardness Attention seeking Dirty	Do you need me to help you find the toilet? Are you having difficulty taking off some of your clothing? Are you in pain?
Eating everything Hyperorality	He's worse than a child	Are you still hungry? Is there an underlying physical problem? Is this fronto-temporal lobe dementia?
Stealing other people's drinks	Greedy, childish	Are you still thirsty? Has the person got an underlying physical problem? Is the person developing diabetes?
Taking other people's clothes, grabbing at curtains	He is so naughty I wish he would leave them alone	Are you cold? Are you disorientated Are you trying to find something that is important to you?
Taking off clothing Disinhibition	Stripper Pervert	Are you too hot? Does the person want to take a bath or a shower but does not realise where they are? Does the person want to change their clothing?
Wandering Repetitive	Attention seeking Nuisance	Are you worried about something? Are you looking for something/somebody? Do you know where you are? Do you need to get outside to get some fresh air?
Trying to get out of the door, shouting	Troublesome Always wants to 'escape'	Is the noise in here bothering you? Is there somewhere that you would like to go?
Curling up on the floor Trying to get into bedrooms	He's a liability He gets on other people's nerves	Are you feeling tired? Do you need some time alone?
Becomes withdrawn, uncommunicative, unresponsive	He's being lazy	Are you unwell? Are you tired? Are you feeling depressed? Is this person experiencing delirium?

How do we assess in a person-centred way?

In dementia care the starting place for assessment is the Mini-Mental State Examination (MMSE) (Folstein et al. 1975). The tool is helpful to establish, to an extent, the degree of cognitive impairment and will provide guidance as to whether the person is able or unable to be considered for treatment with cognitive enhancers. The tool can identify specific difficulties with recall and higher cortical function, but in view of the person's needs, what does that actually tell us?

Based on clinical experience, the MMSE can provoke immense anxiety in people who, with an awareness that they are experiencing some memory difficulties, desperately try to 'get it right' and can become upset if they are unable to produce the required answer. Assessment tools can be useful for providing measurable outcomes but to get to the heart of the person's needs, we need to get the perspective of the person with dementia first and foremost. All too often, assessment tools are carried out by practitioners who assess the current functioning and do not take into consideration how the information they have gathered is presented in relation to how the person has been in the past. Files contain numerous pieces of paper but often they are not viewed in an analytical way. They provide a measure of each area but how is that combined and utilized to view the whole picture?

Dementia Care Mapping (DCM) was developed by the late Professor Tom Kitwood and his co-worker Kathleen Bredin (Kitwood and Bredin 1992). The coding frames were developed through ethological observations over many hours spent in nursing homes and hospital facilities. In his final book, *Dementia Reconsidered*, Kitwood described DCM as 'a serious attempt to take the standpoint of the person with dementia, using a combination of empathy and observational skill' (1997: 4). In spite of Tom Kitwood's untimely death in 1998, the Bradford Dementia Group has continued to train practitioners, to conduct research and to support people using the DCM in practice (Brooker 2005). DCM has been through a number of changes since its inception. The 8th edition (DCM 8) was launched in the UK in 2005. DCM is only available through licensed trainers who undergo a rigorous preparation for their role. DCM training is now available in the USA, Germany, Denmark, Australia, Switzerland and Japan. All DCM practitioners take the same assessment of competence wherever they undertake their training. This has been accomplished by the development of Strategic Partnerships with organizations around the world who meet the specific criteria for establishing DCM training and support within their respective countries. There are 35 DCM trainers and approximately six thousand people trained at basic level worldwide.

During a DCM evaluation the observer (mapper) tracks between five to ten people with dementia continuously over a representative time period (e.g. six hours during the waking day). The mapper attempts to blend in with the care environment. Mapping only takes place in communal areas of care facilities. Mappers may use DCM in care environments in which they work (Barnett 1995; Neel 2002) or more usually in a place where they are not responsible for the provision of direct care (Brooker et al. 1998; Muller-Hergl 2004). Mappers may be qualified nurses or other professionals (Brooker et al. 1998), nursing assistants (Packer 1996) or family carers (Fossey 1999).

After each five minute period (a time frame), four coding frames are used to record what has happened to each individual being observed in that time frame. The Behavioral Category Code (BCC) is a description of the behaviour that has occurred in a five-minute time frame. There are twenty-three BCC's to choose from altogether.

The mapper also makes a judgement for each time frame, based on behavioural indicators, on the level of mood and engagement that the person is experiencing. This is called an ME (Mood and Engagement) Value. This is usually rated on a six-point scale, −5, −3 and −1 representing disengagement and negative mood and +1, +3 and +5 representing positive engagement and mood. Over a few hours of observation, these ME values can tell us about the relative state of ill-being or well-being experienced by the person with dementia. ME values can be averaged to arrive at a WIB (Well/Ill Being) Score for a particular time period for an individual or a group.

Personal Detractions and Personal Enhancers are recorded whenever they occur. Personal Detractions are any episodes of Malignant Social Psychology (Kitwood 1997) that are observed. These personal detractions are devaluing interpersonal interactions from care workers that are thought to undermine the personhood of those with dementia. Personal Enhancers that support personhood are also recorded systematically. Kitwood developed the concept of Positive Person Work (Kitwood 1997) to improve personhood and enable practitioners to be able to capture and record positive events as well as episodes of malignant social psychology. Positive Person Work was developed further as part of the 8th Edition of DCM to provide feedback for staff teams on examples of good practice.

DCM can be used in a series of developmental evaluations in care settings in order to improve care practice generally. Through such a process staff are empowered to consider care from the point of view of the person with dementia. Its effective use in such developmental evaluation requires careful preparation, feedback and monitoring (Brooker et al. 2004). DCM is used to monitor change and provides positive reinforcement for the provision of person-centred care when used as part of a continuous quality improvement cycle (Brooker et al. 1998; Younger and Martin 2000). The Audit Commission (2000) recommended the use of DCM as a means of improving the quality of care in formal care settings and it has been the subject of a number of positive reports from the Commission for Health Improvement.

DCM can also be used to assess individuals who are displaying so-called challenging behaviour. By carrying out the detailed observations within DCM, an observer can often shed light on the underlying reasons for the behaviour. DCM provides a way for practitioners to heighten their empathy with the perspective of the person with dementia. This is the starting point in developing the interventions that we need to increase (Positive Person Work) and those we need to revise or eliminate from practice (Malignant Social Psychology).

DCM can also be useful in assessing the training needs within a care team. In Walsall, the Dementia Care Team used DCM in this way. Baseline maps were carried out within all the nursing homes that cared for people with dementia. The information obtained from these maps helped to develop a two-day training package in direct relation to the needs and wishes of the care teams within the homes. Training was developed in consultation with practitioners themselves. Following DCM feedback, staff within the homes or day centres recognized their need for knowledge, particularly in relation to Malignant Social Psychology and Positive Person Work. This, in turn, developed further interest in DCM and how it could be used to improve care and there are now 80 staff trained within these units in the use of DCM to enable us to work in partnership and move dementia care forward. DCM is used generally to assess care practice and, on an individual basis, to clarify care planning needs.

Case studies

The following case studies demonstrate how the needs of a person with dementia can be met. These case studies are all based on real-life examples of working with people with dementia within care homes in the past few years.

Case example 1: Removing the challenge – introducing the person

'Welcome to the "Challenging Behaviour" Unit.' A member of staff showed me around the unit, a huge expanse of darkened corridors and rooms. Residents milling around, heads down, some sitting in their chairs, some crying, some screaming. Others were simply staring ahead into the apparent void before them. And the staff? They appeared tired, but dedicated to their mission in what appeared to be a military operation. The job was being done.

I explained to the staff about DCM and how we might use it to assess the needs of the residents within the unit and work towards improving well-being. I was met with some scepticism initially surrounding the possibility of people with advancing dementia being able to move forward from where they were. After all, this is why people were placed within the unit, wasn't it? However, staff were keen to try it out and to see what the outcomes of the assessment were.

My initial fear turned into reality as I spent time observing the residents within the unit. Half of the residents were disengaged, withdrawn, sleepy. Interactions between the remainder of the residents were volatile. Staff attempted to 'jolly' people along. There was no evidence of malicious malignant social psychology, merely attempts at 'improving the residents' lot'. Attempts at Positive Person Work were turning into Personal Detractions. I remember feeling distinctly uncomfortable, wondering how I was going to feedback my observations and move forward with the team in a positive way.

When it was time to feedback the DCM results, I entered the unit with trepidation, report in hand, practising my feedback verbatim. It transpired that my fear was unfounded, staff were eager to listen and more importantly, willing to contribute. Empathic skills were boundless and the team drew much from their realization of the things that I had observed from the residents' point of view. Staff identified their need to update their skills in person-centred care and communication. They were also keen to develop their knowledge surrounding engagement and occupation. During our discussion on the environment of the unit, staff identified that they too felt that it was not conducive to a positive atmosphere. The main lounge was vast but barren of visual stimulation and although it gave people a great expanse of area to move around in, the overall view was that the unit was not homely. Staff felt that their residents were being excluded from the improvement plans for the remainder of the units and felt let down that other units within the home had been decorated and revamped.

A one-day training plan was carried out at the home, the formulation of which was developed by the staff. Training following a map can be extremely beneficial as we are able to relate some of the content of the training to the residents involved in the assessment, enabling us to make the link between theory and practice. Following the training sessions, we then dedicated an hour to developing a vision and an action plan. Staff were enthused, they wanted to make a difference and DCM had provided the vehicle to begin their journey.

We planned a further DCM evaluation in three months' time. During that time, staff would approach the management about a redesign of the unit and purchase some sensory activities to carry out with the residents.

The follow-up DCM evaluation revealed a different picture. Staff were using positive person work to negotiate and facilitate former 'task-orientated' procedures, valuing the person rather than the job and validating feelings. At this point, the environment had not undergone a physical restructure, but had taken on a completely fresh psychological structure. Internal changes in approach were beginning to make a huge impact both for the residents being supported in the unit and for the staff as individuals and as a team. Individual sensory work proved to be beneficial for residents who were experiencing difficulty communicating and well-being levels were increasing.

Behaviour previously seen as 'challenging' was now being viewed as an expression of need, validated and supported.

The unit has continued to develop over the past two years. Structural changes have taken place, smaller lounges have been created and a snoezelen room introduced. A smaller six-bed unit has been created, to prepare residents for discharge to 'standard' nursing homes or residential care.

DCM was a catalyst in this unit and its regular use continues to provide a sense of achievement and self-reflection and, perhaps more importantly, a continual effort to improve things further.

Case example 2: Life in a cardboard box

Winnie and I had never met before. My first encounter with Winnie was when I heard her screaming outside the residential home, calling for the police. Staff (who had little experience of working with people with dementia at that time) were trying to prevent Winnie from leaving the building. Understandably, staff were concerned. Winnie had only been admitted to the home a few hours previously for a period of respite care. Winnie was extremely agitated and staff feared that she would run across the very busy road. Winnie, however, just wanted to go home. Prior to my arrival, staff had placed a call to the duty social worker, their feeling at this time (and that of the social worker) was that Winnie would have to be sectioned under the Mental Health Act and removed to a place of safety.

The scene as I arrived can only be described as chaotic. Four members of staff with Winnie in the middle, desperately trying to pull away, hitting out at the members of staff trying to restrain her and shouting at the staff, who in turn, were shouting at Winnie in an attempt to calm her down.

As I approached, and asked the lady's name, staff clearly 'warned' me to keep my distance as Winnie would be liable to hit me, as she had been physically aggressive with all the staff. I asked the staff to release Winnie and approached her and introduced myself. Winnie continued to shout, although she did not attempt to leave at this point. I asked Winnie to try and explain to me what she wanted, at which point, she also appeared to think that I was one of her 'enemies'. She appeared paranoid and initially, was extremely suspicious of my motives for wanting to talk to her.

I asked Winnie if she would come and sit with me outside on the bench and talk to me. Again, Winnie appeared quite hostile, demanding to know why I was interfering. Winnie agreed to sit by me but sat aloof, with piercing eyes, maintaining total eye contact. I recall her making derogatory comments about my appearance, following on with 'so what do you think of that'. I replied that it was okay, if that was how Winnie felt, then she must tell me. At which point, Winnie laughed out loud and began to visibly relax. We spoke about Winnie's home, about the garden, about my incompetence as a gardener, which is where Winnie felt that she then had the 'upper hand'. She spoke with confidence about her hobby and laughed at my lack of knowledge. She began 'teaching' me, give me tips and hints on what I should plant and when. She then began to cry.

I sat quietly and listened as Winnie told me that she shared a bedroom with her daughter at home and that the 'man' that had brought her here had told her that he would call by before he went home. She went on to explain that she had been burgled at home, and the lengths that she had taken to ensure that this would never happen again. It transpired that it was an aggressive burglary, the perpetrators having knives, and although this was several years ago, Winnie still found it difficult to come to terms with. I tentatively offered to place my hand on Winnie's and her eyes met mine as she took hold of my hand. Winnie then began to tell me about the loss of her husband and that she had his picture on her bedroom wall at night. Every night, Winnie would kiss the picture before she went to bed. Winnie held my hand tighter and told me that she was frightened. She did not recognize the room and she did not want to sleep on her own. She did not want to stay.

I asked Winnie if she could show me her room. Winnie agreed and took me to where she would be staying for the next ten days. On the chair, beside the bed, Winnie's 'life' was in a cardboard box. The box contained a nightdress, some slippers and a change of clothing.

By now, it was ten o'clock and Winnie appeared to be extremely tired. I asked her if she would like me to help her wash and change for bed. She agreed that she was tired and said that she would stay if I stayed with her. I explained that I would have to go home shortly but that I would arrange for another nurse to sit with her.

Together, we unpacked Winnie's belongings, and Winnie started to get ready for bed, asking me for assistance when she needed it. She asked me to sit on the bed and hold her. I introduced Winnie to the member of care staff that would be taking over when I left and reassured her that she would be by her side all night, at which point Winnie made me promise that I would stay with her until she fell asleep, to which I agreed. Winnie was exhausted, she so desperately needed to sleep but as I sat stroking her hand, every small noise would cause her to waken and she would look at me with startled eyes, squeeze my hand and then return to sleep. I left Winnie at midnight, sleeping peacefully in the knowledge that somebody was with her in her time of need.

I spoke to the staff and asked them to ask the social worker to bring in some of Winnie's personal belongings in the morning, in particular, the picture of her husband. We talked through the approach when Winnie had first attempted to leave and why she may have become resistive.

Winnie was anxious, she wanted to be at home with her daughter. At the time, staff had not found out why Winnie was attempting to leave and the situation had spiralled out of control, for Winnie, and for the staff. Several elements of Malignant Social Psychology were apparent (Kitwood 1997). Winnie was disempowered, staff had used treachery by telling Winnie she could go home tomorrow. The social worker had told Winnie that he would call by before he went home and had not, leaving Winnie distrustful and anxious. There were elements of infantalization whereupon Winnie was clearly being treated as a child. Winnie was ignored; nobody actually listened to what Winnie was actually trying to say. However, by using Positive Person Work (Kitwood 1997), Winnie felt reassured and that her needs were being met.

Table 15.2 Malignant social psychology and positive person work with Winnie

MSP	What happened to Winnie?	PPW	What helped Winnie?
Labelling	'She's physically aggressive'	Recognition	Winnie was anxious and needed reassurance
Outpacing	Staff took decisions out of Winnie's hands and their rapid approach contributed to increased confusion and anxiety	Negotiation	Winnie discussed what she wanted and how it could be achieved
Intimidation	Winnie was physically restrained and 'threatened' with hospital	Facilitation	Winnie was encouraged to identify the problem herself and show the nurse the root of her anxiety
Disempowerment	Winnie had all decisions taken away from her. Her voice was not listened to	Empowerment	Winnie was encouraged to express her concerns
Withholding	As staff had not recognized Winnie's anxiety they were unable to provide psychological or physical support	Holding	Winnie was provided with both psychological and physical support
Invalidation	Staff did not enter Winnie's space. Her anxieties were disregarded	Validation	Winnie's anxieties were acknowledged and validated as real concerns for her

Some may argue that it would be impossible to carry out four hours of Positive Person work for one person within a residential home. We might agree with this statement but would add that the time spent in this particular instance was actually to unravel the implications of Malignant Social Psychology. If Recognition and Validation had been used initially, how might the picture have looked, what pathway would Winnie have taken?

Brief DCM snapshots that helped to develop the full picture

Annie

One of the first maps in Walsall provided a real insight into how DCM can be used to provide a very different picture to the one that staff are viewing while carrying out care within a very busy environment. Annie was perceived by staff as 'attention-seeking'. She was described as constantly putting herself on the floor and being resistive. During the map, it became quite apparent that Annie was quite purposeful in her mission. She did indeed get onto the floor, but then proceeded to pick up all the little bits off the carpet and used her hands to 'dust down' the skirting board. When staff came across her on the floor, she was lifted up and placed on the chair. Annie looked bored and would then place herself on the floor once more, on her hands and knees, carrying out her job.

Staff were truly amazed when they heard the feedback from the map and now encourage and facilitate Annie to carry out her 'task'.

Nancy

Nancy was reported to be resistive to nursing intervention, constantly screaming out and generally 'unmanageable'. It transpired that Nancy had always had difficulty taking medication. An individual DCM assessment was carried out and the information obtained married with an observation chart from the previous seven days revealed that Nancy was only becoming resistive when she was being mobilized or transferred. Nancy was taking some pain relief for her severe arthritis but it appeared that she was still having pain breakthrough. Following the map, we contacted the GP and Nancy was prescribed an analgesia patch. Staff at the home report that Nancy is much happier.

Jack

A care manager approached us to see if we could carry out an individual map for Jack, a 67-year-old gentleman, whom they felt would benefit from day care but seemed to become 'agitated and restless' while he was there. Staff at the day centre had informed the care manager that they could not look after him any longer.

During a DCM evaluation, Jack appeared to enjoy the activities in the morning and presented in a moderate to high level of well-being. However, shortly after lunch, Jack walked across to the window and looked out stating that he wanted to go home. Staff kindly informed him that it wasn't time yet and sat him down. Again, Jack went across to the window and then to the door, explaining that he wanted to go home. Again staff informed him that the transport would collect him later. The scenario developed and escalated, a repetitive transaction from both parties until Jack became really frustrated and shouted.

Why did Jack want to go home when he had been quite content in the morning? While talking with Jack, it transpired that after lunch, he always walked his dog and he was worried that he was not at home to take him out. It was difficult to reassure Jack that his wife would walk the dog as he felt it was his 'duty'. We spoke to staff and arranged for Jack to attend in the morning only.

Reflections on our success

The process of Dementia Care Mapping is a continual learning curve for both the Mapper and the staff engaging within the developmental process. For Dementia Care Mapping to be effective, we have found that 'groundwork' with the staff is a crucial component to enable us to gain the trust of the staff and develop their willingness to engage with the DCM process. Staff are encouraged to enter into a relationship with the 'trusted stranger' as described by Muller-Hergl (2004). We are an outsider to the care home. We are rooted in the belief that changes are always possible. We work with the staff, not telling them what to do, but we use DCM to achieve objectivity and mentoring for the team through the process of development.

DCM is a powerful tool and requires a high level of expertise to maintain a person-centred approach with both residents and staff. We have used each other in the team for our support and development but also the wider DCM network. We have 80 staff trained at Basic Level and four to advanced level, one at evaluator level and we also have an in-house DCM trainer (Innes et al. 2000). We have peer support through Regional DCM Networks (Edwards 2005) and through the Bradford Dementia Group DCM Trainers' group. This has helped to sustain and nourish our journey with DCM.

Summary

There are now 80 staff trained in the DCM method within the borough. All these staff are developing smaller networks to improve person-centred care and rethink 'challenging behaviour'. Initially, it was thought that DCM would be too time-consuming to make a real difference, that the tool itself cannot change the world and that there were too many 'potholes' for us to fall into. Colleagues were very dismissive of DCM initially. Those colleagues, who are now trained in DCM, think very differently about the impact of DCM. Those who have been trained are highly motivated and want to work with each other to develop a real person-centred approach to care.

Our champions have been the leaders in our service, both in health and social services, who grasped DCM with both hands and proactively supported our quest to improve care. Person-centred care is a whole systems approach. Staff need to be supported to maintain their enthusiasm, capture their ideas and enable them to deliver those ideas to continue to improve care for people with dementia. The establishment of Dementia Care Team has enabled us to provide this support.

Lessons for CMHN practice

- The importance of engaging with staff to look for the underlying reasons for challenging behaviour.
- Being sensitive to staff needs and concerns and working in partnership to achieve goals. Adopting a position of negotiation and collaboration when working with staff teams as an external evaluator.
- Being open and honest to the ideas and solutions that staff bring, knowing that we are all experts in life and that none of us have all the answers.

- Recognizing that people with dementia living in residential and nursing homes are part of the community and have just as many rights to our expertise.

- DCM can provide a vehicle for engaging with the private sector in working with people with dementia and challenging behaviour.

References

Audit Commission (2000) *Forget-me-not*. London: The Audit Commission. Available at www.audit-commission.gov.uk

Ballard, C., Fossey, J., Chithramohan, R., Howard, R., Burns, A., Thompson, P., Tadros, G. and Fairbairn, A. (2001) Quality of care in private sector and NHS facilities for people with dementia: cross-sectional survey, *British Medical Journal*, 323: 426–7.

Barnett, E. (1995) A window of insight into quality of care, *Journal of Dementia Care*, 3(4): 23–6.

Bowman, C., Whistler, J. and Ellerby, M. (2004) A national census of care home residents, *Age and Ageing*, 33(6): 561–6.

Bradford Dementia Group (2005) *Dementia Care Mapping- DCM 8th Edition*. Bradford: University of Bradford (available only as part of the basic DCM 8 course).

Brooker, D. (2004) What is person-centred care for people with dementia? *Reviews in Clinical Gerontology*, 13: 212–22.

Brooker, D. (2005) Dementia Care Mapping (DCM): A Review of the research literature. *The Gerontologist*, 45 (1): 11–18.

Brooker, D., Edwards, P., Benson, S. (eds) (2004) *DCM: Experience and Insights into Practice*, London: Hawker Publications.

Brooker, D., Foster, N., Banner, A., Payne, M., Jackson, L. (1998). The efficacy of Dementia Care Mapping as an audit tool: report of a 3-year British NHS evaluation, *Aging and Mental Health*, 2(1): 60–70.

Department of Heath (1999) *Fit for the Future: National required standards for residential and nursing homes for older people.* London: Department of Health.

Department of Health (2001) *The National Service Framework for Older People*. London: HMSO.

Department of Health (2002) *Consent and Capacity: A Guide for Relatives and Carers*. London: HMSO.

Edwards, P. (2005) Putting Dementia Care Mapping on the map, *Journal of Dementia Care*, 13(1): 16.

Folstein, M., Folstein, S. and McHugh, P. (1975) Mini-mental state: a practical method for grading the cognitive state of patients for the clinician, *Journal of Psychiatric Research*, 12: 189–98.

Fossey, J. (1999) A carer on the team, *Journal of Dementia Care*, 7(2): 10.

Innes, A., Capstick, A. and Surr, C. (2000) Mapping out the framework: Journal of Dementia Care, in D. Brooker, P. Edwards, S. Benson (eds) (2004) *DCM: Experience and Insights into Practice*. London: Hawker Publications.

Kitwood, T. (1997) *Dementia Reconsidered: The Person Comes First*. Buckingham: Open University Press.

Kitwood, T. and Bredin, K. (1992) A new approach to the evaluation of dementia care, *Journal of Advances in Health and Nursing Care*, 1(5): 41–60.

Knapp, M., Wilkinson, D. and Wigglesworth, R. (1998) The economic consequences of Alzheimer's Disease in the context of new drug developments, *International Journal of Geriatric Psychiatry*, 13: 531–43.

Margallo-Lana, M., Swann, A., O'Brien, J., Fairbairn, A., Reichelt, K., Potkins, D., Mynt, P. and Ballard, C.G. (2001) Prevalence and pharmacological management of behavioural and psychological symptoms among Dementia sufferers living in care environments, *International Journal of Geriatric Psychiatry*, 16: 39–44.

Muller-Hergl, C. (2004) The role of the trusted stranger in DCM feedback, *Journal of Dementia Care*, 12(2): 18–20.

Neel, A. (2002) How DCM may affect caregiver mappers, *Journal of Dementia Care*, 10(4): 26–8.

Packer, T. (1996) Shining a light on simple, crucial details, *Journal of Dementia Care*, 4(6): 22–3.

Ronch, J.L., Bradley, A.M., Pohlmann, E., Cummings, N. Howells, D., O'Brien, M.E. and Beria, J. (2004) The Electronic Dementia Guide for Excellence (EDGE): an internet-based education programme for care of residents with dementia in nursing homes, *Alzheimer's Care Quarterly*, 5(3): 230 40.

Smyth, C. (2000) EQUAL: working in partnership with the Independent sector, *Signpost*, 5(2): 13–14.

Steele, C., Rovner, B., Chase, G.A., Folstein, M. (1990) Psychiatric symptoms and nursing home placement of patients' with Alzheimer's Disease. *American Journal of Psychiatry*, 147: 1049–51.

Stokes, G. (2000) *Challenging Behaviour in Dementia: A Person-centred Approach*. Bicester: Speechmark Publishing.

Whyte A. (2003) Creative care for older people, *Nursing Times*, 99(47): 24–5.

Woods, R.T. (2001) Discovering the person with Alzheimer's disease: cognitive, emotional and behavioural aspects, *Ageing and Mental Health*, 5(1): 7–16.

Younger, D. and Martin, G. (2000) Dementia Care Mapping: an approach to quality audit of services for people with dementia in two health districts, *Journal of Advanced Nursing*, 32(5): 1206–12.

16

Assertive outreach and the CMHN

A role for the future?

Caroline Cantley and Peter Caswell

Introduction

This chapter draws on an evaluation of an intensive community treatment team (ICTT) pilot project to explore the role of the community mental health nurse (CMHN) in assertive outreach services for people with dementia. The chapter begins by outlining the key features of assertive outreach and the background to the ICTT service and its evaluation. We then describe how the ICTT project operated in practice. In the section that follows, we discuss key dimensions of the role played by the ICTT staff. We conclude with some observations about how this pilot project can inform the CMHN's potential role in providing assertive outreach in dementia care.

Background

Assertive outreach, sometimes referred to as assertive community treatment or intensive case management (Ryan 1999), is a cornerstone of mental health policy in the UK. Assertive outreach services provide intensive support in the community for working-age adults who are severely disabled by their mental health problems and who are difficult to engage with services. A common aim of assertive outreach services is to reduce hospital admissions and enable people to remain in their own homes. Services take a variety of forms and key characteristics of successful assertive outreach have been identified (Hemming et al. 1999; The Sainsbury Centre for Mental Health 2003) as including:

- a multi-disciplinary team approach;
- working with clients in their own environment;
- frequent contact with clients and commitment to being proactive in maintaining contact even when this is difficult;
- a key worker who is responsible for the overall package of care for each service user;
- a low ratio of service users to workers, around 10:1;
- provision of services to meet basic needs and assist with practical everyday tasks;
- emphasis on developing trusting relationships with service users;
- no time limits to the service;

- provision of crisis intervention or links with existing crisis services; and,
- provision of specific evidence-based interventions.

It is also important that assertive outreach services are integrated into the wider system of services.

Origins and development of the ICTT project

The ICTT project was established by an NHS organization in the north of England, the Hull and East Riding Community Health NHS Trust. It was developed in a local service context in which higher than average care home placements in some areas covered by the Trust had provided an imperative for health and social services to find ways to better support older people in their own homes. Integrated intermediate care services for older people had gone some way towards addressing this need, but there had been no development of early, proactive and preventative services for people with dementia. In this context, the ICTT project was conceived as a means of promoting the health and quality of life of people with dementia and their families, and of avoiding over-dependence on services and unnecessary admissions to care homes and hospitals.

From the outset it was planned that the ICTT project would pilot the use of a model of 'assertive outreach' in older people's mental health services. The assertive outreach approach had hitherto been developed mainly in working-age adult mental health services. However, the Trust identified that this method of working could be applied in older people's mental health services where it would be consistent with the aims of intermediate care and of the National Service Framework for Older People (Department of Health 2001).

The project was established to cover one part of the Trust's catchment area, a geographically large patch with a population of approximately 130,000 (approximately 10,400 aged 75 years or more) living in small towns, villages and dispersed rural areas. The project's services were intended for people aged over 65 years, with new or existing memory difficulties, in situations where 'a higher and more intensive level of community treatment is required'. Key components of assertive outreach that the Trust identified as underpinning the project were more frequent and intensive support than was available from the standard CMHT service, and a focus on working with difficult-to-engage clients. More specifically, the aims of the project were:

- to provide timely, realistic and coordinated packages of care;
- to maximize the individual's well-being, independence, choice and dignity;
- to prevent admissions to hospital or care homes;
- to facilitate a planned approach to necessary admissions as a means of ensuring the best possible outcome for people with dementia and their carers.

As the service evolved, the following additional aim was identified:

- to provide comprehensive packages of therapeutic interventions to enable people with dementia to return home from hospital sooner than would otherwise be possible.

The project was staffed by one F grade community psychiatric nurse (CPN) and one B grade health-care support worker (HCSW). The service operated Monday to Friday from 9 a.m. to 5 p.m. Outwith these hours, support for clients was available from the main-stream out-of-hours service (comprising telephone support from an inpatient unit with access to an on-call CPN as required). The project staff were line managed within the Trust's Older People's Mental Health Services and remained closely linked with the Community Mental Health Team (CMHT) for the area.

The ICTT project was set up initially for two years and was subsequently extended for around nine months before being discontinued and the staff returned to mainstream CMHT duties.

The evaluation

An evaluation of the project was undertaken by the ICTT staff in collaboration with Dementia North, the regional dementia services development centre (Cantley and Caswell 2004). This chapter draws on the following data collected during that evaluation:

- Data on case activity over 16 months collected using structured referral/initial assessment and discharge forms designed specifically for this purpose. This comprised 48 referral/initial assessment forms and 34 post-discharge forms.

- Data on staff perspectives and activities collected through reflective practice diaries, kept by members of the team for approximately 12 months, and time diaries, kept by both staff for a total of 15 weeks in three separate periods.

- Data on the perspectives of 32 other service providers, who had contact with the project, obtained by postal questionnaire. The questionnaire contained pre-coded ratings of the ICTT, as well as open questions about the strengths and limitations of the service and suggestions for future development. To protect the anonymity of respondents the questionnaires were sent out from, and returned to, Dementia North.

Dementia North undertook most of the data analysis. It was evident from the analysis that the ICTT staff strove to ensure that, in their reflections and assessments of the project, they included problems and limitations as well as achievements and strengths.

The ICTT in practice

Needs and problems

The project operated an open referral system with referrals being channelled through the existing CMHT bases. The team provided a prompt response with approximately one-third of cases being seen on the same day or next working day, and almost 60 per cent within four working days. The vast majority of initial assessments were undertaken in the client's own home.

Most referrals included at least one of the following problems:

- deterioration in the client's mental health and/or increasing cognitive impairment;
- aggressive or disruptive behaviour;
- evident risks;
- carer struggling to cope;

- poor compliance with medication;
- client resisting service input.

The ICTT case-load, which on average comprised six cases, was characterized by:

- a high proportion of clients aged over 80 years;
- a very high proportion of clients with coexisting physical and mental health difficulties;
- a high proportion of clients with social support needs;
- carer stress in almost all cases;
- clients almost all receiving a complex mix of service inputs from across the NHS, social services and the independent sector.

The team assessed all clients as having significant memory and other cognitive difficulties, although many had not had a diagnosis of dementia confirmed by a medical practitioner. They assessed almost three-quarters of their clients as experiencing mental health problems in addition to dementia, quite frequently multiple problems or needs, and just over half of their clients as having behaviour that challenged others. They also assessed almost three-quarters of their clients as being 'at risk' of abuse, of non-deliberate self-harm, or of harming others.

Outcomes

Based on the team's assessment, across their case-load there was improvement in:

- a small proportion of physical health problems;
- a moderate proportion of problems with activities of daily living, social issues (housing, leisure, finance and social support), continence, sleep and risk of abuse or harm to self;
- a high proportion of problems with carers' stress, mental health needs, challenging behaviour, use of medication, risk of harm to others, and dressing and diet.

In the team's assessment, they achieved overall or partial success in achieving their aims in almost two-thirds of their cases. They identified a wide range of factors that contributed to them not achieving their aims in other cases, including: the client's, and sometimes the carer's, lack of insight or resistance to service involvement; the intractable nature of some problems; and limitations in the availability of other support services. On discharge from the project, approximately two-thirds of clients remained at home, with almost half having some increase in their care package.

The team was involved for over 12 weeks in almost half of its cases. The average duration of contact for cases that exceeded the project's 12-week limit was 18 weeks with a maximum contact time of 34 weeks. The vast majority of these longer-term cases (80 per cent) were closed within 18 weeks. We comment further on the team's duration of contact with clients below.

CPN and HCSW roles

The team reported that they worked directly with the person with dementia in all of their cases and that in most cases they also worked with a family member. In different cases, there was considerable variation in the number of contacts which involved only the client with dementia; some cases involved a high level of contact with the person with dementia on their own. Contacts involving relatives and not the person with dementia were usually infrequent. In a large number of cases, intervention involved occasional joint working with clients and their relatives; extensive joint work with clients and relatives occurred much less frequently.

In the vast majority of cases the team undertook five main interventions with the person with dementia, which they described as: 'being with'; emotional support; practical support; reminiscence and orientation. In approximately 40 per cent of cases, they also provided one or more of the following interventions: education, coping strategy enhancement, and developing problem-solving skills. Although the team identified life storybook work and validation therapy as potential interventions to be used with people with dementia, these were not used in practice.

The team reported interventions with carers in 30 cases. In almost three-quarters of these cases, the team undertook at least four interventions including: emotional support, practical support, 'being with', and education. Interventions focusing on coping strategy enhancement and problem-solving skills were undertaken with fewer carers and almost always in combination with this broader 'package' of support.

Direct contact with clients or their families accounted for an estimated 30 per cent of the ICTT workers' total working hours. Almost all cases involved a combination of individual input from the CPN, individual input from the Health Care Support Worker, plus some joint work. The HCSW spent about one-third more time working with people with dementia alone than did the CPN. Family work was generally undertaken jointly and the time spent on this was relatively limited; joint work was usually for specific tasks such as assessment or care planning. However, there were also a small number of cases in which there was a very considerable joint input from both workers; one case involving 21–30 hours joint input and one over 60 hours.

In almost three-quarters of their cases, the team reported collaboration or joint working with a combination of other NHS, social services and independent sector services. Both workers were involved, generally jointly, in activities related to working with other services.

Perceptions of the team's role

This section describes key dimensions of the roles of the ICTT staff, as we identified them from the comments of the staff and other service providers.

Providing therapeutic expertise

The ICTT staff did not generally see themselves as using highly specialized techniques or therapies. The following is a typical description of their perceptions of the essentially 'low tech' nature of the work:

> We have made contact with [a couple] every day this week. His wife, the main carer, is struggling with a marked deterioration in her husband's behaviour. Offered advice and support during these visits. I feel that being able to be present in the home at least daily helped his wife feel more able to cope and eased her worry over their future. On

occasions this week [she] has spoken of 'feeling near the end of my caring role' but with daily support and practical help she reported feeling more positive about her continuing role and the demands that will be made of her. Again it appears that 'being with' is very much the 'positive' that people required.

Overall, the team's perspective was summarized in the comment that 'our work is about time and patience rather than the application of specialized therapeutic techniques'.

The team's 'low tech' approach to practice was based in large part on their experience of their clients' reactions. For example, they found that clients were often distressed or uncomfortable with the use of the standardized cognitive or mental health assessment tools that underpin much CMHN practice. This led the team to question, and to a large extent, abandon, the use of these instruments.

Despite the team's very modest assessment of its expertise, other service providers rated the team's specialist knowledge and skills in working with clients very highly, for example, three service providers summarized the team's strengths as follows:

> Their strengths are their obvious and thorough knowledge of dementia. Also their interpersonal skills with patients and carers.

> They have undertaken some difficult and sensitive work and have always achieved a positive outcome.

> Very positive responses and action in crisis situations.

The team was acutely aware that many of the problems with which they were dealing were intractable and that the success or failure of their interventions was often the result of factors other than their expertise. For example, often an accident or the client's failing physical health limited what the team could achieve.

Having time

As noted above, the staff saw it as crucial that their role included 'having time' to allow for intensive work with people with dementia and carers. The following case example illustrates the importance of time and just how much time was sometimes involved:

> [We] are working with a lady to facilitate her return home after a long spell in hospital. Our current plan means we have to transport her home and back [to hospital] again at the end of the day. And further we are providing a lunchtime call as well. This takes approximately four hours of our working day.

The staff aimed to work within the 12-week time limit of the project and accepted the underpinning rationale of not promoting over-dependency on an intensive service input. However, they found that having a time-limited role did not always sit comfortably with the nature of the task that confronted them, for example:

> It is a classic situation with a person who has quite significant memory difficulties and no insight into the fact. The carer is very stressed and desperately in need of help and support. The person with the memory difficulties will not accept any support coming into the house, and maintains they are coping fine. The person attends day care 2 days per week but this is in danger of collapse. Any attempt to introduce support

services into this environment does nothing more than provoke anger and distress. What to do? Our view is to approach this situation very slowly so that in time we can hopefully develop a trusting therapeutic relationship. Unfortunately time is a luxury we do not have, however, we will see what we can achieve in our twelve(ish) week window of opportunity.

The team were realistic that time was not in itself a panacea and they did on occasion note cases that took up a lot of their time to limited effect. For example:

Our lady [in hospital] who I was taking home all week has become physically unwell again over the weekend and is now back on a general ward. We have spent a lot of time with this client but even with our high level of input we are unable to cover all the risks and eventualities.

The team 'having time' featured frequently in other services providers' comments about the benefits of the ICTT service. Other service providers identified the importance of the promptness of the ICTT response to referrals and in ongoing work. They particularly stressed the importance of the amount of time available to the team that enabled them to work intensively and in a person-centred way.

A number of service providers pointed out that the additional time available to the team was a function of having a smaller case-load than mainstream services, and some implied that it was this, rather than specialist expertise, that comprised the difference between the ICTT role and that of mainstream CMHT services. For example:

'Ability to provide the more intensive work required for a client which is not always possible for individual community psychiatric nurses to become involved in due to time/large caseloads.'

The team was aware that other service providers perceived them as being 'time rich' and this created some tensions for staff who at times felt under pressure to increase their case-load beyond what they felt was consistent with the intensive service that they aimed to provide.

Responding to service users' views and wishes

Being responsive to, and promoting, the views and wishes of people with dementia and their carers was central to the team's perceptions of their role. For example, the following extract illustrates the significance that the team attached to carer responses:

Another visit to another day care site with a different client today. Again I am trying to establish day care as a form of respite for a carer . . . Carer very pleased with positive outcome today. I feel I used my skills today with success and received recognition of this through the carer's obvious relief that all had gone well.

Permeating the team's accounts of its work was a strong awareness of the importance of respecting the views and wishes of the person with dementia and of their families/carers. This inevitably on occasion gave rise to dilemmas when the views of family members were not in accord with the views of the person with dementia. With some family conflicts, the team was able to work with the family to reach a resolution that met the person with dementia's needs, for example:

Although we did initially receive quite a hostile reception from the . . . lady's family, we eventually found a common ground from where we could work forward. I think the family was more reassured when they realized that [we] would be visiting on a very frequent basis.

The team also faced dilemmas about how they should respond to the expressed views of the person with dementia if these views ran counter to their professional assessments of the person's best interests. For example, there were a number of cases in which the staff thought that the person with dementia's rejection of services was detrimental to their diet, hygiene or health.

Sometimes the team judged client refusal of services to be a result of the person's lack of insight. Their aim in these cases was that 'ways can be found to move forward' through 'assessment of capacity and ability to make informed choice and duty of care' combined with 'time, patience and creativity'. This could, however, prove very difficult, for example:

[We] are continuing to work with a lady who is provoking a high degree of concern because it is felt that her needs are not being met appropriately. What is compounding our difficulties at the moment is the lady's absolute lack of insight into her current situation. Despite our persistent attempts to raise our concerns in as sensitive and tactful manner as possible, we are meeting with very little success.

In some cases the client's initial reluctance was overcome and the staff felt comfortable that the outcome had both respected their client's wishes and met their best interests, for example:

I succeeded in getting one of our lady clients to day care. She has been very resistive to this but today she decided to accompany me there. I had decided to stay with her for a while to offer support but she was soon immersed in conversation with others and I was soon forgotten.

In other cases, however, the team felt that the person with dementia's refusal to use services simply reflected their dislike of what was being offered. In such cases, the team respected the wishes of clients who, having been persuaded to try a service, still rejected it. For example:

A visit with a gentleman client to a day care facility. He is not keen to attend but agrees to visit. I felt this morning went well but the client does not wish to go again. Again we are back to square one.

Other service providers generally rated the team's responsiveness to service users and carers very highly. They particularly commented on the team's ability to engage with people with dementia and their families, to keep the client at the centre of assessments, and to support carers, for example:

Has definitely helped a few of my patients to return home when without ICTT they would have had to go into residential care against their wishes. ICTT have established a rapport with patients who have refused all contact with social services/health services.

(Hospital ward staff)

One aspect of the team's role was in acting as an advocate for the person with dementia and sometimes their relatives, particularly in enabling them to take calculated risks. This role was not always well accepted by other service providers, for example:

At the ward round today it was made abundantly clear that [man known to team] would not be returning home, and it was the family's wish that he go into residential care. I believe I provoked quite a degree of irritation when I asked what was the gentleman's view in this matter. I received some curious looks and mutterings about risks and being realistic.

Managing risks

A recurring theme in the team's accounts of their work was their role in the assessment and management of risk. The team sometimes acted as an advocate for their clients in taking risks, for example:

> This lady and her son are adamant that she should go home but staff on the ward and her social worker feel that residential care would be more appropriate. It was agreed that she would return home with a home care package and our support. [We] felt that she should be given the chance to go back home but we both acknowledged the high risk of falls and that medication compliance may be a problem.

Staff reflected that as their experience grew, they became more comfortable about living with, and enabling their clients to live with, a higher level of risk than would usually be acceptable to other service providers.

Other service providers rated the team's role in the management of risk very highly. Social services staff in particular valued the way the ICTT team shared responsibilities with them in assessing and managing risks.

Promoting independent living

The team saw part of their role, in line with the formal aims of the project, to be about enabling people with dementia to remain in their own homes or to return to their home from hospital. In the team's view, assisting with hospital discharges was an area in which they could make a particularly positive impact, for example:

> The end of a week attempting to re-establish a client back home following a period of time on a general ward. All has gone well. Family are concerned over her abilities but she has managed very well this week with our support. This type of work with clients appears to be a successful side of the project in that we are able to dedicate a large period of time in order to assist with any difficulties. My time has been well spent this week.

However, admission to a care home or hospital was not necessarily seen as failure by the team if they felt they had respected the person's wishes and assisted them to stay at home for longer than would otherwise have been possible. The following diary extract illustrates this point:

> [We] have had two opposite results with two clients recently. One chap has returned home and is coping well. Another lady has entered residential care with her husband and is coping very well. It may seem strange but I consider both these outcomes to be good results. Why? Because each of these people is happy to be where they are. Yes it would always be nice to help someone remain in their own home but certainly there are times when this is not the only and appropriate option open to us.

Other service providers generally rated the team highly in respect of its role in helping people to remain in, or return to, their own home. The following comments illustrate these positive views:

> Excellent service which I feel helped maintain my client in living in the community.
>
> (Social worker)

> Intensive support provided maintaining independence at home. Extra level of support/care I am not able to provide, avoiding in some cases (most) hospitalization.
>
> (Community psychiatric nurse)

Influencing and supporting other services

The ICTT team worked closely with other services, for example in facilitating clients' access to other services and monitoring the support provided. One of the main challenges for the team was to influence other services, particularly when their practice skills or approach of these services, or their resources, were inadequate to meet client needs.

The team noted some success in influencing other services, particularly traditional nursing–medical hierarchies and the extent to which consultant colleagues listened to their views and respected their opinions. They also noted cases in which they negotiated an agreed definition of the 'problem' based on discussing different perceptions of risk issues and appropriate standards, for example:

> Referral from social services expressing lots of concern about a lady very much at risk. When did joint visit found lady who hoarded newspaper and tins of cat food. Agreed that living environment not ideal but lady had lived like this for years and thought it a social matter rather than a mental health crisis.

However, other service providers sometimes resisted the team's input and advice. For example, some care home staff were anxious that the team might be critical or interfering. In such instances the team's approach was to try to persuade staff that they wanted to support them and work in partnership with them. In some settings the team found it difficult to have as much influence as they would have liked. They described, for example, how at a case review with '15 people present all offering opinions in a noisy and confusing meeting', their suggestion to discuss the possible options with the client and relative in a more private and calm environment was ignored.

Sometimes the team felt that referrals to the ICTT were left 'too late', that they were picking up problems at a stage when other services had not been able to meet their objectives, and that it was difficult to see how the ICTT could retrieve the situation. The team felt that, as the ICTT was a pilot project and required to demonstrate its value, they had to take these cases on and 'give it a go', even though they were sometimes doubtful from the outset about the prospects of success.

Other service providers appreciated the team for its optimism, objectivity, flexibility and reliability in working with them on individual cases. They also identified the team as having a valuable role in providing them with support and advice, for example:

> I have enjoyed working with the team and my own practice/insight has also benefited.
>
> (Community social work team member)

The ICTT gives support in very difficult circumstances at times. Always on hand to offer help to [CMHT] team members. An invaluable service.

(Mental health practitioner)

They have been totally supportive to me as a colleague . . . I have been so grateful for their professionalism and support.

(Hospital social work team member)

The only critical comments about the team's role in working with other services came from two social services respondents who commented that the team had limited understanding of what social services could realistically provide in care packages and that this sometimes led service users or carers to expect more than could be offered.

Summary

Overall, it is clear that the staff involved in the ICTT, and other service providers thought that the project made some very positive contributions in individual cases and in providing specialist expertise and support in the service system.

The ICTT project demonstrated a number of dimensions of the role that CMHNs can play in the provision of assertive outreach: providing expertise, having time, responding to service users, managing risk, promoting independence and, influencing and supporting other services. This role has much in common with the roles that have been identified more generally as being undertaken by CMHNs in dementia care (Keady and Adams 2001). The area in which the ICTT role was most distinctive was in the time available for staff to work directly and intensively with people with dementia and with family members. The ICTT role was also distinctive in the strong emphasis that staff placed on understanding, respecting and responding to service users' views and wishes, particularly those of people with dementia themselves.

The experiences of the ICTT pilot project provide some pointers for other CMHNs embarking upon the development of assertive outreach in dementia care. In particular, the ICTT experience suggests the importance of the following:

- Working intensively with the person with dementia alone as well as, in most cases, with a family member.
- Having input from both CMHNs and support workers.
- Having staff with knowledge and expertise in assessment and the use of a range of interventions (although not necessarily very specialist therapeutic techniques).
- 'Having time' to work intensively in each case and build relationships with people with dementia and their carers.
- Taking very seriously, and responding to, the views and wishes of people with dementia and their families.
- Advocating for people with dementia.
- Supporting, advising and influencing other services.
- Sharing risk management responsibilities with other services.
- Being committed to supporting people with dementia in their own homes but not necessarily seeing admission to a care home or hospital as a failure.

However, there are many questions about the role of CMHNs in developing assertive outreach teams in dementia care that this project has highlighted as requiring further investigation. These questions include:

- How do people with dementia and their carers view this model of intensive service intervention?
- Should not assertive outreach teams be multi-disciplinary (cf. Ryan 1999)?
- What is the optimal ratio of support worker time to professionally qualified CMHN time?
- What services should be provided out of office hours?
- Should intensive services of this kind be provided without time limit?
- Is it necessary, or desirable, to have a separate assertive outreach team or could the benefits of the team be achieved as effectively through other service structures, for example, by increasing the staffing in mainstream CMHT services to allow for more intensive working (cf. The Sainsbury Centre for Mental Health 2003)?

The ICTT project adopted some, but not all, of the key characteristics of assertive outreach as developed in working-age adult services. The experience of the ICTT project suggests that there is great potential in learning from and adapting assertive outreach to fit the specific needs and circumstances of people with dementia and their families. However, the ICTT project was a small-scale development and more work is needed on implementation and evaluation of assertive outreach before we can with confidence identify the model or models that are effective in dementia care. There is also a need to examine how assertive outreach compares with other approaches to delivering intensive support for people with dementia, for example, intensive care management (Challis et al. 2002). Most importantly, any development of assertive outreach must be undertaken as part of a coordinated, multi-disciplinary and multi-agency response to the needs of people with dementia and their families (Audit Commission 2000; Department of Health 2001; Lingard and Milne 2004).

Lessons for CMHN practice

- Assertive outreach has been little used in dementia care. While its potential is clear, there is a need for further piloting and evaluation of service models, including multi-disciplinary models.
- Key aspects of the CMHN role in assertive outreach demonstrated by the ICTT project were: providing expertise, having time, responding to service users' views and wishes, managing risk, promoting independence and influencing and supporting other services.
- There remain many unanswered questions about the role of CMHNs in assertive outreach in dementia care.
- There is a need to examine how assertive outreach compares with other approaches to delivering intensive support for people with dementia.
- It is important that any development of assertive outreach is undertaken as part of a coordinated, multi-disciplinary and multi-agency response to the needs of people with dementia and their families.

Acknowledgements

The study on which this chapter is based was supported by the Hull and East Riding Community Health NHS Trust and Dementia North (Trust). We are particularly grateful to Nicola Burton for her contribution to the work of the ICTT and to collecting data for the evaluation; and to Monica Smith for her help throughout the evaluation. We are also grateful for the assistance of the many service providers who shared their views and experiences of the project.

References

Audit Commission (2000) *Forget Me Not: Mental Health Services for Older People*. London: Department of Health.

Cantley, C. and Caswell, P. (2004) *An Evaluation of the Intensive Community Treatment Team (ICTT) Project: Confidential Report to the Hull and East Riding Community Health NHS Trust.* Newcastle: Dementia North, Northumbria University.

Challis, D., von Abendorff, R., Brown, P., Chesterman, J. and Hughes, J. (2002) Case management, dementia care and specialist mental health services: an evaluation, *International Journal of Geriatric Psychiatry*, 17(4): 315–25.

Department of Health (2001) *Older People: National Service Framework for Older People*. London: Department of Health.

Hemming, M., Morgan, S. and O'Halloran, P. (1999) Assertive outreach: implications for the development of the model in the United Kingdom, *Journal of Mental Health*, 8(2): 141–7.

Keady, J. and Adams, T. (2001) Community mental health nurses in dementia care: their role and future, *Journal of Dementia Care*, 9(2): 33–7.

Lingard, J. and Milne, A. (2004) *Integrating Older People's Mental Health Services: Community Mental Health Teams for Older People. A Commentary and Resource Document.* Commissioned by the Children, Older People and Social Care Policy Directorate, London: Department of Health.

Ryan, P. (1999) *Assertive Outreach in Mental Health*. London: Nursing Times Clinical Monograph, Emap Healthcare.

The Sainsbury Centre for Mental Health (2003) *Mental Health Topics: Assertive Outreach*. London: The Sainsbury Centre for Mental Health.

17

'A third way?' Challenging behaviour and the development of CMHN services

Case site examples from Hong Kong, China and Manchester, UK

Cordelia Man-Yuk Kwok and Philip Hardman

Introduction

In one way or another, the lived experience of dementia levies a toll on all of those involved. That toll becomes progressively more pronounced when the person with dementia becomes challenging in their behaviour and unpredictable in their response to emotional, physical and environmental stimuli. In such circumstances, family carers may be driven to the point when their own health suffers and their relationship with the person with dementia sours. The person with dementia finds that the unmet need being communicated through their behaviour goes unrecognized and the response may well be punitive and damaging to their well-being. Care staff can struggle to cope with challenging behaviour and the struggle is often exacerbated by a lack of training in techniques that may ameliorate and contextualize such behaviour. Presented with such a scenario, and usually not having access to appropriate support or supervision, care workers are put in an invidious position and may deliver care that is below expected standards.

As highlighted in the first book (Pugh and Keady 2003), there is a clear need to interpret and respond to challenging behaviour, to understand the nature and meaning of the 'challenge' and to develop person-centred methods of response. In meeting these needs, it becomes important to consider the cultural context of the individuals concerned, an issue that was overlooked in Pugh and Keady's (2003) previous review of challenging behaviour and the role of the community mental health nurse (CMHN). Cultural beliefs and values often shape how a disease is perceived or understood and, in turn, influence when and why families seek help and how clinicians respond (Wang 2004). In an attempt to broaden the debate and set cultural influence (and CMHN practice) within an international setting, this chapter reviews traditional Eastern and Western beliefs about dementia and the meaning that 'challenging behaviour' has within these cultures. Instinctively, it would be expected that CMHN practice within these two cultures would be divergent but, using Hong Kong Special Administrative Region (HKSAR), China and Manchester, UK, as comparative case study sites, we found that this is not necessarily the case. Indeed, by and large, Western approaches to dementia care are philosophically influenced by the 'best' of holistic values found in traditional Chinese culture and practically influenced by Western concepts of education and systematic intervention. It is this combination that provides the unique flavour and practice context of CMHN work irrespective of country, or culture, of origin.

From this synthesis what emerges is a 'third way' wherein there is a 'joining together' of the best elements of each worldview; the joining together also reveals gaps in the stitching and glimpses of where additional padding is required. For instance, the challenge to the CMHN in HKSAR is to confront some traditional cultural beliefs and to introduce aspects of the Western paradigm, particularly related to early diagnosis and treatment. On the other hand, the challenge to the CMHN in the UK is in continuing to move away from the dominance of the bio-medical model, to develop person-centred dementia care in the community and advocate for better understanding of the cultural, psychological and social roots of challenging behaviour. The nature of these challenges starts to focus attention upon the role of a CMHN in dementia care and particularly in relation to challenging behaviour and cultural influences. This is now discussed in relation to two CMHN services, one in HKSAR, China, and the other in Manchester, UK.

Case site: HKSAR, China

China is the largest developing country in the world, and its population of those aged over 60 years has reached more than one hundred million, about 10 per cent of the total population (Zhang 1998). There are about five million people with dementia living in China, with some 300,000 new cases each year and the incidence of dementia has become regarded as a significant 'threat' to the well-being of the older population (Sheng 2003). The Hong Kong Special Administrative Region (HKSAR) has a population of 6.7 million, 96 per cent of whom are ethnic Chinese and has a rapidly ageing population with 11 per cent of the total population being older people. By 2016, it is projected that the older population will reach 1.9 million, which will approximate to 13 per cent of the total population and by 2029 one in every five of the population will be aged 65 or above. In a 1995 community-based study, the prevalence of moderate to severe dementia in HKSAR was found to be 4 per cent for those aged 65 or above, a percentage that doubled every five years until around the age of 90 (Chiu et al. 1998).

With changes in demography and technology, and increasingly expensive health care, dementia care is one of the challenges facing caregivers, clinicians, practitioners, researchers, managers and policy-makers in HKSAR, as well as in other developed countries. The government policy of HKSAR is aiming to be responsive to the changing needs of the growing ageing population and to the provision of appropriate services to those with care needs. In reality, service development for dementia care has been a neglected area in China and HKSAR until the last few years. Mental health services for older people in HKSAR are in their infancy and dementia care has started late compared with services in the UK; however, the pace of development in recent years has been remarkable. In the past decade, several studies on the prevalence of dementia in China have been published, and since HK reverted to Chinese rule in 1997, an 'Elderly Commission' has been established to focus on the strategic direction of elderly care services (Elderly Commission 2001). Additionally, medical services, community support services and new initiatives are being established to address the inadequacies in quantity and quality of existing service (Chiu and Zhang 2000).

Cultural influences

Chinese traditional medicine, influenced by the philosophy of Confucianism, Taoism and Buddhism, is centuries old and by Western standards highly abstract. It focuses on the integration of a person's entire being: physical, mental, emotional, spiritual, and the close relationship between the human and his or her day-to-day lifestyle in the context of the social and natural environment. The Chinese tradition of medicine has a unique physiology in understanding the human body and a unique pathology for understanding its disorders.

At the heart of this unique tradition is the belief that health and illness may be defined within a broader understanding of the universe itself. The body is a small-scale physical representation of the large-scale cosmos and both are inherently connected through the force of *chi*, a form of energy that permeates both the universe and the body, the rhythm of which can affect the functioning of the body. Health exists when there is a balance between: the rhythmic working of the body; its adjustment to the environment; and its harmony between function and emotion. Illness occurs either as a consequence of internal imbalance or where malign and demonic spirits possess that body. The key concept in understanding beliefs about balance and imbalance is the relationship between *yin* and *yang*, or forces that are at one and the same time both opposing and complementary. *Yin* means shadow, and is a passive, non-aggressive feminine force, while *yang* means sunlight, and is a hard, active and aggressive masculine force. *Yin* and *yang* are forces that exist together and are at the same time both opposing and complementary. The degree to which the forces are balanced is fundamental to understanding both the nature and phase of disease.

There is a distinction between *Kuang* and *Dian*, where *Kuang* (excess of *yang*) leads to excitatory behaviours, restlessness, agitation, hallucinations, and so on, and *Dian* to a more passive psychotic presentation. Importance is placed upon the observation and description of behaviour with successful treatment outcomes being dependent upon how well the behaviour or imbalance is understood. Traditional Chinese medicine is therefore a subjective discipline, based more on a philosophical model and the experiences of the practitioner than on the proven scientific rigour of Western modern medicine, and from this subjectivity cultural beliefs regarding health have developed over many centuries. Box 17.1 outlines the commonest Chinese cultural beliefs about dementia.

Such beliefs and values often shape how a disease is perceived or understood. These generally negative responses by caregivers and patients interfere with their willingness to

---

Box 17.1 Chinese cultural beliefs about dementia

- Dementia is a form of normal ageing.
- Dementia is a form of mental illness.
- Dementia is a source of shame.
- Dementia is a result of fate.
- Dementia is a retribution for the sins of the family or the actions of the ancestors.
- Dementia is an imbalance between the *yin* and the *yang*.

seek appropriate medical assessment and intervention; consequently, there have often been delays in seeking treatment and care. Challenging behaviours emerging within dementia are subject to these same beliefs, and their presentation may often be the factor that brings the person with dementia to the attention of health services. Commonly the person with dementia will be maintained within the family for extended periods of time, being deliberately isolated from the outside world, and only when the family feel unable to cope, usually due to excessive or disruptive behaviour, will outside help be considered. It is at this point that family support breaks down and the person is blamed, scapegoated and ultimately rejected. Such a response reflects the 'shame culture' of Chinese society and the perpetrator of challenging behaviour is regarded as bringing shame not only to the immediate family but also to the ancestors.

BPSD: a guided care protocol approach

In HK, challenging behaviour falls under the wider labelling of the 'Behavioural and Psychological Symptoms of Dementia' (BPSD). To stop such labels simply stigmatizing people with dementia, it is crucial to view symptoms as multi-factorial in nature and encompassing a number of modalities. BPSD occur in up to 90 per cent of people with dementia at some time during their experience of living with dementia (Herrmann et al. 2000) and they are the most common reason for psychiatric referral, treatment with psychotropic drugs and admission into continuing care (Steele et al. 1990). They are also one of the main causes of caregiver stress, excess disability and diminishing quality-of-life for both the caregiver and the person with dementia (Steele et al. 1990; O'Donnel et al. 1992; Stoppe et al. 1999).

There is usually no one best treatment for any behavioural disturbance (Rabins et al. 1999), but it is advocated that non-pharmacological interventions should be considered as the first line in dealing with BPSD (International Psychogeriatric Association 1998) as often the negative impact of using a 'pharmacology only' intervention illustrates that drugs are often inappropriate or ineffective (Ballard and O'Brien 1999). Moreover, neuroleptics may lead to deterioration in the cognition of persons with dementia and increased risk of falls (McShane et al. 1997). Careful assessment and analysis, which culminate in individualized programmes and draw on knowledge of the person's biography, offer the greatest prospect for therapeutic success (Burns 1999; Ballard et al. 2001; Pugh and Keady 2003).

Hong Kong is a juxtaposition of Eastern and Western culture where both Chinese tradition and Western paradigm coexist to maximize the positive effects of interventions. In addition to the traditional holistic approach, there is an increasing emphasis placed upon evidence-based practice and the application of standardized tools to help in the assimilation and evaluation of information about behaviour. It is important to address the limitations of long-held traditional beliefs and clinical practices which are based upon subjective opinions and experiences. This is a major challenge to the CMHN in the dissemination of knowledge and the raising of standards of care in the community.

Frequent difficulties in dementia care can arise because the person with dementia may not be able to verbally communicate their needs and instead rely upon behaviour to do so. Unfortunately, this may lead to these behaviours being misinterpreted and their underlying needs remaining unrecognized and unmet. The CMHNs, based at the Kwai Chung Hospital, are presented with the difficulty of confronting traditional beliefs among care staff while educating them about responding appropriately to BPSD. To do so they utilize a 'guided care' protocol to facilitate and support caregivers in the community to identify the underlying causes of BPSD through systematic assessment and then to make choices about appropriate interventions related to validated techniques (Kwok 2004). Guided care draws others into a process that the wider community mental health team has developed through a systematic literature search review of papers, clinical practice guidelines and advice from recognized experts.

Guided care aims to provide a standard, semi-structured approach to support care staff, who often have only a basic level of training, to understand the need of people with dementia who experience symptoms of BPSD. Such an approach is important for improving the standard of individualized dementia care and the well-being of people with dementia. The principles of the care protocol are based on the concept of personhood (Kitwood and Benson 1997) and the '4D approach' which focuses attention upon carers to: *define* the problem, *decode* the unmet need, *devise* a treatment plan, and *determine* if it works (Rabins et al. 1999).

The CMHNs of the psychogeriatric team adopt the guided care protocol as an intensive educational intervention. By doing so they aim to introduce a conceptual framework for the management of BPSD; to assist care staff in analysing and decoding the causes of BPSD, step by step; and teaching them how to review the care plan in such a way that individual interventions begin to suggest themselves. A 'guided care' protocol is utilized to help less experienced care workers identify the core information and skills required to implement evidence-based individualized care. When devising a treatment plan, the interventions for BPSD are based, to some extent, on traditional beliefs which emphasize the required balance for the whole body, allowing care staff or family members some familiarity with the approach.

Taking an educational approach is probably wise when it is remembered that the CMHN is addressing deeply rooted traditional beliefs about dementia and without doubt the CMHN faces a significant challenge in educating the wider population about dementia, its diagnosis and treatment (Chow 2000). Certainly most of the staff working in residential facilities in HKSAR do not have prior education or experience in mental health, and at best some may only have unsophisticated training to help them attempt to cope. The care workers' inability to cope might itself exacerbate behaviour problems, which in turn could increase the care workers' feeling of being overwhelmed by the situation. This is perhaps the same for family carers and for both involvement with the CMHN is crucial.

It is the nurses' role to act as a skilled and knowledgeable helper to family members providing care in the community and staff in care homes. In the HKSAR carers will receive written materials and information regarding the causes of BPSD for individual patients, and it is vital for the CMHN to support care staff as they learn to implement the appropriate interventions while also providing skills training in behaviour management. Achieving a successful outcome in the management of BPSD requires humane, empathetic and skilful application of evidenced-based interventions. Appropriate interventions are those that are broad-based or multifaceted; they consist of different components which have to be flexible, creative and consistent (Mahoney et al. 2000). Most of the applied interventions focus upon modifying the role of care worker or family carer to become the 'interventionist' when symptoms of BPSD occur. Placing a growing awareness on how they, as care staff or family member, interact with patients is crucial to understanding interaction as being a common antecedent of behavioural disturbances.

Overall this guided care protocol approach has an emphasis on the involvement and education of the carer. It actually creates the logic for caregiver involvement and it is a highly structured method of intervention that recognizes caregivers playing an important role in behavioural treatment to alleviate BPSD in people with dementia. Interventions occur in a logical sequence of steps or phases and these are: (1) identification; (2) assessment; (3) treatment; and (4) evaluation. As carers are in the best position to impact upon the person with dementia's behaviour, they are taught to identify, and respond to, specific behavioural problems. The guided care protocol is necessary to identify the core information and skills required by carer workers to implement evidence-based individualized care. Hopefully, it can help to reduce the stress and strain in caring for people with dementia, and the quality of life for both patients and caregivers can be improved. The following case exemplar illustrates this.

Case example 1: Mr Y.

Mr Y. a 58-year-old retired administrator, first presented to the mental health service in 2000, although the family first noted changes in 1998 when he was still working. He was tidy, well-groomed and polite, although rather flat, lacking in spontaneity and presenting with significant word-finding difficulty. His MMSE was 16/30. Over the subsequent year, gradual deterioration was noted despite his treatment with a cholinesterase inhibitor. As his condition had become worse significantly within several months, his wife felt unable to cope and he was sent to reside in a private old-age home in 2004.

Following admission, he was referred to the CMHN, as he paced around aimlessly, tried to leave the nursing home and entered the female toilet and someone else's bedroom at night. He had poor sleep and outbursts of aggression to staff were reported. The CMHN implemented the guided care protocol and supported care staff to better understanding the causes of behaviours and their underlying needs. His wife was assisted to reframe her beliefs about his condition and to gradually, although never wholly, accept their relationship to neurological damage.

First, delirium was excluded as Mr Y. did not present the acute onset or relevant symptoms, and there were normal findings of laboratory tests. There was no other sign of physical problems such as pain and discomfort, or the side effect of medications. The frequency and severity of the neuropsychiatric symptoms and the level of distress to the caregivers were carefully assessed and recorded by the CMHN. Mr Y. was found to see things that were not there and to grasp at imaginary objects on the table. The main concern was his agitation; it was severe and very prominent presenting as a dramatic change and distressing for the caregivers. He resisted help, was uncooperative, cursing angrily and even hit his wife.

The carers were assisted to understand the impact of transition upon Mr Y. His move into the nursing home had created sudden and unexpected changes in both his routine and environment. The CMHN identified carer behaviours such as placing demands on the patient that exceeded his capabilities, overreacting towards his disorientation (e.g. when he went into the female toilet). The CMHN then worked with the care staff to develop and implement a care plan, with defined goals described in a positive way and based on the best combination of interventions.

The strategies encouraged by the CMHN were for care staff to be patient, allowing Mr Y. ample time to complete tasks or when he refused to cooperate to try again later, to think about their communication and simply state instructions one step at a time, to offer him reassurance, comfort and appropriate structured activities. The CMHN demonstrated each action or task allowing Mr. Y. to perform parts of the task that could still be accomplished.

Despite guiding the care of the staff there were no improvement in cognitive functioning or reduction in frequency of the hallucination, however the frequency and severity of agitation of Mr Y. improved considerably and the distress of caregivers was significantly reduced.

Case site: Manchester, UK

If the Western bio-medical model was influenced by the Industrial Revolution, then its very heart has historically been in the northwest of England. Now suffering from the loss of its industrial base, Manchester has some of the highest levels of social and economic deprivation in the UK. The Manchester Mental Health and Social Care Trust (MMHSCT), Older Peoples Services provide a range of secondary care in patient and community mental health and social care services to people over 65 years, and is mindful of the changing demography of this group. The population of the UK is increasing and ageing. By 2020 the numbers of people over 65 years will increase from 9 million to 14.5 million, or 25 per cent of the adult population. It is further estimated that the number of people in the UK who have a dementia will increase from a current 600,000 to 855,000 (Department of Health 1997). The need to respond to this demographic shift poses challenges and opportunities to society and as older people are the greatest consumers of health and social care, public policy will need to reflect this reality. At a local (city) level, Manchester is no exception to this need for new pathways of understanding and response and has acknowledged this through the development of a specialist Elderly Dementia Intervention Team (EDIT). This section will describe how EDIT developed from 1998 at a time when little research or information was available to inform service provision and development.

EDIT: team development and structure

The need for the EDIT team was identified, and its development prompted, by the experiences of a variety of health and social care professionals who worked in the existing services for older people and who had experienced a gap in service provision manifested through patterns of repeated readmissions to the assessment unit of people with a diagnosis of dementia but who displayed 'challenging behaviour'. EDIT developed from the streamlining of long-term care services for older people with mental illness in the then North Manchester Healthcare NHS Trust.

The original team consisted of staff who had previously worked in long-term care settings of two continuing care wards. At its onset, EDIT comprised a team manager, four CMHNs, and seven senior support workers (SSW). The clinical nurse specialist who worked with the team on a weekly sessional basis provided leadership in the areas of clinical practice and team development. This larger team is divided into two smaller teams who each work in identified geographical areas. All staff expressed a preference to work in the field of challenging behaviour and dementia. From its outset the challenge for the team was to work within the principles of personhood and the social model of dementia as advocated by Kitwood and Benson (1997) and to adhere to those principles in the reality of day-to-day CMHN practice. The team are one element of a multi-professional community mental health service. EDIT provides a service to those people living in any type of residential care setting and their own homes that have a diagnosis of dementia, are over 65 years of age and are described by referrers as presenting with challenging behaviour. Referral criteria exist, of which a key element is that the person must have a diagnosis of a dementia, a diagnosis made by a consultant psychiatrist to ensure the diagnosis is reliable. This ensures the referred person has been involved in a 'gold standard' diagnostic process. The team works with informal and formal carers, working in partnership with the patient and those in the caring role. The results of the pilot indicated the main referrers were consultant psychiatrists (38 per cent) and that 66 per cent of people referred were from residential homes and nursing homes, including specialist Elderly Mentally Ill (EMI) homes.

Cornerstones and principles

The cornerstones of the EDIT team are built on five principles, which are briefly considered below:

1   *Personhood and the social model of dementia.* Kitwood (1995) suggests:

> We should understand a person's dementia as being the result of a complex interaction between the personality, their physical health, their biography or life history, their social psychology (the network of their social relationships) and their neurological impairment (the dementia).

He continues to say that all these factors combine to make a person who they are, and to concentrate on one of the factors only without proper regard for the others is to treat the person as less than a whole person.

2   *Challenging behaviour as a form of communication.* 'All so-called "problem" behaviours should be viewed primarily as an attempt at communication related to unmet need. It is necessary to seek to understand the message being conveyed and so engage with the need that is not being met.' (Kitwood and Benson 1995)

3   *Risk taking.* Kemshall and Pritchard (1997) suggest that a person-centred approach to care is essential to both understand and manage risk taking in the person with dementia: 'People with disabilities are frequently trapped in other people's perceptions of risk and their negative images.'

4   *Empowerment, choice and autonomy.* Dementia is not a *normal* part of ageing. It can have a colossal impact on a person's life and the life of their carer. The person with dementia can be disempowered in two ways, first, by the illness itself and second, by other people's reactions to the illness *and* the person concerned (Goldsmith 1997). The practice of the team is to evoke the principles of personhood while recognizing that the ability of the person with dementia to make decisions will deteriorate over time and may be variable from day to day or hour to hour, however, they will be empowered to make decisions wherever possible.

5   *Challenging ageist attitudes and practice.* Older people are one of the most marginalized groups of people in our society, and those who have a mental health problem such as dementia experience a double jeopardy. The effects of negative stereotyping and ageist attitudes can be harmful for older people both as individuals and as a whole group. Effects can range from denial of services and amenities to withdrawal and depression.

EDIT staged process of working

The role of the CMHN within EDIT is best summarized in Figure 17.1 as it is their clinical responsibility to lead at each stage of the process as it applies to individual clients within their own case-load. The CMHN will direct the interventions of the SSW within the staged

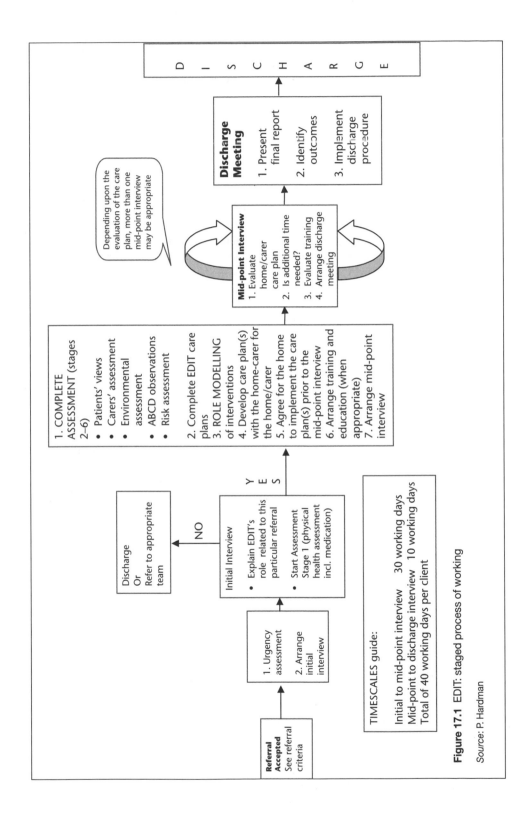

Figure 17.1 EDIT: staged process of working

Source: P. Hardman

working process. An essential element of the work of the CMHN is their ability to develop relationships and partnerships with people. Recent changes in legislation and policy have attempted to place users of services at the centre of their own care. This shift of emphasis seeks to enable the user of the service to become an active consumer of health care rather than a passive recipient. The CMHN needs to reflect upon their practice and, if needed, develop alternative ways of working that fully engage in collaborative arrangements to care founded upon genuine therapeutic partnerships that optimize the person's well-being. The essence of the work is to identify causatory factors of 'challenging behaviour' and formulate a strategy to assist those in the caring role.

CMHN practice interventions begin with a comprehensive assessment of the person as a unique individual, including their life review. Further detailed assessment follows to identify any external, environmental influences or internal factors, such as physical or mental health needs which could affect the individual's well-being and contribute to the occurrence of challenging behaviours. The needs of the carer and their perceptions of the issues are recorded verbatim to prevent assumptions or misinterpretations from the nurse. Attempts are always made to record the views of the person with dementia and this exercise has been revealing and insightful.

Team members undertake a period of observation within the individual's environment. Observations are recorded using an ABCD chart; 'D' represents the decision made based upon the observations. Assessment is complemented by care plans written in partnership with patients and carers. Interventions identified in care plans are implemented and evaluated. Team members role model interventions to carers and this has become an important technique to demonstrate approaches and to maintain clinical integrity. Nursing practice will focus upon the achievement of care plan outcomes that demonstrate a health gain for the patient. The nurse will use the indicators of well and ill being as proposed by Kitwood and Bredin (1992) to objectively reflect upon the effectiveness of their work. The team work to prevent hospital admission, and evaluation of the pilot project has shown that this occurs, but recognize that on occasions it may be unavoidable. Where admission is required, the team follow the patient and work with them in the ward setting.

To measure the outcome of nursing interventions, information from the following sources is taken and collated:

- registered nurse clinical opinion;
- patient's opinion (whenever possible);
- carer's opinion;
- use of verified tools;
- reflective practice;
- clinical supervision;
- audit.

The CMHN work towards the achievement of the following outcomes:

- The individual's distress is relieved.
- The individual's behaviour becomes less challenging.
- The carer's level of distress is relieved.

- Carer's knowledge increases.
- The individual remains in their own environment.

The model reflects a psychosocial approach as the main thrust is about changing attitudes and providing a consistent, individualized, person-centred approach to people who are distressed by dementia. A psychosocial approach would gather information, hypothesize, test an approach. Interventions would be individualized and consist of a 'package' best suited to the profile built from the information gathered about the circumstances of the person with dementia and their carer. The work of the CMHN in EDIT is now elaborated through the following case exemplar.

Case example 2: Mrs B.

Mrs B., an 87-year-old lady, moved from her family home of some 40 years into full-time residential care six months ago. Following the death of Mrs B.'s husband, she came to the attention of the local older age mental health services when her family became concerned about her memory problems, her ability to self-care and to keep herself safe. Mrs B. was diagnosed as having Alzheimer's disease. Several care packages failed to meet her self-care needs and maintain her safety within her own home. Mrs B. was physically active and independently mobile. She was able to use verbal communication but the content and flow often became disjointed. She needed some assistance to maintain her self-care.

A first referral had been made to EDIT and their interventions had assisted the staff within the home in responding to meet Mrs B.'s needs during the initial period of her stay in the home. Some months later the care staff were describing difficulties that they encountered while trying to assist Mrs B. in meeting her self-care needs. She was described as becoming 'restless' and of 'wandering' around the home. On reaching the doors she would often attempt to leave the home, stating she needed to go home. At such times confrontations would take place, which left Mrs B. and care staff feeling anxious and upset. The home manager felt that if Mrs B.'s current behaviour continued, then reluctantly a transfer to another establishment would have to take place.

The home had begun to make a high number of repeat referrals to EDIT. Rather than continue to accept the referrals on an individual basis a more structured approach was taken regarding the home as a 'whole' unit. EDIT would continue to work with individual residents and staff but underpinning this work the team would develop, deliver and evaluate a programme of staff education and skills development. The aims of the work were jointly agreed between the home management team and EDIT. The aims of the work were to raise awareness of dementia and to demonstrate a positive impact on the delivery of care to residents. The programme delivered 16 hours of presented sessional time running in parallel to the individual working with referred residents and care staff using the Staged Working Process. Advice and discussions were had with the home management as to the development of support systems for staff within the home.

The evaluation of the programme was positive. In brief, care staff valued the programme, feeling it was both necessary and relevant. The manager stated that the whole approach had had a positive effect upon client care and went on to add that:

- Staff feel more confident about working with people with dementia and are not afraid any more.
- Staff support systems have been identified and altered to provide more and easier access to supervision.
- The staff had been able to utilize information from the course, i.e. the use of life review in order to build upon a relationship with the clients instead of their previous way of interacting with them.

Returning to Mrs B., the most important person at the centre of all this activity, she remained at the home and staff became more accepting of her as a person as they developed their knowledge of her past life and of her individual experience of dementia. Following the programme for a period of 12 months, it was noted that referrals from the home reduced considerably almost to zero.

Discussion

As in many other places around the world, CMHN teams in HKSAR and Manchester are working to improve the care of people with dementia who present with challenging behaviour. If achieving a holistic person-centred understanding of challenging behaviour is the destination, then both teams are heading in the right direction by placing emphasis upon supporting and training carers. The pace of travel differs between the teams, although this probably reflects the age difference between the services involved, and in HKSAR there are additional pressures regarding the targeting of community nursing resources, particularly as the development of services for the early recognition and diagnosis of dementia is limited. Consequently, there may be as much pressure for the role of the CMHN to develop in this area as there is to directly respond to challenging behaviour. The case of Mr. Y. highlights the impact of this delayed referral and the negative influence of traditional beliefs about dementia. He presented to the CMHN service only when he was very disturbed, and when his behaviour had became intolerable to his caregivers. In Manchester, there are similar pressures, evaluation of EDIT concluded that the model of working should be replicated across Manchester. Today, the challenge to the team is to retain the specialist focus of its work during a time of significant changes in the provision of community services and furthermore to counter pressures to move towards a generic model of delivering community mental health nursing care.

The experience of Manchester is also that when resources are targeted towards the resolution of challenging behaviour, the CMHN can find him or herself very much in demand. In the case study of Mrs B., it is clear that the home in question was making many repeat referrals to EDIT, suggesting, not only the extent of the problem, but also that once support is offered, it is often outstripped by demand. It is often difficult to work out how much input, and how comprehensive, intensive and frequent the training and education, are required to support formal caregivers should be.

Both teams are therefore aiming to develop the skill base of care staff, aiming for them to better identify, understand and intervene in challenging behaviour and to do so through a systematic process. The Kwai Chung hospital team use the term 'guided care' which acts to define the role of the CMHN as one of advising, educating and supporting other care workers to respond appropriately to BPSD, literally to 'guide the care'. Overall, there is the belief that successful resolution of BPSD requires the skilful application of interventions that are humane and empathic but also very much evidence-based. EDIT call this staged working and in Manchester the CMHN is seeking to focus attention upon the well-being of the person with dementia, with much of the work being around changing of attitudes through education, effective joint care planning and role modelling interventions.

Developing an efficacious and practical approach towards the care of older people in these homes is desirable but equally valuable are the positive benefits of augmenting community care by using nurses as advisers/educators to the family caregiver. These benefits include reducing admissions to hospitals, reducing emergency room usage, and improving patients' ability to perform activities of daily living (Chappell and Dickey 1993; Kane 1989; Mezey 1990). In Hong Kong there is the wider, and sensitive, challenge of confronting cultural beliefs about dementia that often lead to families feeling such a great sense of shame that they may refuse to seek help until it is too late and a crisis occurs. EDIT are faced with the same kind of challenges and, as a more mature service, are deliberately working towards a goal of empowerment for people with dementia and a reduction in discrimination. By addressing these issues, both teams of nurses are aiming to enhance well-being and quality of life for people with dementia.

It is important that the needs of the CMHN are not overlooked. To work effectively in this rewarding but psychologically demanding area of practice, effective clinical leadership is essential to provide an overall vision and a focus for the day-to-day work while ensuring reflective practice, and clinical supervision; case management and education deliver effective support. Leadership and team support systems should be underpinned by a culture of audit and reflection which together can positively challenge the effectiveness of nursing interventions and thus push the boundaries of nursing practice.

Summary

In HKSAR, the development of 'psychogeriatric' teams is in infancy and, akin to many Asia-Pacific regions, whereas the clinical practice is heavily influenced by the globalizing concept of the evidence-based medicine and evidence-based health care. The interventions are structured and systematic approaches are based on the scientific inquiries: systematic reviews of a panel of experts and the needs of the individuals. This is one of the options for facing the challenges in delivering consistent, appropriate and high quality health care with the available resources. In Manchester, old age psychiatry services are now, at the age of nearly 30 years, starting to reach maturity and EDIT, as a nurse-led development, reflects this. EDIT has successfully risen to the challenge of moving away from the bio-medical model and demonstrates innovation in nursing practice.

Both teams are clearly trying to achieve the desired 'third way'. In HKSAR, there remains a leaning towards the bio-medical model and care must be taken to avoid establishing an old culture of dementia care that would do little to influence some of the traditional health beliefs about dementia and those affected by it. In Manchester, there has been a drive towards achieving a fully psychosocial model but care should be taken not to exclude the physical entirely but to identify its place within true holistic practice.

Lessons for CMHN practice

- In preparing others to work with challenging behaviour, the fundamental principle is to start with yourself, examining your belief system, in order to become comfortable working within a psychosocial model.
- The role of the CMHN is not to directly intervene in challenging behaviour but to role model, educate, advise and support other health-care workers and families to do so in a person-centred way.

- Challenging behaviour is best understood from within a holistic and humanistic 'new culture of care' rather than reliance upon the soulless use of mechanistic assessment tools and structures.

- Successful outcomes should be demonstrable improvements in well-being for people with dementia and stress reduction for those providing care.

- Practice by the CMHN has to be supported by a robust structure of clinical leadership, supervision and reflective practice.

References

Ballard, C. and O'Brien, J. (1999) Pharmacological treatment for behavioural and psychological signs in Alzheimer's disease: how good is the evidence for current pharmacological treatments? *British Medical Journal*, 319: 138–9.

Ballard, C., O'Brien, J., James, I. and Swann, A. (2001) *Dementia: Management of Behavioural and Psychological Symptoms*. Oxford: Oxford University Press.

Burns, A. (1999) Non-pharmacological treatment of BPSD in dementia: report on behavioural and psychological symptoms of dementia (BPSD): a clinical and research update, *International Psychogeriatrics*, 11 (Suppl. 1): 88.

Chappell, H. and Dickey, C. (1993) Decreased rehospitalization costs through intermittent nursing visits to nursing home patients, *J Nurs Admin*, 23: 49–52.

Chiu, H.F.K., Lam, L.C.W., Chi, I. et al. (1998) Prevalence of dementia in Chinese elderly in Hong Kong, *Neurology*, 50: 1002–9.

Chiu, H.F.K. and Zhang, M. (2000) A Chinese view, in J. O'Brien, D. Ames and A. Burns (eds) *Dementia*, 2nd edn. London: Hodder, pp. 345–52.

Chow, T.T. (2000) Diagnosis and treatment of dementia in Chinese patients, paper presented at the 10th conference on health problems related to the Chinese, 30 June–1 July 2000.

Department of Health (1997) *A Handbook on the Mental Health of Older People: The Health of the Nation*. London: HMSO.

Elderly Commission (2001) 23rd Meeting of the Elderly Commission (24 April 2001). URL http://www.info.gov.hk/hwb/text/english/advise/ summ23.htm

Goldsmith, M. (1997) *Hearing the Voice of People with Dementia: Opportunities and Obstacles*. London: Jessica Kingsley Publishers.

Herrmann, N. and Black, S.E. (2000) Behavioral disturbance in dementia: will the real treatment please stand up? *Neurology*, 55(9): 1247–8.

International Psychogeriatric Association (1998) *Behavioral Psychological Symptoms of Dementia (BPSD) Educational Pack*. Macclesfield: Gardiner-Caldwell Communications Ltd.

Kane, R.L., Garrad, K., Skay, B.A. et al. (1989) Effects of a geriatric nursing practitioner on process and outcome of nursing home care, *American Journal of Public Health*, 79: 1271–7.

Kemshall, H. and Pritchard, J. (1997) Introduction, in H. Kemshall and J. Pritchard (eds) *Good Practice in Risk Assessment and Management*, vol. 2. *Protection, Rights and Responsibilities*. London: Jessica Kingsley Publishers.

Kitwood, T. (1995) Cultures of care: tradition and change, in T. Kitwood and S. Benson, *The New Culture of Dementia Care*. London: Hawker Publications.

Kitwood, T. and Benson, S. (1997) *The New Culture of Dementia Care*. London: Hawker Publications.

Kitwood, T. and Bredin, K. (1992) Towards a theory of dementia care: personhood and well-being. *Ageing and Society*, 12: 269–87.

Kwok, C. (2004) A guided care protocol for management of behaviour and Psychological Problem of

Dementia (BPSD) in care facilities, in *Abstract Proceedings of the International Psychogeriatric Association*, Asia Pacific Regional Meeting in Seoul, Korea.

Mahoney, E., Volicer, L. and Hurley, A. (2000) *Management of Challenging Behaviors in Dementia*. Baltimore, MD. Health Professions Press.

McShane, R., Keene, J. and Fairburn, C. (1997) Issues in the drug treatment for Alzheimer's disease, *The Lancet*, 350: 886–8.

Mezey, M.D. (1990) GNPs on staff, *Geriatr Nurs*, 11: 145–7.

O'Donnel, D.F., Diachman, D.A., Barnes, H.J., Peterson, K.E., Swearer, J.M. and Lew, R.A. (1992) Incontinence and troublesome behaviour predict institutionalization in dementia, *Journal Geriatr Psychiatry Neurol*, 5: 45–52.

Pugh, M. and Keady, J. (2003) Assessing and responding to challenging behaviour in dementia, in J. Keady, C. Clarke and T. Adams (eds) Maidenhead: *Community Mental Health Nursing and Dementia Care: Practice Perspectives*. Open University Press.

Rabins, P., Lyketsos, C. and Steele, C. (1999) *Practical Dementia Care*. Oxford: Oxford University Press.

Sheng, S. (2003) Senile dementia becomes major threat to Chinese elderly, *People's Daily*, Beijing.

Steele, C., Rouner, B., Chase, G.A., and Folstein, M. (1990) Psychiatric symptoms and nursing home placement of patients with Alzheimer's disease, *American Journal of Psychiatry*, 147: 1049–51.

Stoppe, G., Brandt, C.A. and Staedt, J.H. (1999) Behavioural problems associated with dementia: the role of newer antipsychotic drugs, *Ageing*, 14(1): 41–54.

Wang, H. (2004) *Dementia caregiving and care seeking experiences in Chinese culture*. Alzheimer's Association. Available at: www.alz.org/04china_wang.asp

Zhang, M.Y. and Guo, Q.H. (1998) An epidemic review on dementia in China, *Chinese Mental Health Journal*, 12: 9–12.

18

Matters of the heart
The CMHN and palliative care

Kay de Vries

> You should have seen her face when she saw the house.
> (Husband of a woman with Creutzfeldt-Jakob disease, speaking
> of his wife's reaction when she came home after
> a respite admission in a hospice)

Introduction

One of the certainties of life is that every person must die and yet death remains a subject feared and avoided by many. Bereavement experiences and responses are highly influenced by the manner in which people came to know of their illness and how the time was spent between diagnosis and death (Shuchter and Zisook 1993; Parkes 1996). An important element within these events is the place of death, and home is often cited as the place that most people would prefer to die. However, few are actually able to achieve this (Hunt 1997; Higginson 2003). For various reasons many dying people spend the last days of their life in a hospital, hospice or other care environments, such as a nursing home, rather than remaining at home. Reasons for this include family members or significant others not being able maintain care as the illness advances and the person becomes more and more incapacitated (Neale 1993), or that the dying person may not wish to die at home or may not have been consulted on preferred place of death (Pemberton et al. 2003). The literature on preferred place of death has, however, focused on the cancer death, and there has been little research on end-of-life wishes for people with dementia.

There is a large literature on the experience of caring for a person with dementia at home, often referred to as 'carer burden', that will not be addressed in this chapter. What is lacking within the literature is specific discussion and research on the end-of-life experiences of the person with dementia, the carers and the community services that may be accessed when the dying person remains at home, and perhaps one of the most overlooked areas of CMHN practice is their role in caring for people with end-stage dementia. This chapter will review the available literature on the subject and draw upon a study that involved people with Creutzfeldt-Jakob disease (CJD) and their palliative care experience (de Vries 2006). Data appertaining to the role of the CMHN will be drawn out of the study to provide a framework for practice.

Place of death

An increasing number of older people are now living alone and a 1987 interview survey of end-of-life experiences of 639 people, as reported by carers, found that the group living alone were much more likely to progress to institutional care, and this group were largely those of the frail and confused older people (Seale 1990). Comparing this study to a 1969 survey (Cartwright et al. 1973), Seale (1990) identified that the duration of time over which mental confusion, depression and incontinence were experienced has risen and these increases can be related to the greater proportion of older people in the 1987 study.

Using the data from a retrospective national population-based interview survey of relatives or officials of 3696 people who had died in the last quarter of 1990 from 20 English Health Districts (Addington-Hall and McCarthy 1995), a secondary analysis was conducted to investigate how many patients die from causes other than cancer (Addington-Hall et al. 1998). From this, 170 people with dementia were identified and these were compared with 1513 people with cancer (McCarthy et al. 1997). The authors concluded that people dying with dementia have symptoms and health-care needs comparable to those with cancer. The most frequent symptoms reported for dementia patients were mental confusion, urinary incontinence, pain, low mood, constipation and loss of appetite. These were of similar frequency as those reported for cancer patients but people with dementia experienced them for longer. This factor of 'protracted' death was also the conclusion of Black and Jolley (1990) in a review of the characteristics of 97 patients dying during one year while under the care of psychiatry for old age services.

Seale (1990) found that those who were the most poorly serviced and supported at the end of life were the older cognitively impaired. Most of the group providing care for the dying person with a diagnosis other than cancer and in old age lived alone, or in small family units, and resources were general poor. The services for those people dying at home with a non-malignant disease were, overall, less than those with a cancer diagnosis and the burden of care often fell directly onto a frail elderly spouse (Seale 1990). While these surveys are retrospective carer views, they do provide insight into the problems experienced by this group. It has been clearly identified that the progressive neurological and functional decline of the person with dementia causes a great deal of stress on families and caregivers (Mace et al. 1999), however, little research has been conducted that directly addresses the experiences of the person with dementia. Also, in discussing the support mechanisms in place for this group at the end of life, no mention is made of the role of the CMHN in relation to the end-of-life experiences of those who died at home or moved into institutional care near the end of life.

The role of the CMHN and palliative care

The role of the CMHN in care provision of people with dementia has been little explored (Adams 1996; Pickard 1999; Nolan et al. 2002). Advanced skills of the CMHN in providing continuity of support for both the dementia sufferer and their family/carers, particularly in relation to the early recognition of dementia, have been identified (Grace 1993; Ineichen 1994; Manthorpe et al. 2003) and the diversity of the work of the CMHN highlights the issue of whether the role should have a social or health orientation (Gunstone 1999). It is consistently emphasized that the CMHN role is not to provide personal care for people with dementia but that their role is primarily to carry out assessments, provide carer education and service liaison (Pickard and Glendinning 2001; Manthorpe et al. 2003). The physical needs of people with dementia have been a neglected area of care (Adams 1999; de Vries et al. 2003; de Vries 2006). This has been due to the focus on carer needs that has dominated the literature on dementia care (Adams 1999). This focus on carer needs is not confined to CMHNs. It has also been identified that GPs focus on the needs of the carer over that of the needs of the dementia sufferer (Blunden and Long 2002).

As the illness progresses, the physical needs of the person with dementia become increasingly more important. Although Keady and Nolan (1995) identified that a key component of a care package is the need for continuity of care, where care provision is proactive as the dementia progresses, Pickard (1999) points out that a holistic view of care for this group remains undeveloped, particularly in relation to who should or does provide the physical care. The need for coordinated care for older people with dementia within primary care has been highlighted (Keady and Nolan 1995; Pickard 1999; Pickard and Glendinning 2001), however, the end-of-life issues for this group are not specifically addressed within the discussion.

In an investigation carried out in Sweden, comparing perceptions of good support, between 316 staff working closely with people caring for a person with dementia to 121 staff working with carers of people in palliative cancer care, Albinsson and Strang (2003) highlight providing support at the time of death and after as a major difference between dementia and palliative care staff. Dementia care staff placed this of lowest importance on a 10-point item list of categories identified by the researchers, this, despite late-stage dementia clearly meeting WHO criteria for palliative care. There are equally important issues in the ability of palliative care staff to communicate with and understand the specific needs of people with dementia (de Vries et al. 2003; de Vries 2006) and Albinsson and Strang (2003) identified that trying to relieve the family's feelings of guilt was an important factor for dementia care staff but not for palliative care staff, which further emphasizes the focus of care on carers rather than on the person with dementia. The non-generalizability of these findings to all staff is addressed by the researchers.

The attitude of nurses towards death and dying is a significant factor in enabling them to work with large numbers of dying people and the hospice model and environment offers an opportunity for sharing in the experience of dying with dying people themselves. The importance of this shared experience is identified by Addington-Hall (2000) as one of the barriers to the integration of people with dementia to the hospice environment. However, there has recently emerged discussion on the integration of palliative care and dementia care education in recognition of dementia as a terminal illness. Within the UK, initiatives to forge collaborations between mental health and palliative care services have been proposed, following research on the palliative care needs of people with dementia (Addington-Hall 2000; de Vries et al. 2003; de Vries 2006), and it has been shown that collaboration and multi-disciplinary work between palliative care and psychiatry for older people teams can have a positive impact on the end-of-life care for people with dementia (Lloyd-Williams and Payne 2002). However, this work is significantly underdeveloped.

Specialist palliative care teams rarely become involved in the end-of-life care of a person with dementia, unless the person also has a cancer diagnosis (Lloyd-Williams 1996). They do not have the expertise, or the capacity to meet the needs of this patient group and their carers within the community at present. Surveys of the views of family doctors support the move to extend the remit of this team beyond cancer and to provide a 24-hour care service, and the need for improving liaison within the teams and making it clear who was responsible for what type of care when patients were discharged home was highlighted (Boyd 1993, 1995; Higginson 1999). The CMHN is in a position to take a key role in coordinating the palliative care needs of people with dementia in collaboration with other members of the primary care team.

Team collaboration

Nolan et al. (2002) highlight the challenge of providing dementia care and the need to develop partnerships between providers and users at an early stage of the illness. This need for collaboration is further highlighted for end-of-life care for people with dementia (Addington-Hall 2000; de Vries et al. 2003; de Vries 2006). Within the CJD study (de Vries 2006), the earlier cases (1997–2002) did not access or utilize community dementia care services. Due to the age of the variant CJD group and some of the symptoms of CJD, they have been frequently referred to psychiatric services in the early stages of the disease, a situation also found by other researchers on the experience of people with CJD (Douglas et al. 1999; Spenser et al. 2002; de Vries et al. 2003), but not necessarily to dementia care services in the later stage.

In a later case (2003) the family utilized a large and sophisticated multi-disciplinary team, of which one member was a CMHN, in this case an Admiral Nurse (AN) – see also Chapter 20 in this book by Emma Pritchard and Sue Ashcroft-Simpson for additional discussion on the role of the Admiral Nurse. This team also consisted of the following: specialist community palliative care nurse (SCPCN), district nurses, GP, physiotherapist, wheelchair therapist, occupational therapist, dietician, speech therapist and the liaison nurse from the CJD Surveillance Unit. The care package for this case was complex and elaborate and it was the assertiveness of the carer (also considered a member of the team) that was pivotal in much of the decision-making of the team, as indicated in the following quote from the SCPCN:

> [H]e knows who to contact, he taps into each one of us now, individually as he wants, he knows who to contact with each one. And sometimes if he doesn't want to he won't contact any of us . . . I suspect if she stopped swallowing it would be (CJD UNIT) that he contacts, not the speech therapist or the dietician, she tends to be his main [contact] because he's involved with the CJD Society.

Carers of people with CJD have been heavily funded and supported following the government responses to the emergence of variant CJD in 1996 and many, as in this case, are closely involved with CJD groups. Grants are offered to help with cost (Turner 2004) as the following example of a care package demonstrates. The family had nine carers providing 21 hours a day, seven days a week care, including two carers during the day. They had a wheelchair, hospital bed, fully adjusted armchair, hoist and a specially adapted vehicle. Also included in the package was counselling for the family and friends, complementary therapies and a team to help clear the downstairs room ready for adaptations to be made (CJD Support Network 2004).

The CJD group support bears no similarities to that which is in place for other people dying at home and this difference is further commented on by the SCPCN:

I've not known of any care to be so well formulated and so well coordinated as this package of care, it's quite unusual. I dread to think how much it costs, to be honest, because it would be so nice to get everybody this care.

This further opens the charge by Douglas (1992) that deluxe dying is provided for a few while ignoring the needs of the majority, or a service Field (1994) describes as 'five star' dying. While these comments are made in relation to cancer, dying and hospice, it applies equally to the 'elitist' support to the CJD group. Due to the youth of the victims and the distressing nature of the clinical progress of variant CJD, it could become defined as a 'dreaded disease' in the future (de Vries 2004, 2006) with irrational fear driving policy without consideration of the large number of older people with dementia who cannot access these services.

The success of the CJD home-care package is such that most people with CJD are now cared for at home until death and could provide a template for developing care packages for the wider dementia group (de Vries 2006). The effectiveness of a comprehensive home-care package for people with dementia was demonstrated in a US study by Volicer et al. (2003). The researchers found that care recipients who received psychiatric care, were involved in hospice programmes, and had effective pain relief for chronic conditions that caused chronic pain, particularly arthritis, were more likely to die at home, or stay at home significantly longer than those who did not receive this input. It was recognized that chronic pain worsened behavioural symptoms of the dementia and made it more difficult to keep the person at home.

Moving from familiar surroundings

Little empirical study has been carried out on the transition of a person with dementia from home to an acute environment or into institutional care. The role of the CMHN in managing such a transition, whether an inpatient service, nursing home or use of a respite facility is important, but is also under-researched. Referral to palliative care services, including the community services, has been determined in large by the cancer death experience and cancer care is the focus of palliative care within the present model, with limited admission criteria for people with non-malignant diseases such as motor neurone disease and multiple sclerosis.

Specialist palliative care is deemed an 'acute' service within the category and definition of the service and admission into the service of a person with dementia, who may have a 'long' and unpredictable prognosis, become a matter of concern, where 'long term' has a negative connotation for acute areas of health care (de Vries 2006). Making a prognosis for the progress of dementia to end stage is problematic due to the variability of the disease trajectory for the different types of dementia and accurate predictions remain one of the difficulties in determining an admission to palliative care services for people with dementia (Luchins et al. 1997; Hanrahan et al. 1999).

Respite care

Respite in palliative care is an under-researched area (Ingleton et al. 2003), even though it is considered good practice to use respite as part of a package that would enable patients and carers to make choices about preferred place of death, a factor that has been advocated in UK government policies (Department of Health 2000, 2001; Pemberton et al. 2003). It has been recognized that CJD cases do benefit from input from palliative care services (Douglas et al. 1999; Bailey et al. 2000; Barnett 2002; de Vries et al. 2003; de Vries 2003, 2006), however, the philosophy of palliative care, day care and inpatient respite facilities raise issues of the suitability of the environment for people with dementia.

Respite services are an integral part of many packages of care that are developed to enable a person with chronic or acute illnesses to support carers in maintaining care at home. The findings from the CJD study (de Vries 2006) confirmed that carers will take up services only if they are consistent with their perceived needs or they consider them to be of a suitable quality (Braithwaite 2000). Two attempts at using the respite services offered by a local hospice were unsuccessful in the view of a carer of one of the cases of CJD. The removal from her home for a period of respite was likened to 'abuse' by the carer and she had her first major myoclonic fit during this admission. In this case it was not that the quality of the hospice care was poor, but that the traumatic and stressful experience of being taken from home to a strange environment was seen as unacceptable to the carer:

> [I]t's like child abuse, it's somebody left out in the park by themselves and something . . . I can only react on her experience in the hospice. She was alright in the hospice, there was no distraught kind of thing. But there must have been a reaction for her to have a deep, to have a first spasm and then to, you know, the facial expression I saw when she came back . . . so there must have been a reaction and that's why, you know, as long as I can keep going I'll keep her in the house.

In another case, where the person with CJD was cared for at home by her husband, one of his greatest fears was that she would be admitted to hospital.

Day hospice care

While it is well established that respite and day care services are an important part of a strategy to maintain care of the person with dementia at home, the appropriateness of the use of palliative care respite and day care for this group needs to be carefully considered. Palliative care day services have been largely under-researched. The type of activity that is conducted generally includes a review of patients' symptoms, some treatments and a variation of activities such as complementary therapies and art and music therapy (Higginson et al. 2000). There was no evidence of people with dementia being admitted to this service in the survey carried out by Higginson et al. (2000).

Comparing activities carried out in day care for people with dementia and hospice day care suggests that hospice day care does not provide activities that would be appropriate for the dementia group. An attempt to utilize the day care for one of the CJD cases who was at an advanced stage of the illness, was extremely traumatic for the day hospice staff, other patients attending the day hospice and, most significantly, for the person with CJD. She demonstrated extreme distress and agitation throughout the visit, refusing to eat or speak and spent the entire time trying to struggle out of her chair. Responses of the other patients to the person with dementia highlight the 'novelty' aspect of the CJD experience (de Vries 2004, 2006) as described by the manager.

And she rocked and rocked and rocked to try and tip the wheelchair over. We had to have a nurse with her doing one-to-one all the time. And even in the wheelchair she'd try and slide out of that. And she just looked such a frightened lady and I just thought ... the other patients were obviously distressed ... The, the conversation, the whispering, there wasn't ... they were just focused on her all the time and they couldn't ... I suppose they didn't want to stare, but they couldn't help it. And it just, the whole day just was focusing on this lady. And they were scared to move out of their chairs.

As long as they were able to give one-to-one support she was calmer, however, before the end of the visit it was clear to the day hospice manager that they would not be able to repeat the visit. The poignancy of her description of the experience cannot be adequately expressed simply in the words used below, when she describes just *how* the patient uttered 'Why?' as both a question and an accusation 'and I told him that we could not accommodate their need. And when he first came back, she just looked at him, and said 'Why?' That was really the first word she'd uttered all day. 'Why?'

The experience of another CJD admission to a day hospice was also traumatic for the staff and patient, however, the team managed to accommodate the person for a number of admissions. This was managed by a family member staying with the person with CJD for a number of initial visits, and then leaving her handbag behind when she did leave. In both of these cases the person with CJD was described by the day care staff as having 'a fear of abandonment', confirming findings on the respite experience of people with dementia by Pickard and Glendinning (2001).

Clearly there needs to be a balance between the support for the carer and the impact of being moved from a familiar environment for the person with dementia, albeit for a short period of respite. Research on the use of respite for carers of people with dementia has focused predominantly on carer experience but very little on post-respite impact on the person with dementia. In one study, Burdz et al. (1988) found that the problematic behaviour of the person with dementia improved with respite care but paradoxically the caregivers reported a significant post-respite worsening of the relationship. This confirms how the person with dementia may experience bereavement both as a manifestation of the illness and as a result of the move from home and it has been shown that people with dementia of the Alzheimer's type still respond to their illness, even after their 'illness-insight' has disappeared, expressing a chronic trauma related to separation, loss, powerlessness, displacement and homelessness (Miesen 1997). A similar response was identified for the person with variant CJD (de Vries et al. 2003; de Vries 2006).

The importance of the diverse and individual circumstances of all cases of CJD (and of dementia) cannot be understated and family members of some people with CJD who were admitted to a hospice for end-of-life care could not speak highly enough of the care they received, referring to the hospice environment as 'Shangri-La' in one case and it was clear that the hospice environment stabilized the psychological state of the person with CJD in two cases of inpatient admission (de Vries 2004, 2006).

Discharge from hospital

There is little research on the admission and discharge of people with dementia between hospital and the community and the CMHN should be a key team member in any admission or discharge plan for people with dementia, whether to an acute unit or for long-term care. The need for hospital admission often indicates that the person is reaching the terminal stage of the dementia (Black and Jolley 1990; Lyketsos et al. 2000) and it is an opportunity to plan end-of-life care with other team members such as the community palliative care service. Lyketsos et al. (2000) suggest that admission and discharge of people with dementia between hospital and community are areas of care in urgent need of investigation and policy development, particularly in relation to costs, length of stay and mortality rates. In their survey of the discharges of 21,251 people (from one hospital in the USA) aged 60 or older at the time of admission, they found (overall) 3.9 per cent of the group had a dementia, with 8.9 per cent in the age group 85 years and older. Of significance, the researchers report that many of the conditions that were more prevalent in the group with dementia, such as urinary tract infections, drug psychoses, organic psychotic conditions, and behavioural, functional or social complications of dementia could have been prevented, recognized earlier, or managed in other settings, reducing the need for acute hospitalization.

Admission for long-term care

Placing a family member in a nursing home is one of the most difficult decisions that family caregivers may have to address and the need for support in the decision-making required of family members/carers of people with dementia has been highlighted in a number of studies (Gessert et al. 2001; Forbes et al. 2000; Kramer 2000). Challenges faced by families of people with late-stage dementia are complex. They may experience guilt associated with the institutionalization of the family member, unfamiliarity with death in general and death due to advancing dementia, and have limited understanding of the natural cause of late-stage dementia. In these cases they need support in coming to terms with some of the events that occur during dying and after death such as admission to an acute unit or a nursing home or the introduction of artificial feeding and other end-of-life interventions (Gessert et al. 2001).

What is the involvement in palliative care for CMHN?

The absence of research on the CMHN experience of palliative care allows only anecdotal report within this chapter. These were gained through informal discussions with a number of CMHNs and indicate consistency of experience. CMHNs reported that they were finding more frequently that the person with dementia is remaining at home until death. Reasons for this vary. There is a general expectation that the carer will look after the person with dementia at home and they have often made significant adaptations at home at an earlier stage of the dementia trajectory. The team composition will depend on the condition or type of illness and, as death approaches, the role of the CMHN becomes less easy to define, particularly when the district nurse or SCPCN take on more and more responsibility for the physical care of the dying person. CMHNs report a range of team composition, often with a large membership, as was found with the CJD case, with up to 15 members sometimes. The family then receive many visitors, all with their own agendas, often carrying out repeated assessments with poor consistency in the messages being given to the family. Further confusion to the issue is that key worker roles are divided between social services and the health-care team. Proposed changes in this approach to a single assessment procedure are locally managed and have yet to be evaluated.

Although the importance of collaborative team work is highlighted, support and care for people with dementia and their carers are problematic when a large team is involved, and undermines the recognized importance of carers requiring a person they know and trust to assist them in dealing with crises as they occur. Keady and Nolan (1995) suggest that the CMHN often provides this role due to the relationship that has evolved over a period of time. This trust relationship can be of crucial importance if the need to negotiate the use of a respite service, or admission to a care environment near the end of life arises.

It is of particular importance to enable people with dementia to be supported, maintained and cared for in their own homes until death, if that is their wish. That it *is* their wish is also an important consideration, and while the issue of advanced directives have not been addressed in this chapter, there is a need for further research and policy development on the issue of how and where people with dementia wish to end their lives. While 'The Preferred Place of Care' Document (Pemberton et al. 2003) was specifically designed for planning end-of-life care for people with cancer, it does offer a framework/template for the CMHN that may be used in collaboration with other primary care team members, to explore the end-of-life wishes of people with dementia and their carers. The nature of the dementia experience and disease process would suggest that the initiation of discussions about death and dying should take place at an early assessment stage, at a stage when the person with dementia could participate meaningfully in any discussion about death and dying with their carers and health-care team members. Gessert et al. (2001) recommend that advance care planning would both improve end-of-life care for dying people with dementia and improve the experience of family members involved in end-of-life decision-making and bereavement experiences. If the opportunity to include the person with dementia in end-of-life discussions is missed due to disease progression, it is still important that these are discussed with carers at an early stage.

Summary

In this chapter I have attempted to draw together a selection of palliative care and dementia care literature (of which there is a vast amount), focusing on the end-of-life events and experiences of people with dementia, and drawing on data from a study on the palliative care experiences of people with CJD (de Vries 2006). The support and funding for people with CJD cannot be compared to that which may be accessed by carers of people with other dementias, however, the CJD experience does offer a framework/template for potential policy and funding developments in dementia care at the end of life.

There is a vast literature on the carer experience of the person with dementia. However, in recent literature it has been highlighted that the physical needs of people with dementia are marginalized, as are the views and voices of the dementia sufferers themselves. CMHNs do not offer 'hands-on' care, but their position in caring for the person with dementia remains crucial as the coordinator of this care, as they become physically more and more incapacitated. The CMHN may be the one health-care professional who has the complete trust and confidence of the carer, and as the advocate for the person with dementia can ensure that only the best palliative care services and support are provided for them.

Lessons for CMHN practice

- Recognizing that dementia is a terminal illness and within the assessment process making preparation for the management of dying through early discussion and documentation of preferred place of care at the end of life, so that support mechanisms can be put in place as the dementia progresses.

- Single assessment process that identifies the CMHN as the key worker for the coordination of all care at an early stage so that a relationship of trust can be developed with the person with dementia and their carer.

- Collaboration with palliative care community services (and other primary care workers) in putting support systems in place and ensuring a streamlined service, making it more clear who is responsible for what type of care.

- A system of hospital liaison for discharges from hospital of people with dementia who may not be known to the CMHN.

- Ensure as little as possible disruption of the person with dementia from environments of familiarity and security.

- Being involved in support, education and training initiatives for district nurses, SCPCNs, GPs and other primary care workers in caring for people with dementia at the end of life.

References

Adams, T. (1996) Informal family caregiving to older people with dementia: research priorities for community psychiatric nursing, *Journal of Advanced Nursing*, 24: 703–10.

Adams, T. (1999) *Recent Developments in Dementia Care*. London: EMAP Publications.

Addington-Hall, J.M. (2000) *Positive Partnerships: Palliative Care for Adults with Severe Mental Health Problems*. London: NCHSPC and SPAPCC.

Addington-Hall, J.M., Fakhoury, W. and McCarthy, M. (1998) Specialist palliative care in non-malignant disease, *Palliative Medicine*, 12: 417–27.

Addington-Hall, J.M. and McCarthy, M. (1995) Dying from cancer: results of a national population-based investigation, *Palliative Medicine*, 9: 295–305.

Albinsson, L. and Strang, P. (2003) Differences in supporting families of dementia patients and cancer patients: a palliative perspective, *Palliative Medicine*, 17: 359–67.

Bailey, B., Aranda, S., Quinn, K. and Kean, H. (2000) Creutzfeldt-Jakob disease: extending palliative care nursing knowledge, *International Journal of Palliative Nursing*, 6(3): 131–9.

Barnett, F. (2002) Nursing patients with variant Creutzfeldt-Jakob disease at home, *British Journal of Community Nursing*, 7(9): 445–50.

Black, D. and Jolley, D. (1990) Slow euthanasia? The deaths of psychogeriatric patients, *British Medical Journal*, 300: 1321–3.

Blunden, P. and Long, R. (2002) Dementia and GP referrals to CPNs, *Mental Health Nursing*, 22(4): 8–12.

Boyd, K.J. (1993) Palliative care in the community: views of general practitioners and district nurses in east London, *Journal of Palliative Care*, 9: 33–40.

Boyd, K.J. (1995) The role of specialist home care teams: views of general practitioners in south London, *Palliative Medicine*, 9: 134–44.

Braithwaite, V. (2000) Contextual or general stress outcomes: making choices through caregiving appraisals, *The Gerontologist*, 40(6): 706–17.

Burdz, M.P., Eaton, W.O. and Bond, J.B. (1988) Effect of respite care on dementia and nondementia patients and their caregivers, *Psychology and Aging*, 3: 38–42.

Cartwright, A., Hockey, L. and Anderson, J.L. (1973) *Life Before Death*. London: Routledge and Kegan Paul.

CJD Support Network (2004) www.cjdsupport.net.help.html.

Department of Health (2000) *The NHS Cancer Plan: A Plan for Investment, A Plan for Reform*. London: HMSO.

Department of Health (2001) *National Service Framework for Older People*. London: HMSO.

de Vries, K. (2003) Nursing patients with variant Creutzfeldt-Jakob disease, *European Journal of Palliative Care*, 10(1): 9–12.

de Vries, K. (2004) 'Dealing with the unknown': a sociological perspective on variant Creutzfeldt-Jakob disease, paper presented at the British Sociological Association Annual Conference, York.

de Vries, K. (2006) Caring for the person with variant Creutzfeldt-Jakob disease within the hospice service, PhD thesis, University of Surrey.

de Vries, K., Sque, M.R., Bryan, K. and Abu-Saad, H. (2003) Variant Creutzfeldt-Jakob disease: need for mental health and palliative care team collaboration, *International Journal of Palliative Nursing*, 9(12): 512–20.

Douglas, C. (1992) For all the Saints, *British Medical Journal*, 304: 479.

Douglas, M.J., Campbell, H. and Will, R.G. (1999) *Patients with New Variant Creutzfeldt-Jakob Disease and their Families: Care and Information Needs*. Edinburgh: National Surveillance Unit for CJD.

Field, D. (1994) Palliative medicine and the medicalization of death, *European Journal of Cancer Care*, 3: 58–62.

Forbes, S., Bern-Klug, M. and Gessert, C. (2000) End-of-life decision making for nursing home residents with dementia, *Journal of Nursing Scholarship*, 32(3): 251–8.

Gessert, C.E., Forbes, S. and Bern-Klug, M. (2001) Planning end-of-life care for families with dementia: roles of families and health professionals, *OMEGA*, 42(4): 273–91.

Grace, J. (1993) Alzheimer's disease: your views, *Geriatric Medicine*, 1: 39–41.

Gunstone, S. (1999) Expert practice: the interventions used by a Community Mental Health Nurse with carers of dementia sufferers, *Journal of Psychiatric and Mental Health Nursing*, 6: 21–7.

Hanrahan, P., Raymond, M., McGowan, E. and Luchins, D.J. (1999) Criteria for enrolling dementia patients in hospice: a replication, *American Journal of Hospice and Palliative Care*, 16(1): 395–400.

Higginson, I.J. (1999) Palliative care services in the community: what do family doctors want? *Journal of Palliative Care*, 15(2): 21–5.

Higginson, I.J. (2003) *Priorities and Preferences for End of Life Care in England, Wales and Scotland*. London: National Council for Hospice and Specialist Palliative Care Services.

Higginson, I.J., Hearn, J., Myers, K. and Naysmith, A. (2000) Palliative day care: what do services do? *Palliative Medicine*, 14: 277–86.

Hunt, R. (1997) Place of death of cancer patients: choice versus constraints, *Prog Palliative Care*, 5: 238–41.

Ineichen, B. (1994) Managing demented old people in the community: a review, *Family Practice*, 11(2): 210–15.

Ingleton, C., Payne, S., Nolan, M. and Carey, I. (2003) Respite in palliative care: a review and discussion of the literature, *Palliative Medicine*, 17: 567–75.

Keady, J. and Nolan, M. (1995) A stitch in time: facilitating proactive interventions with dementia caregivers: the role of community practitioners, *Journal of Psychiatric and Mental Health Nursing*, 2: 33–40.

Kramer, B.J. (2000) Husbands caring for wives with dementia: a longitudinal study of continuity and change, *Health and Social Work*, 25(2): 97–108.

Lloyd-Williams, M. (1996) An audit of palliative care in dementia, *European Journal of Cancer Care*, 5: 53–5.

Lloyd-Williams, M. and Payne, S. (2002) Can multidisciplinary guidelines improve the palliation of symptoms in the terminal phase of dementia? *International Journal of Palliative Nursing*, 8(8): 370–5.

Luchins, D.J., Hanrahan, P. and Murphy, K. (1997) Criteria for enrolling dementia patients in hospice, *Journal of the American Geriatrics Society*, 45: 1054–9,

Lyketsos, C., Sheppard, J., and Rabins, P.V. (2000) Dementia in elderly persons in a general hospital, *The American Journal of Psychiatry*, 157(5): 704–7.

Mace, N.L., Rabins, P.V. and McHugh, P.R. (1999) *The 36-Hour Day: A Family Guide to Caring for Persons with Alzheimer Disease: Related Dementing Illnesses, and Memory Loss in Later Life*, 3rd edn. Baltimore, MD: Johns Hopkins University Press.

Manthorpe, J., Iliffe, S. and Eden, A. (2003) Early recognition of dementia by nurses, *Journal of Advanced Nursing*, 44(2): 183–91.

McCarthy, M., Addington-Hall, J. and Altmann, D. (1997) The experience of dying with dementia: a retrospective study, *International Journal of Geriatric Psychiatry*, 12: 404–9.

Miesen, B.M.L. (1997) Awareness in dementia patients and family grieving: a practical perspective, in B.M.L. Miesen and G.M.M. Jones (eds) *Care-Giving in Dementia: Research and Applications*, Vol. 2. London: Routledge, pp. 67–79.

Neale, B. (1993) Informal care and community care, in D. Clarke (ed.) *The Future for Palliative Care: Issues of Policy and Practice*. Buckingham: Open University Press, pp. 52–67.

Nolan, M., Ryan, T., Enderby, P. and Reid, D. (2002) Towards a more inclusive vision of dementia care practice and research, *Dementia*, 1(2): 193–211.

Parkes, C.M. (1996) *Bereavement: Studies of Grief in Adult Life*, 3rd edn. London: Routledge.

Pemberton, C., Storey, L. and Howard, A. (2003) The Preferred Place of Care document: an opportunity for communication, *International Journal of Palliative Nursing*, 9(10): 439–41.

Pickard, S. (1999) Co-ordinated care for older people with dementia, *Journal of Interprofessional Care*, 13(4): 345–54.

Pickard, S. and Glendinning, C. (2001) Caring for a relative with dementia: the perceptions of carers and CPNs, *Quality in Ageing: Policy, Practice and Research*, 2(4): 3–11.

Seale, C. (1990) Caring for people who die: the experience of family and friends, *Ageing and Society*, 10: 413–28.

Shuchter, S.R. and Zisook, S. (1993) The course of normal grief, in M.S. Stroebe, W. Stroede and R.O. Hansson (eds) *Handbook of Bereavement*. Cambridge: Cambridge University Press, pp. 23–43.

Spencer, M.D., Knight, R.S.G. and Will, R.G. (2002) First hundred cases of variant Creutzfeldt-Jakob disease: retrospective case note review of early psychiatric and neurological features, *British Medical Journal*, 324(7352): 1479–82.

Turner, G. (2004) Emerging concerns related to CJD, *Nursing Times*, 100(34): 28–30.

Volicer, L., Hurley, A.C. and Blasi, Z.V. (2003) Characteristics of dementia end-of-life care across care settings, *American Journal of Hospice and Palliative Care*, 20(3): 191–200.

19

At the margins of society

Social exclusion and the experience of dementia: some reflections and challenges to CMHN practice

Sean Page and Philip Hardman

Introduction

This chapter explores the social exclusion of people with organic and cognitive impairments who are marginalized from society to the point of policy, practice and research invisibility. Accordingly, this chapter is descriptive and free thinking in its construction and begins with a broad overview of three main areas of concern before drilling down into the experience of people with dementia and exploring issues raised for CMHN practice. The three issues selected for discussion in this chapter are: (1) being homeless with dementia; (2) being in prison with dementia; and (3) being an older asylum seeker with cognitive deficits – life experiences that are all associated, in some form or another, with social exclusion. For all it is believed, possible inaccurately, that relatively small numbers of people with dementia are involved; however, these people are so disadvantaged, and their experience so divergent from mainstream dementia care provision, that attempting to understand this experience requires new ways of practice and more integrated patterns of community support. As we make our way through this chapter we have drawn on literature that is more generic in its focus although we believe that there is much to be learnt and applied in this process to people with dementia and their support network. We will start with an overview of social exclusion and its sociological meaning and relevance to dementia.

Social exclusion

Dementia is now well recognized as being a much more complex phenomenon than simply an 'organic illness'. It is a lived experience that is generally damaging to both physical and psychological health. Much of the psychological damage occurs as a consequence of the way in which society denigrates, diminishes, dehumanizes and discriminates against people with dementia; a process eloquently captured within Kitwood's (1997) concept of 'malignant social psychology'. Malignant social psychology is essentially a description of the elements of social exclusion and, by connecting the two we can place the needs of extremely marginalized people with dementia within a more mainstream framework allied, in the United Kingdom, to a current political imperative:

Millions of people suffer from mental health conditions some time in their lives. For a minority, these can be severe and long lasting. Even now with welcome new attitudes in society, those suffering mental distress still find themselves excluded from many aspects of life the rest of us take for granted.

(Tony Blair cited in Social Exclusion Unit 2004)

Among those things that may be taken for granted are employment, financial security, a place to live, good health and the support and regard derived from positive relationships with family and friends. When a person, for whatever reason, is deprived of these things, then the potential to become socially excluded is increased. When an individual is faced with multiple social deprivations, then social exclusion may well become a way of life. The dominant characteristic of social exclusion is that the problems an individual encounters are linked, mutually reinforced and combine to impact significantly upon quality of life, self-esteem and the regard society has for the individual.

Given the right set of circumstances, everyone is potentially 'at risk' of social exclusion, and older people who present with an array of vulnerabilities are no exception to this (see Box 19.1). In considering some of these vulnerabilities we may pause to remember that two million people of pension age live below the poverty line and that the sole source of income for one quarter of people with dementia is the state pension.

Many older people are socially isolated, usually through bereavement or family moving away, and it is suggested that 154,000 people with dementia live alone (Alzheimer's Society 1994), most of these being older women with no close family support (Wenger 1994). Even in sheltered housing, people with dementia can become isolated because they either withdraw from community activities or are rejected by other tenants. Through this rejection the stigma which taints the lives of people with dementia becomes a visible and a real experience. Goffman (1961) described stigma as being very much a relationship of 'devaluation' in which one individual is disqualified from full social acceptance. People with dementia can become stigmatized as they are seen to present 'differently' to others in society; these differences, particularly in behaviour and poor cognitive performance, may challenge the accepted social norms and act to legitimize actions that in any other circumstances would be deemed unacceptable.

This same stigma is very much a part of life for the homeless, the prison inmate and the asylum seeker. It is to their lived experiences that we now turn our attention.

Box 19.1 Vulnerabilities for social exclusion in older people

- High incidence of ill health.
- High incidence of physical disability.
- Mental impairment.
- Poverty.
- Isolation and loneliness.
- Bereavement.
- Poor housing.
- Problems of ageing carers.

(Social Exclusion Unit 1994)

Being homeless

> The sight of a rough sleeper bedding down for the night in a shop doorway or on a park bench is one of the most potent symbols of social exclusion in Britain today.
>
> (Foord 1999)

This is particularly striking if one considers that the person sleeping rough is probably not recognized as 'homeless' by statutory services, may well have recently completed a custodial sentence or service with the Armed Forces, may well be an older person and experience a more deleterious mental and physical health status than the general population. However, we tend not to consider, or be aware of, such facts, and much of society's perception of homeless people is rooted in deep-seated stereotypes and prejudices, as the following quotation from the early 1930s illustrates:

> When one comes to think about it, tramps are a queer product and worth thinking over. It is queer that a tribe of men, tens of thousands in number, should be marching up and down England. But though the case obviously wants considering, one cannot even start to consider it until one has got rid of certain prejudices. These prejudices are rooted in the idea that every tramp is . . . a blackguard . . . a repulsive, rather dangerous character, who would die rather than work or wash and who wants nothing but to beg, drink and rob.
>
> (Orwell 1933: 178)

Times change but prejudices, stigma and ignorance remain. Finding a definition of homelessness which sits comfortably with both the objective legal and the subjectively psychological is not easy. To define a person as 'homeless' is probably not enough, some people sleep rough on the streets, some are resident in a shelter or hostel, others are vulnerably housed or sleeping on the floor or sofa of a friend and many are in a constant state of transition between all these states. It can be argued that homelessness is a universal, social and political phenomenon and an issue about which everyone holds an opinion, although, as previously rehearsed, too often that opinion is based upon ignorance or stereotypical images of homelessness.

While the nature of homelessness has moved away from traditional images of 'the tramp' travelling from town to town, the 'idle vagrant', the 'dangerous vagabond' or the 'alcoholic bag lady', the legacy of those images remain embedded within our psyche. To be homeless is to engage in deviant behaviour, the most extreme and observable example of which is to become a rough sleeper on the streets of any town or city in the UK (Crane 1999). It is no wonder that many try to become less observable whether this be the estimated 5,000 'mole people' hiding away in tunnels beneath Manhattan as described by Toth (1993), or the older homeless people who avoid town centres, sleep rough in secluded places and are too ashamed or despondent to seek help.

In the UK, the homeless fall into one of two groups: those who are described as 'statutory homeless people' and consequently recognized by local authorities as deserving of help, and 'non-statutory homeless people' who are not recognized and consequently not deserving of assistance (Warnes et al. 2003). Statutory homeless person status is awarded by virtue of that person becoming unintentionally homeless, having dependent children or being in some other way recognized as being sufficiently vulnerable (Box 19.2) to trigger

Box 19.2 The vulnerable homeless

- Pregnant woman.
- People with dependent children.
- Vulnerability due to old age.
- Vulnerability due to mental illness or physical disability.
- Homeless as a consequence of disaster.
- Aged below 21 years and previously looked after or fostered.
- Ex-member of the armed services.
- Homeless following completion of custodial or remand sentence.

priority-housing need. The non-statutory homeless fall outside of this, are generally single without dependent children and belong to specific groups (Box 19.3).

Agreeing on the size of the total homeless population is somewhat contentious as there are no official figures for those regarded as the non-statutory homeless. Despite this, it is known that the annual rate of applications to local authority housing departments is fairly stable at around 250,000, of which 30 per cent are not recognized as homeless, and Crisis (a national charity for homeless people) have suggested a figure of 400,000 for the non-statutory homeless, which is broadly accepted. In respect of the most obvious of these, the rough sleepers, numbers have in recent years been falling, due largely to the impact of political will, and currently it is estimated that on any given night there are in the region of 596 rough sleepers in the UK.

This chapter is concerned with the non-statutory homeless population and accepts that although definitions are often uncomfortable and incorrect, we will attempt to make distinctions by use of the terms:

'Rough sleeper' (to refers to those people living outside any form of housing).

'Vulnerably housed' (to refer to those people currently sleeping elsewhere than on the streets).

'Homeless' (to refer to the non-statutory population as a whole).

Pathways into homelessness

Reasons as to why people become homeless are often complex and reflect inter-related patterns of personal vulnerability sometimes occurring acutely, sometimes following a predictable series of events and sometimes as a deliberate choice. Orwell stated that the life of the tramp in 1930s England was a world which awaited anyone who ever had the misfortune to become penniless and, when one considers the pathways into becoming homeless, it remains as true today that, given a particular set of circumstances, many of us are potentially at risk of experiencing homelessness.

Homelessness due to retirement or unemployment is not uncommon. There is a well-documented and historical correlation between the itinerant casual worker and future homelessness. Many such workers employed in transient labouring jobs living in transit camps, never settling, never marrying, losing contact with family, drinking heavily and

Box 19.3 The non-statutory homeless

Group	Estimated number
Those who have been provided with supported housing (hostels/YMCAs/shelters) and not considered statutory homeless	Around 25,000
Bed and breakfast and other boarded accommodation and in receipt of Housing Benefit	Around 50,000
People at imminent risk of eviction due to rent arrears	Around 2,000
Squatters	Up to 10,000
Concealed households sharing overcrowded accommodation with family or friends: (people who neither own nor rent the property they are living in and are neither the spouse, partner nor dependent child of the owner/renter)	170,000–220,000
Concealed households sharing accommodation with family or friends which is not overcrowded but where the head of household deems the arrangement unsatisfactory	55,000–70,000
Total numbers	310,000 to 380,000

Source: Crisis (2004)

saving little, ultimately find themselves, when the work stops, mainly due to old age, not only homeless but not recognized as such by any local authority. Retirement may also lead to loss of tied accommodation particularly among the low paid or to loss of income, which leads to debt, arrears and eviction.

The commonest vulnerability is that which follows breakdown of family or relationship usually as a consequence of bereavement or related to marriage, or partnership, disintegration. The breakdown of a relationship is cited by some 40 per cent of homeless people as the most significant factor altering their social circumstances.

Bereavement triggers homelessness in two significant groups, first, in middle-aged people unable to cope with the demands of life, perhaps as a consequence of mental health problems, and supported by ageing parents until their ultimate death. Second, by older widowed men affected by depression who simply abandon the family home or who lose it because of financial mismanagement, usually related to depression-fuelled alcohol abuse.

A considerable number of those discharged from a custodial sentence find themselves homeless. Up to 40 per cent of those sent to prison lose their homes while serving their sentence and in 2001 one-third of those due for release had no home to go to, consequently, of 87,000 prisoners released, 28,500 became homeless. Of the other significant ex-institutional group, the chronically mentally ill, many became homeless as an effect of the psychiatric hospital closure programme in the 1980s, while more specifically, but in smaller numbers, those with paranoia may abandon their homes and those with an undiagnosed dementia may simply 'wander away', never return and somehow live on the streets. Despite the recognition that people may simply, and through no fault of their own, fall into homelessness, it remains a shameful scar upon a civilized Western society that those people continue to be regarded at best as deliberately choosing to remove themselves from society, and therefore undeserving of the benefits enjoyed by the rest of that society, or at worst rough sleepers becoming an object for abuse or derision: 'These are the people one steps over on the way into the opera' (Sir George Young, Minister of Housing 1989, cited by Foord 1999).

Homelessness and health

Without doubt becoming homeless greatly increases an individual's risk of suffering ill health, of aggravating a pre-existing condition and of dying at an early age. The greatest risks are presented to rough sleepers who commonly experience skin infestations, nutritional deficiencies or circulatory problems. Most of these are treatable, however, circumstances often dictate that they go untreated and add to the misery of day-to-day existence.

The vulnerably housed are more likely to be registered with a GP, a luxury denied the rough sleeper, and are therefore better placed to have physical health problems noticed and addressed, and yet they still experience a greater proportion of ill-health than the general population. Common chronic problems are those related to respiratory disease, usually pneumonia and bronchitis, although tuberculosis is not unknown, and cirrhosis of the liver due to alcohol abuse. Additionally, injury from accident or malicious assault is not uncommon, particularly for older homeless men who, for many reasons, are more vulnerable to violence.

Rough sleepers are up to fifty times more likely to be fatally injured due to violent assault than the general population, and twice as likely to die in an accident. Equally striking is the fact that they die earlier, the average recorded age at death ranging from 42 to 53 years in coroner studies, and overall homeless men find that their average life expectancy is reduced by some twenty years.

Homelessness and mental health

In promoting a social model of dementia care over the past decade or so, many have come to recognize the degrading and dehumanizing aspects of life for many of those who are affected by a dementia. Although the culture is starting to change for the better, we continue to recognize that people with dementia remain largely marginalized, excluded and disadvantaged. Parallels may be drawn with the lot of the average rough sleeper and when one listens to the voice of the homeless, through their own words (cited in Warnes et al. 2003: 75), one begins to capture a sense of their world:

> It's the lowest low. I felt like something that's been thrown away, disregarded. I didn't feel like I was worth anything.
>
> (boy aged 16 years)

> Unclean, unwanted. Outcast, actually. As if you didn't belong any more. It's as if no one really wants to know.
>
> (man aged 45 years)

These are powerful statements conveying a sense of hopelessness, of rejection, of disempowerment and disregard, which serves to provide a view of homelessness those statistical reports alone cannot achieve. Indeed, many research studies exploring the mental health of homeless people are somewhat controversial in their findings. Their wide variance of incidence in respect of psychiatric morbidity may lead to them being regarded as unreliable or invalid particularly as there are inherent methodological flaws in respect of the recognition, detection and diagnosis among sample populations.

Despite these concerns, the available evidence does suggest that mental illness is something of a growing problem among the homeless and particularly so for the rough sleeper. Studies suggest that the proportion of homeless people with any mental health problem is in the region of 30–50 per cent, at least double that found in the general adult population. For serious mental illness, such as schizophrenia, the incidence is in the region of 12–26 per cent, which is up to six times greater than the general population, and around 11 per cent of rough sleepers have schizophrenia, which is seven times higher than the general population (Folsom and Jeste 2002). Mental health problems are consistently reported as more prevalent among homeless women, the elderly and the very young. The incidence of mental illness appears to be increasing. In part, this may be due to the changing profile of the homeless population, particularly the increasing use of illegal street drugs.

Older homeless people

> Homelessness is a problem that is all too often associated with young people, yet there are more over-50s than teenagers on our streets. While there are 22 projects for young people in London, there are none for older rough sleepers.
>
> (Charles Fraser, Chief Executive, St Mungo's)

In the literature on homelessness, the term 'older' is used to describe people over the age of 50 years and is a reflection of the fact that rough sleepers and long-term vulnerably housed present with health problems that one would usually expect to see in someone 10–20 years older.

Charles Fraser suggests that there are a sizeable number of older homeless people and all the evidence does lend itself to the reality that this is a wide-scale problem. While the statutory homeless population is seeing fewer older people, the problem lies in the increasing numbers in the non-statutory group. By the very nature of the cohort it is difficult to fully understand the extent of the problem as many older rough sleepers hide away, refuse contact with services or deny that they are homeless. Most recent estimates are based upon researchers or outreach workers purposely going out to find older people living on the streets.

Crane and Warnes (2001) found 834 older rough sleepers in London in the period 1999 to 2000, of whom 186 were aged in their 60s and 43 were over 70 years of age. There are equally sizeable numbers living in hostels. A one night survey of London hostels found 700 (23 per cent) residents aged over 50 years, and 94 who were over 70, suggesting that there are three times as many older than younger people resident in hostels. Interestingly, despite this, many of the older homeless refuse to consider hostels as an option. Often this is because they are perceived as isolating or less sociable or inhabited by young people who by their use of alcohol or drugs are regarded as a threat to the older person. Of further interest appears to be the fact that once an older person moves into a hostel, they tend to stay there (see Table 19.1) and the fact that 30 per cent of residents in 'first contact' hostels have lived there for more than ten years does reinforce the belief that resettlement programmes are generally ineffective or simply that those concerned become rapidly institutionalized.

Table 19.1 Length of stay in hostel for people aged over 60 years

Length of stay in hostel	Percent of older hostel residents
Up to 6 months	18
6 to 12 months	06
12 months to 2 years	12
Two to five years	26
5 to 10 years	09
More than 10 years	30

Homelessness and cognitive impairment

Crane and Warnes (2003) describe the work of the Lancefield Street Centre, a project whereby street outreach workers intensively go looking for older homeless people in order to gradually introduce them to the services they require. They cite a case study of 'Tom', 70 years old, and a 20-year veteran of life on the streets characterized by heavy drinking and eating from litter bins. On moving to the centre Tom presented with a variety of cognitive impairments, needed help with basic activities of daily living, could not find his own room and always got lost if he went out alone. Subsequently a psychiatrist confirmed his severe memory problems and he was admitted into residential care.

Tom's experience may not be uncommon. Among those older people assisted by the Lancefield Street Centre, 16 per cent have memory problems, of whom 12 per cent are sufficiently severe to require assistance with activities of daily living, executive functioning and frequent memory prompts or reminders. Some report a higher incidence of cognitive problems, Gonzalez et al. (2001) found 80 per cent of their sample to have an established neuropsychological deficit and 35 per cent to have impairment as rated by the Mini-mental State Examination. Crane (1994) reports 54 per cent of her sample as having a memory problem ranging in severity from slight to severe.

It is not by no means certain that the symptoms presented equate to dementia. For many they may represent an unavoidable consequence of life on the streets whereby orientation is less important, attention to news or current affairs often meaningless, previous standards of hygiene or toileting behaviour compromised and social interaction diminished. While many report or claim to have a memory problem, those who meet the criteria for dementia will invariably be fewer, and Cohen et al. (1988) place the figure at around 9 per cent for mild to moderate dementia and 5 per cent for moderate to severe dementia.

Summary

Available evidence clearly suggests that the lived experience of homelessness in old age is unenviable, firmly rooted in social exclusion and mostly focused upon the basic act of survival. Many older homeless people are sleeping rough and, in fear of their security, they tend to choose secluded places, such as parks, woods or disused toilets, or public places open through the night, such as hospitals or cafés, where they can largely be anonymous. Almost all live in poverty, most are socially isolated and estranged from relatives or friends, and very few have access to the kind of services which can help.

Being in prison

> The prison service has no policy on the elderly at all and 'when I discover an 87-year-old on a Zimmer frame with Alzheimer's in a high-security prison, I'm sorry, but I think that is a nonsense'.
>
> (Sir David Ramsbotham, then Chief Inspector of Prisons, as cited by the *Guardian* 2001)

There are 137 prisons in Britain (Parrish 2003) and between 1990 and 2000 the number of people held in prisons in England and Wales increased by 42 per cent from 45,636 to 64,602, increasing again to 74,000 by July 2003. The prison population has an age-sex distribution different from the general population in that 95 per cent are male and relatively young, 79 per cent are 15–39 years compared to only 35 per cent in the general population (Howse 2003).

It is becoming more recognized that the population of older people in prison in England and Wales is increasing and there are strong indications their physical and a mental health needs are greater than that of the general population. Despite this, the focus of policy-makers and researchers from within the criminal justice field remains almost exclusively focused on persistent youth offending, particularly the 18–20 age group. Frazer (2003) refers to this as 'The Policy Gap'.

Health-care provision within the UK prison service

The UK government's policy for prison health care is based upon the principle of 'equivalence of care'. Prisoners should receive the same level of health care as they would were they not in prison and that care would be equitable in terms of policy, standards and delivery. Such services are expected to be equivalent to primary care with access to specialist outpatient services. Prisoners needing more than primary care are expected to be transferred from prison to hospital to receive appropriate care (Health Advisory Commission for the Prison Service 1997).

Debate has arisen over the principle of 'equivalence of care' as to the adequacy of health-care provision for prisoners, particularly mental health care. Wilson (2004) represents the view of many commentators that prisoners with mental health problems require adequately equipped and staffed hospital facilities whether inside or outside the prison walls. In December 1999, a working party was established by the Health Minister to consider the development of nursing in HM prisons and the effective reintroduction of prison health-care officers as part of a multi-disciplinary health-care team. The outcome of this work is the report *Nursing in Prisons* (NHS Executive 2000) and it recommended a partnership be established between the NHS and the prison service to provide joint training, benchmarking and to develop a framework for clinical governance. The two organizations working together would provide access to a wider resource of professional support and supervision. Occupational standards were to be introduced to ensure that a competency framework underpinned the role of prison health-care officer. Specialist knowledge and skills would be developed among staff, beyond the standard level three competences, according to the needs of individual establishments.

Health-care services are provided through contractual arrangements with third party providers (Marshall et al. 2000). The involvement of the DOH in prison health care provided a timely opportunity to re-examine models of service delivery. The work of mental health in reach teams is seen as a vehicle to effect positive change to the physical and psychological well-being of prisoners.

The greying of the prison population

Compared with the statistics for the UK adult population, older people are under-represented within the prison population. In comparison, minority ethnic groups are over-represented in the prison population, making up 25 per cent of the prison population, and older people from minority ethnic groups are more heavily over-represented. In November 2001, 11 per cent of prisoners aged 60 years or more being held in English and Welsh prisons were known to belong to a minority ethnic group (Frazel et al. 2001a). Howse (2003) cites Home Office statistics for 2001, which show that those under sentence and aged 60 or over represented 2.4 per cent of the male prison population and 0.7 per cent of the female prison population. Between 1990 and 2000 the proportion of prisoners under sentence who were aged 60 or over increased from 1 per cent to 2.3 per cent.

In 1990, 412 men and women aged 60 or over were received into English and Welsh prisons (0.8 per cent of total number of adult receptions). By 2000, this figure had increased almost twofold to 808 (1.1 per cent of the total). Most are male (97 per cent in 1990 and 96 per cent in 2000) and the majority of older prisoners aged 60 or above are in their 60s (81 per cent). The ratio of male to female in the prison population aged 60 or over has hardly changed in 10 years hence in 2000, 16 of 1154 sentenced prisoners aged 60 or more were female (less than 2 per cent) (Howse 2003).

The literature points to the provision of prison wings specifically for older prisoners as being only a recent phenomenon. As an example, H wing in Kingston Prison is one of very few facilities adapted for older prisoners. The idea behind H wing was to provide vulnerable, older 'lifers' with protection from other prisoners. The wing was described as having many of the trappings of a care home (Katz 2001) and during an interview with the *Guardian* newspaper, Stuart McLean, retired Governor of the prison, provided an insight into the dilemma faced by the prison services as to where to place older prisoners as they become physically and mentally frail. He indicated the difficulty of releasing such prisoners or transferring them into nursing homes: 'There is a delicate balancing act between compassion and risk and the scales are tipped heavily against compassion' (McLean, cited in Katz 2001).

Types of crime committed by older people

> The research shows that New Labour's commitment to tougher sentencing for serious offenders had a disproportionate effect on the size of the older male prison population, and on the number of all female prisoners aged 21–59. This is largely attributable to the accumulation of ageing male prisoners and older sentenced men serving longer sentences for sexual offences, and growing numbers of female offenders of all imprisoned for drugs offences.
>
> (Frazer 2003)

Older people are more likely to be serving longer sentences than younger prisoners. Twenty per cent of older people under sentence are lifers compared to 9 per cent in the general prison population. The National Prison Survey (1991) indicated a high proportion of older prisoners (29 per cent) had been convicted of serious violent crimes such as murder, manslaughter or rape (OPCS 1992).

There is a disproportionate high number of sex offenders who are 60 years and over within the prison population, about half of older male prisoners under sentence are sex offenders (Frazel et al. 2002a). The proportion of sexual offenders in prison increases with age whereas the proportion of offences against property (includes burglary, robbery and theft and handling) decreases with age. Theft is the most common of the offences against property committed by older people. In 2000, 6 per cent of older people sent to prison were convicted of drug offences – this may be as high as 14 per cent. Fraud and drug offences are the most common offences for which older people are imprisoned, but overall the numbers are very small (Frazel et al. 2001b).

Prisons, mental health and dementia

The Home Office does not routinely collect information on the health and disability status of prisoners in England and Wales, however, it is recognized that the health of prisoners of all ages is worse than that of the general population.

The principles and direction for the delivery of mental health services in England and Wales were laid out in the National Service Framework (NSF) for Mental Health (DOH 2000) and the National Service Framework for Older People (DOH 2000). The NSF for Older People contains no direct standards relevant to older prisoners. A joint Prison Service and Department of Health report from a working group on 'Doctors Working in Prisons' recommended that

> As part of the health needs assessment process, prisons, health authorities and primary care groups/trusts review the needs of older prisoners and those with a disability and take steps to ensure that they have access to the same range of professionals and services that are available to these groups in the community. There needs to be greater emphasis placed on providing both groups with a healthy and suitable regime.
>
> (DoH and HMPS 2001)

Frazel et al. (2001a) studied 203 male sentenced prisoners over the age of 59 years from 15 prisons in England and Wales and found high rates of severe, but hidden, psychiatric morbidity. Thirty per cent of older prisoners had clinical depression and if the finding from the study were extrapolated to all elderly prisoners, then about 50 older sentenced men would be experiencing psychosis at any one time. This study indicated the poor rates of detection and treatment due to a lack of resources and training of staff at that time.

Frazel et al. (2001b) and work from the USA by McShane and Williams (1990) have found that older prisoners report much higher levels of chronic ill health compared with older people in the community. The work from the USA suggests that the health profiles of older prisoners mirror that of the homeless, with both exhibiting 'accelerated biological ageing' and prison inmates being found 'to have aged roughly 10 years beyond the average citizen'.

The presence of older prisoners who have developed dementia during their sentence (it is assumed that a person with dementia would be unlikely to be deemed fit to stand trial) raises both practical problems in providing appropriate care in environments fit for purpose as well as important ethical dilemmas. Frazel et al. (2002a) explore in depth the ethical dilemma in the context of the role and purpose of prison and punishment. They suggest that prolonging the imprisonment of people with dementia may contravene the 1998 Human Rights Act. More research is needed to examine the philosophy and standards of care received by older prisoners who have dementia and the environments in which that care is given.

Summary

The prison population is growing older and as it does so, the potential for dementing illness to occur behind bars increases. At present, prison health services do not regard dementia as a priority and acts of compassion, even basic unconditional positive regard, are likely to be misunderstood by society when applied to a population of people serving time for serious crimes against that society. While human rights legislation may influence the situation and lead to the greater discharge of older prisoners, this in itself will not necessarily lead to a reintegration into society.

The 'ex-offender' remains stigmatized and largely disadvantaged, as an example of this and a parallel to the earlier part of this chapter many people on completion of a custodial prison sentence find themselves homeless, despite the best efforts of the probation service. One also has to question if we are person-centred enough to deliver equitable care to people with dementia whose very biographies may make us feel uncomfortable.

Being an asylum seeker

The United Nations Convention of Refugees (United Nations 1951) places nation states under an obligation to permit persons from another country to seek asylum and become recognized as refugees. Under this convention the status of refugee has been defined as:

> A person who, owing to fear of persecution for reasons of race, religion, nationality, social position or political beliefs, seeks refuge outside of his/her country of origin and is unable to return to that country.
>
> (United Nations 1951)

Over the past two decades the number of those seeking refugee status has increased significantly. This is mostly the consequence of large-scale population displacement, in the region of 50 million persons, related to conflicts characterized by policies of 'ethnic cleansing' and brutality directed towards the civilian population. Secondary to this has been the increasing 'economic migration' of those seeking to escape poverty and lack of opportunity.

Countries in the developed world have not responded well to such pressures and there has been the appearance of battle lines being drawn between asylum seekers and Western governments. In an increasingly xenophobic and hostile environment marked by contra-dictory public responses towards asylum seekers (Hargreaves 2000), state policies seem to be increasingly intent upon the exclusion of all uninvited immigrants, regardless of their reason for seeking asylum (Silove et al. 2000).

In the UK, the Nationality, Immigration and Asylum Act 2002 has denied asylum seekers access to state benefits including housing, promoted a policy of forced dispersal, or detention, and introduced a voucher system which leads to significant financial hardship and poverty (Hargreaves 2000). Oxfam and the Refugee Council (2002) report that more than 80 per cent of asylum seekers experience hunger, cannot afford to buy clothing or footwear and cannot maintain good health.

Within such a climate the process of seeking to attain refugee status is an experience tainted by insecurity, uncertainty, social exclusion and stigma. It is therefore not surprising that in the UK there is a recent trend towards a fall in the number of asylum seekers. During 2003 there were 49,405 applications made which is some 41 per cent lower than the number for 2002, and at the close of 2003 the UK hosted 270,000 asylum seekers repre-senting 0.4 per cent of the total population (Office of National Statistics 2004).

Older asylum seekers

Older people are less likely to seek asylum in another country. In part, this is because they are more likely to have a greater attachment to their homeland and in part because they may perceive the challenges of the journey involved as being too great to attempt (Burton and Breen 2002). Those who do apply for asylum are therefore likely to be in dire need of help and protection.

Unfortunately, older asylum seekers are also less able to derive a positive outcome from the experience. Many find their basic needs being compromised by physical disability, mental impairment and the loss of status and social support networks. There are also fewer opportunities to recover from trauma, or to rebuild lives.

Perhaps because of this, asylum seekers aged over 60 years represent only 2 per cent of that particular population, while those aged below 30 years represent the majority at 67 per cent (BBC News online 2004). Despite this, the number of older asylum seekers currently exceeds the number of older homeless people by a considerable margin.

Health, cognition and asylum seekers

Those who seek asylum in this country have many points of origin and have experienced a diverse range of events which impact upon their health status. One-fifth of those from sub-Saharan Africa are chronic carriers of hepatitis B, 5 per cent of migrants entering the United States suffer from tuberculosis while 25 per cent of migrants to Australia have serious gastro-intestinal complaints (Burnett and Peel 2004).

The physical and psychological trauma which triggers the need to seek asylum has a considerable effect upon health. Commonly described trauma includes exposure to

Box 19.4 Factors associated with cognitive impairment in asylum seekers

- Traumatic experiences such as torture or rape.
- Weight loss and malnutrition especially vitamin B deficiencies.
- Traumatic brain injury.
- Excessive production of glucocorticoids in response to stress.
- Post-Traumatic Stress Disorder.
- Sleep deprivation.
- Depression.
- Chronic pain.

torture, rape, imprisonment for political or religious beliefs and the murder of family and friends (Mollica et al. 1987). The very journey towards asylum is itself fraught with hazards which commonly include deprivation of food or water, robbery, exploitation, assault and abandonment by 'people smugglers' (Millbank 2000). The eventual arrival in a 'safe' country does not necessarily lead to improvement in the situation. Even in the UK where, theoretically, the asylum seeker is entitled to access the full range of medical services, the BMA Medical Ethics Committee has expressed concerns: 'If you are an asylum seeker and you come to the UK, there is little chance that your health will improve, in fact, it may well deteriorate' (Wilks 2001). Commonly indicted for this is the relationship between ill health poverty and social deprivation, associated with the UK asylum programme. Health needs are often ignored and there are frequent reports of inequity in accessing health services (Jones and Gill 1998). Forced dispersal leads to a lack of continuity in the treatment of chronic conditions and inadequate interpreting services in primary care compound the difficulties (BBC News 2004).

In addition to this, the scope of, and potential for, mental health problems are both considerable and complex. Not only is the initial trauma and travel to the country of asylum highly correlated with psychiatric morbidity (Anon 2002) but also exposure to asylum programme procedures is seen to generate, or exacerbate, mental health problems. The UK asylum process is reported as perpetuating post-traumatic stress disorder and triggering hopelessness, fear, despair, humiliation, demoralization, diminished self-worth and loss of dignity (Luebben 2003). Such findings are mirrored in the United States where asylum seekers are held in detention. Keller et al. (2003) found incidences of depressive illness at 86 per cent and PTSD at 50 per cent. Both were significantly correlated with length of detention whereas release led to a marked reduction in all psychological symptoms although the subsequent process of long-term resettlement into another country or culture is seen as a further risk factor for mental illness (Luebben 2003).

Without doubt, cognitive functioning is fragile when exposed to the events that many asylum seekers experience. Box 19.4 summarizes those factors which may have a significant impact upon memory functioning. It is therefore something of a paradox that memory performance is one of the most important determinants in achieving a successful outcome in applying for asylum (Anthony et al. 1998). Credibility of testimony is regarded as crucial to making judgements regarding asylum yet testimony is affected by memory dysfunction. Immigration officials have a tendency to be sceptical of information recalled in later interviews which was not recalled in the first interview and lack of credibility is seen to be a frequently recurring issue in refusal notices and appeal determinations (Cohen 2001).

Summary

It is possible to state that the whole refugee experience presents individuals with risk factors for developing a dementing illness. However, in respect of the prevalence of dementia among older asylum seekers, there is simply no evidence in the available literature. We are left in the uncomfortable position of hypothesizing that inherently there must be a number of people affected, that their condition may go unrecognized and that their lived experience, characterized by poverty, social deprivation and stigma is, again, an unenviable one.

Social exclusion and implications for CMHN practice

As mental health nurses who have been both influenced and inspired by the social model of dementia care for most of our careers, researching and writing this chapter has been an experience of mixed emotions. There is the phenomenological fascination that comes from developing some understanding, albeit limited, of lived experiences of dementia that are outside of the 'norm'. Sadly, however, this experience can in no way be regarded as a positive one for those people who live it. People with cognitive impairment who are homeless, in prison or seeking asylum have become so marginalized and excluded by society that we regard them as being invisible. Consequently, their complex needs remain largely unrecognized and unmet. What quickly emerges from this is the uncomfortable realization that such a lived experience is outside not only our clinical practice but also that of most other community mental health nurses who work in dementia care.

While the implications of this should concern us all, it does perhaps offer us an opportunity to begin exploring what it is that the CMHN, as a dementia specialist, could potentially bring to each of the three areas we have discussed.

Evidently, as a society we hold deeply rooted traditional beliefs and attitudes about the homeless, the prison inmate and the asylum seeker. Those agencies and individuals who work to improve things are well acquainted with these beliefs and attitudes and deal daily with the challenges they bring about. We suspect that they would be among the first to acknowledge that the concept of 'person-centred care' is not as all pervading in health and social care as has been suggested (Brooker et al. 2004). In the context of dementia, person-centred care has been criticized as being untenable (McCormack 2004) and misguided (Nolan et al. 2004) and while this is not the place to rehearse those arguments, we suggest it may be too idealistic to impact on the three areas we have chosen to examine.

Each area offers little in the way of an egalitarian experience and it may be pure rhetoric to place emphasis on the autonomy of the individual when any institution (prison, asylum centre, etc.) attempting to do so would experience significant internal tension and external condemnation. We are reminded again of the thoughts of Stuart McLean, retired Governor of HMP Kingston: 'There is a delicate balancing act between compassion and risk and the scales are tipped heavily against compassion.'

For people with dementia in these situations there may be a cogent argument in shifting the emphasis away from person-centred care towards a more balanced concept of 'relationship-centred care'. Within such a concept there is less emphasis placed upon the dynamics of power and control but very real constraints and pressures are still acknowledged. Relationship-centred care promotes interdependence and the pursuit of a meaningful dialogue, which leads to shared, rather than subjective, constructs emerging to define an experience. From these shared constructs emerges a valuable starting point of interactions that may represent a new and powerful defining force for health and social care provision (Nolan et al. 2004).

While some may also regard this as rhetoric, there is real value in seeking to pursue relationships based on interdependence as, in each of our three chosen areas, maintaining the status quo (traditional values) is unacceptable and adopting person-centred principles is largely untenable. The problem, of course, emerges when we recognize that people with dementia have fewer opportunities to engage in the 'meaningful dialogue' that is required and fewer opportunities for their voices to be heard. In part, this may be because of cognitive or language impairment and in part because of the other person's inexperience, reluctance, uncertainty or anxiety about interacting with someone who has dementia. In addition to this, the preconceived ideas about the homeless, the prison inmate and the asylum seeker act as barriers to the required dialogue.

Mike Nolan briefly considered many of these thoughts in the Foreword to the first edition of this book (Nolan 2003). He celebrated the promotion of 'communitarian' values that could focus attention upon the needs of the most vulnerable and disadvantaged members of our society. Here, then, we begin to see the role of the CMHN, as dementia specialist, becoming involved to offer advocacy to people with dementia, and advice, support, assessment and training to the relevant agencies and institutions. In closing this chapter we should briefly consider some potential areas for engagement.

Detection

If we strongly suspect that people with dementia are to be found within each of our three chosen groups, then clearly there is a need for detection and subsequent assessment before we can consider any relevant intervention. The right of older people to have access to assessment that is appropriate to their circumstances is enshrined in the National Service Framework for Older People (DOH 2001). The CMHN has been shown to be increasingly active, and effective, in this area, however, the problem lies very much in ensuring access to assessment. In order to achieve this, for our three groups, there is a need for partnerships to evolve between the providers of specialist mental health services and the other organizations, agencies or institutions.

If we consider the ageing prison inmate as an example, he should receive the same level of health care as he would were he not in prison and the National Service Framework for mental health (DOH 1999) espouses improved assessment to identify unmet or inappropriately met need. As such, subjective concerns regarding cognitive impairment should lead to referral to the appropriate specialist service, such as a memory clinic, which could provide an appropriate response. Attaching the dementia specialist CMHN to any existing prison 'in-reach' service could do much to screen for genuine cases of probable dementia and to address the interdependent implications of the diagnosis. The same potential could be realized if organizations working with the homeless and asylum seekers had the facility to refer directly to an attached CMHN or nursing team.

Intervention

The role of many specialist mental health nurses has changed in recent years, moving away from the emphasis being placed upon helping a psychiatrist to make a diagnosis, towards helping people to cope with the diagnosis that is made (Page 2002). This involves the provision of a whole range of therapeutic interventions from monitoring the efficacy of anti-Alzheimer drugs to the provision of psychological treatments, and certainly this book and its first edition provide overwhelming evidence that this occurs.

Within everyone is the opportunity to establish a relationship and within the relationship rests the real potential for meaningful dialogue that achieves the balance between the pursuit of 'authentic decision making' (McCormack 2004) and the interdependent realities of that person's set of circumstances. In the three areas we have identified the reality of the situation is harsher than for most other people with dementia and the need for shared understanding greater. As an example of this, the involvement of the CMHN with homeless agencies could offer much to promote coping and adjustment for people with dementia who, while being assisted out of homelessness, are struggling to make sense of the process and are at increased risk of disappearing back onto the streets.

Changing attitudes

Although the scope of involvement by a CMHN is wide and the abilities legion, it is in the combating of stigma and discrimination that there is most potential. All three of our chosen areas are characterized by stigma that perpetuates traditional values and, to a large extent, denies those affected the opportunity to have cognitive impairment identified or treated. The CMHN working alongside others and interacting with the particular client group can act as a role model in respect of attitudes and behaviour, towards those affected by dementia.

Summary

The CMHN can provide training and specialist advice which may be particularly beneficial for those other workers who are unfamiliar with dementia and its impact. For example, prison officers may find themselves acting as carers for increasingly ageing and impaired convicts, immigration officers may find themselves interviewing people with fluctuating cognitive functioning and outreach street workers may find themselves needing to interpret agitated or confused behaviour.

Overall, the CMHN probably has much to offer those people with dementia who are increasingly marginalized but appropriate access is required and this can be achieved through inter-agency working, if there is sufficient will to do so, and with this in mind Nolan's closing remarks in the first edition ring loud and true in closing this chapter:

> I believe that this book marks a watershed in the evolution not just of the role of the CMHN, but also of a more holistic and inclusive form of partnership in which no one voice is privileged above another. Read this book, reflect upon the messages it contains and play your own part in shaping a new order of things.

Lessons for CMHN practice

- There is a 'research vacuum' in relation to the needs of people with dementia who may be homeless, in prison or seeking asylum.

- Additionally, there may also be a 'service vacuum' as in researching this chapter we have not found any wholly dedicated CMHN services working specifically to identify or address the needs of people with dementia in these populations.

- Older people exist in these populations, but have become almost invisible, and their unmet needs are both complex and considerable. For many reasons they do not come to us for help, and generally specialist mental health services do not go looking for them.

- The concept of equivalence of care should mean that the skills and clinical experience found within older age CMHN services are applied to develop services that can meet the needs of these populations.

- In promoting a social model of care, the CMHN needs to adopt a phenomenological approach and better understand the lifestyles of the older person who may be homeless, in prison or seeking asylum, and the correlations with mental health problems, especially dementia.

References

Alzheimer's Society (1994) *Home Alone*. London: Alzheimer's Society.

Anon. (2002) Mental health challenges for refugees, *Mental Health Nursing*, 22(3): 12.

Anthony, W.A., Cohen, M., Farkas, M. and Cohen, B.F. (1988) Case management – more than a response to a dysfunctional system, *Community Mental Health Journal*, (24): 219–28.

BBC News (2004) Asylum system damages health. www.news.bbc.co.uk.

Blair, T. (2004 cited in Social Exclusion Unit, 2004) *Mental Health and Social Exclusion: Social Exclusion Unit Report Summary*. London: Office of the Deputy Prime Minister.

Brooker, D., Edwards, P. and Benson, S. (2004) *Dementia Care Mapping: Experience and Insights into Practice*. London: Hawker Publications.

Burnett, A. and Peel, M. (2004) Health needs of asylum seekers and refugees, *British Medical Journal*, 332(7285): 544–7.

Burton, A. and Breen, C. (2002) Older refugees in humanitarian emergencies, *The Lancet*, 360(47): 47–8.

Cohen, J. (2001) Errors in recall and credibility: can omissions and discrepancies in successive statements reasonably be said to undermine credibility of testimony? *Medico-Legal Journal*, 69(1): 25–34.

Cohen, C.I., Teresi, J. and Holmes, D. (1988). The mental health of old homeless men. *Journal of the American Geriatric Society*, 36: 492–501.

Crane, M. (1994) The mental health problems of elderly people living on London's streets, *International Journal of Geriatric Psychiatry*, 9(2): 87–95.

Crane, M. (1999) *Understanding Older Homeless People: Their Circumstances, Problems, and Needs*. Buckinghamshire: Open University Press.

Crane, M. and Warnes, A.M. (2001) *Single Homeless People in London: Profiles of Service Users and Perceptions of Needs*. Sheffield: Sheffield Institute for Studies on Ageing, University of Sheffield.

Crane, M. and Warnes, A.M. (2003) Responding to the needs of older homeless people: the effectiveness and limitations of British services. *Innovation: The European Journal of Social Science Research*, 18: 137–52.

Crisis (2004) *Hidden homelessness: Britain's invisible city*. Background information. London: Crisis.

Department of Health (1999) *National Service Framework for Mental Health*. London: Department of Health.

Department of Health (2001) *National Service Framework for Older People*. London: Department of Health.

Department of Health and Her Majesty's Prison Service (2001) *Report of the Working Group on Doctors Working in Prisons*. London: Department of Health.

Folsom, D. and Jeste, D.V. (2002) Schizophrenia in homeless persons: a systematic review of the literature, *Acta Psychiatr Scand*, 105: 404–13.

Foord, M. (1999) A sustainable approach to planning housing and social care: if not now, when? *Health & Social Care in the Community*, 9(3): 168–76.

Frazel, S., Hope, T., O'Donnell, I. and Jacoby, R. (2001a) Health of elderly male prisoners, worse than the general population, worse than younger prisoners. *Age and Ageing*, 30: 403–7.

Frazel, S., Hope, T., O'Donnell, I. and Jacoby, R. (2002b) Psychiatric, demographic and personality characteristics of elderly sex offenders, *Psychological Medicine*, 32: 219–26.

Frazel, S., McMillan, J. and O'Donnell, I. (2002a) Dementia in prison: ethical and legal implications, *Journal of Medical Ethics*, 28: 156–9.

Frazel, S., O'Donnell, I. and Jacoby, R. (2001b) Hidden psychiatric morbidity in elderly prisoners, *The British Journal of Psychiatry*, 179: 535–9.

Frazer, L. (2003) Ageing Inside. School for Policy Studies Working Paper No. 1. London: School for Policy Studies.

Goffman, E. (1961) *Asylums: Essays on the Social Situation of Mental Patients and Other Inmates*. New York: Anchor Publishing.

Gonzalez, A., Dieter, J., Efrain, A., Natale, R. and Tanner, S. (2001) Neuropsychological evaluation of higher functioning homeless persons: a comparison of an abbreviated test battery to the Mini-Mental State Exam, *Journal of Nervous and Mental Disease*, 189(3): 176–81.

Hargreaves, S. (2000) News, *The Lancet*, 356(9248): 2168.

Health Advisory Committee for the Prison Service (1997) The provision of mental health care in prisons, London prison service, as cited by S. Wilson (2004) The principles of equivalence and the future of mental health care in prisons, *The British Journal of Psychiatry*, 184: 5–7.

Howse, K. (2003) *Growing Old in Prison: A Scoping Study on Older Prisoners*. London: Centre for Policy on Ageing and Prison Reform, Prison Reform Trust.

Jones, D. and Gill, P.S. (1998) Refugees and primary care: tackling the inequalities, *British Medical Journal*, 317: 1144–6.

Katz, I. (2001) 'Grey Area'. *The Guardian*, January 30th 2001.

Keller, A.S., Rosenfield, B., Trinh-Shevrin, C. and Meserve, C. (2003) Mental health of detained asylum seekers, *The Lancet*, 362(9397): 1721.

Kitwood, T. (1997) *Dementia Reconsidered*. Philadelphia, PA: Open University Press.

Luebben, S. (2003) Testimony work with Bosnian refugees: living in legal limbo, *British Journal of Guidance and Counselling*, 31(4): 393.

McCormack, B. (2004) Person-centredness in gerontological nursing: an overview of the literature, *International Journal of Older Peoples Nursing*, 13(3a): 31–8.

McShane, M. and Williams, F. (1990) 'Old and ornery': the disciplinary experiences of elderly prisoners, *International Journal of Offender Therapy and Comparative Criminology*, 34(3): 197–212, as cited by L. Frazer (2003) Ageing Inside. School for Policy Studies Working Paper No. 1. London: School for Policy Studies.

Marshall, T., Simpson, S. and Stevens, A. (2000) *Toolkit for health care needs: assessment in prisons*. Available from www.dh.gov.uk

Millbank, A. (2000) Boat people, illegal migration and asylum seekers in perspective. Canberra: Parliament of Australia.

Mollica, R.F., Wyshak, G. and Lavelle, J. (1987) The psychosocial impact of war trauma and torture on South East Asian refugees. *American Journal of Psychiatry*, 144: 1567–72.

NHS Executive (2000) *Nursing in Prisons: Report by the Working Group Considering the Development of Prison Nursing, with Particular Reference to Health Care Officers*. London: Department of Health.

Nolan, M. (2003) Foreword to J. Keady, C.L. Clarke and T. Adams (eds) *Community Mental Health Nursing and Dementia Care: Practice Perspectives*. Maidenhead: Open University Press.

Nolan, M.R., Davies, S., Brown, J., Keady, J. and Nolan, J. (2004) Beyond person-centred care: a new vision for gerontological nursing, *International Journal of Older Peoples Nursing*, 13(3a): 45–53.

Office of National Statistics (2004) Asylum seekers: applicants fall in latest quarter, available at: www.statistics.gov.uk.

Office of Population Censuses and Surveys (1992) quoted in L. Frazer (2003) *The National Prison. Ageing Inside*. School for Policy Studies Working Paper No. 1. School for Policy Studies.

Orwell, G. (1933) *Down and Out in Paris and London*. London: Penguin Books.

Oxfam and the Refugee Council (2002) *Poverty and Asylum in the UK*. Oxford: Oxfam.

Page, S. (2002) The role of the nurse in a memory clinic, paper presented at 4th National Memory Clinics Conference, Hammersmith Hospital, London.

Parrish, A. (2003) Reaching behind the bars, *Nursing Older People*, 15(3): 10–13.

Refugee Council (2002) Press release: asylum support system institutionalises poverty, available at: www.refugeecouncil.org.uk.

Silove, D., Steel, Z. and Watters, C. (2000) Policies of deterrence and the mental health of asylum seekers, *Journal of the American Medical Association*, 284(5): 604–15.

Social Exclusion Unit (2004) *Mental Health and Social Exclusion: Social Exclusion Unit Report Summary*. London: Office of the Deputy Prime Minister.

Toth, J. (1993) *The Mole People: Life in the Tunnels Beneath New York City*. Chicago: Chicago Review Press.

United Nations (1951) *Convention Relating to Status of Refugees*. New York: UN Publications.

Warnes, A., Crane, M., Whitehead, N. and Fu, R. (2003) *Homelessness Factfile*. London: Crisis.

Wenger, G. (1994) *Understanding Support Networks and Community Care*. Aldershot: Avebury.

Wilks, M. (2001) Chairman of the BMA Medical Ethics Committee, *The Observer*, Sunday 24th June 2001.

Wilson, S. (2004) The principles of equivalence and the future of mental health care in prisons. *British Journal of Psychiatry*, 18(4): 5–7.

PART THREE

Moving forward

Changing and developing CMHN practice

20

The community mental health nurse in dementia care
Educational opportunities and future role preparation

Emma Pritchard and Sue Ashcroft-Simpson

> Alzheimer's makes incredible demands . . . close to the heart of many carers and nurses is the desire to provide care which is humane and protects the dignity of the person . . . not only do healthcare staff need to understand issues relating to this area, but increasingly they need to have knowledge and skills in practice.
>
> (Morrissey 1999)

Introduction

The past decade has seen significant growth in the availability of education and training in dementia. Using key words 'education', 'training', 'community nursing', 'development', and 'dementia' to search the web, yields hundreds of thousands of hits in the UK alone. For community mental health nurses (CMHNs) looking for educational opportunities to develop their skills base, there is much to choose from, although, paradoxically, little guidance available on what constitutes a 'best fit' for their role and practice. For instance, many advertised one-day or sequenced courses on dementia care claim to be relevant for the whole spectrum of those working in this field of practice, including nurses. Moreover, many community nursing courses, although adopting the word 'specialist' in the title, are, on closer inspection, broad-based and contain generic content that is designed to attract nurses from different health-care settings (Coffey and Hannigan 2003).

The chapter suggests some potentially relevant educational opportunities for CMHNs developing their practice. However, it is emphasized throughout that education alone, like training, does not guarantee development or improvement in practice (Lintern et al. 2000). Building up knowledge of dementia and its effects, the range of mental and physical health problems a person may experience, along with the wider sociological factors that can impact on the lives of the person with dementia and their family and carers, is vital. However, being able to identify and work with multiple health and well-being needs requires more than attending the 'right' course. It is the integration of education *into* practice and the demonstration of resulting improvements that are key to the cycle of learning, development and practice change in this field of nursing.

Increasing awareness of the demands dementia can place on health and well-being justifies a focus on the education and development of practitioners working in this area.

295

Despite well-documented advancements in treatment and care in dementia, there is still much to learn. The quote at the beginning of this chapter highlights the importance of continuing to develop knowledge and understanding in dementia, and the value of both theoretical and experiential knowledge. Inherent in this understanding is the challenges of integrating the 'best knowledge' into nursing practice and of developing practice in a systematic and sustained way, working to include and be informed by the views and experiences of people living with dementia.

The chapter begins with a summary of recent changes in nursing education and development. It focuses particularly on supporting CMHNs to develop and demonstrate competency at an advanced level of practice as CMHNs tend to be experienced practitioners. Advanced roles in nursing encompass expert nursing practice and are multi-dimensional, including elements of education, research or consultancy (Manley 1996). Expectations, from both employers and professional bodies, that CMHNs should provide evidence of their knowledge and skills through developing and demonstrating their competency at all levels, are likely to increase (Dewing and Traynor 2003). Therefore, practical guidance for CMHNs follows on building portfolios to develop and demonstrate competency, as having a portfolio is part of the Agenda for Change Knowledge and Skills Framework (Wallis 2004) and is likely to be a requirement of registration as an advanced practitioner (NMC 2004). To illustrate the dynamic movement and integration of education into evidence-based practice, the chapter draws on Admiral Nursing work (see Soliman 2003, for a discussion), developing and demonstrating competency to practise using the Admiral Nurse Competency Framework (Traynor and Dewing 2003). For a brief description of the Admiral Nurse role, see Box 20.1.

A recent history

In 1994, the United Kingdom Central Council (UKCC) (now the Nursing and Midwifery Council) completed its framework for post-registration education and practice. Prior to this, the focus had been solely on developing pre-registration education. The UKCC (1994) framework introduced compulsory re-registration for all practising nurses and graduate-level (or equivalent) entry to specialist practice. For the first time, the importance of learning and development both before and after registration was emphasized. The International Council of Nursing (ICN) and the Royal College of Nursing (RCN) were key influences on this work, emphasizing that patients needed nurses working as generalists, that is, able to care for different patients in a variety of settings; as well as specialists, that is, concerned

---

Box 20.1 A description of the Admiral Nurse role

Admiral Nurses are mental health nurses working in the field of dementia. Admiral Nurses work primarily with carers and supporters of people with dementia and they offer consultancy to professionals providing care for people with dementia. Admiral Nurse clients, therefore, include people who support and/or represent people with dementia and people with dementia themselves. The education and development work undertaken by Admiral Nurses focuses on improving dementia services for all stakeholders.

(Source: for dementia 2004)

with nursing care in a particular area of practice. The UKCC (1994) framework stated that nurses would need to provide evidence, every three years, of participation in a minimum of five days self-directed continuing education. Different educational opportunities have arisen for nurses as a result of these changes, and some of those relevant to community nursing and dementia care are now described.

Certificate and diploma courses in dementia

The English National Board (ENB) N11 post-registration course 'Caring for People with Dementing Illness' was developed in the 1990s and was available for nurses and other dementia practitioners through local academic/educational service providers. This course has been incorporated into many certificate and diploma courses in dementia care run across the UK. Many of these are evaluated positively and are extremely popular. However, wide variation between courses has been reported. There is currently no national standard for training and education in dementia and a lack of clarity exists about what titles such as 'advanced', 'certificate' and 'diploma' actually mean in terms of course content and outcomes for students and their practice (Pulsford et al. 2003).

Community Specialist Practitioner qualifications

Currently, community nurses can opt to study for a 'specialist practitioner' qualification. The first of these programmes began in 1995. The level of study for this qualification is mainly at first degree level with each programme based on 50 per cent practice and 50 per cent theory. According to the UKCC (1995), a specialist practitioner is expected to exercise higher levels of judgement in clinical practice and has a remit to develop care.

A key 'specialist practice' area within this programme is community mental health nursing. CMHNs working with older people with mental health needs are therefore able to gain a qualification that has the potential to integrate theory and practice and to relate to their role. However, criticisms have been levelled at the Community Specialist Practitioner courses (Coffey and Hannigan 2003) such as the variation between courses and the dominance of local educational needs and curriculum designers' interests. The courses attempt to meet the needs of CMHNs who may work with people from across the lifespan. Therefore, a CMHN working with older people with dementia may benefit from developing knowledge of issues such as the effects of ageism or retirement and how these may impact on mental health, or of the complex interplay of sociological and biological factors as we age, as part of such a course. However, these may be less relevant to a CMHN working with children. Accordingly, the generic course content has also been perceived by CMHNs as being largely irrelevant to working with people with mental health needs. There is also reported variation in the standard of practice placements and the support to integrate theory and practice.

Coffey and Hannigan argue that all CMHN education and training should be 'informed by a fundamental mental health nursing ethos which is steeped in the tradition of humanism' (2003: 367). The authors suggest the Community Specialist Practitioner degree needs review and would like to see pre-registration programmes designed to lead to a qualification as a CMHN and then, once this is completed, further courses for preparation as advanced practitioners, working with specific groups of service users such as older people. However, in the wider nursing literature, there seems to be growing support for a more generalist and family-centred pre-registration curriculum, with an opportunity for shared multi-disciplinary learning and specialization taking place following registration (RCN 2004a). For CMHNs, sharing modules or experiences with other mental health professionals could be of benefit as it is likely that CMHNs will spend much of their time working as part of a mental health team. In the case of dementia, this could expand to sharing learning with other key professionals, such as care managers and those working in primary care, as many people with dementia are identified and supported through the provision of social services and primary care.

Higher degrees

More recently, a range of academic courses in dementia, gerontology and nursing at Bachelor and Masters level have been developed. There are also a growing number of options to undertake research degrees (MPhil/PhD) in nursing; and the more recent development of Clinical Doctorates is an exciting opportunity for nurses who wish to explore clinical practice at a Doctorate level. Doctorates in Clinical Practice focus on developing research capability and capacity and aim to improve the quality of professional practice in a particular discipline and clinical domain. They comprise taught modules with a piece of clinically focused research which could explore a particular problem area of community nursing in dementia care, for example, or an area of practice that needs development.

With this growing number of educational options available, CMHNs may find it difficult to choose the most appropriate course. Being aware of the underpinning philosophy, the content, the credits, and the level of different courses course may help when deciding on the course to apply for (see Box 20.2).

However, the move towards nursing becoming a competency-based profession suggests

Box 20.2 Some questions to help CMHNs explore academic courses

- Does the course have a generic or specialized focus or both?
- Is it underpinned by a humanistic philosophy?
- Does it contain the most up-to-date and relevant knowledge?
- Is it informed or influenced by users and carers?
- Is it relevant to clinical practice?
- It is relevant to personal/team/organizational learning and development goals?
- Does it include learning in the workplace, or assessment of integration of knowledge into practice and impact on practice?
- Does it include shared learning with other professionals?
- Does it offer options for recognition and accreditation of prior academic or experiential learning?
- Does it lead to a qualification recognized by NHS and universities in the UK/internationally?

nursing is not something that can be learned purely in the classroom. Whatever educational opportunity CMHNs access, they will need to prove its relevance and impact to their area of practice, particularly if they wish to register as a practitioner at an advanced or higher level.

Advanced practice in community mental health nursing

Education and development opportunities for nurses following registration are constantly under review. In 1999, the UKCC published its intentions in relation to developing Higher Level Practice, and in 2002 they published the model for Higher Level Practice, comprising seven standards that nurses claiming to practise at an advanced or higher level would need to demonstrate their competency. The standard emphasized the importance of developing one's own and others' practice and improving quality through evaluation and research. This setting of a nationally recognized standard reflected the greater emphasis on the need for public protection (UKCC 1999) and outlined a possible framework to support nurses developing and demonstrating competency at a higher or advanced level.

As well as supporting the development of specialist practice in nursing, the UKCC retained the concept of advanced practice, saying it would consider the possibility of recording such qualifications on the register in due course (UKCC 1995). As long ago as 1994, the UKCC stated:

> Advanced nursing practice is concerned with adjusting the boundaries for the development of future practice, pioneering and developing new roles responsive to changing needs, and with advancing clinical practice, research and education to enrich professional practice as a whole.

At that time they suggested that nurses had the option of demonstrating, through their professional portfolios, that they had achieved a level of practice and knowledge that equated with the idea of advanced practice (UKCC 1995). However, nurses had little to assess their progress against, in other words, how could nurses be expected to demonstrate advanced practice when they had no guidance as to the standard to be achieved?

These changes in nursing education and the wider health-care arena gave rise to the development of different nursing roles with different nursing titles, with variations in skills, knowledge, role and grade and some confusion as to what these different titles meant. This lack of clarity was a key driver for the current review. What does being called a 'specialist nurse' really mean? How can I be sure the nurse working with me is practising at an 'advanced level' and what knowledge and skills should he/she have? What do I need to do to prepare myself for advanced practitioner status? What kind of education and development is relevant? All these are reasonable questions to ask.

In 2003, the Nursing and Midwifery Council (NMC) began looking more closely at what practising at a higher or advanced level actually meant. They state:

> The raft of titles that currently exist in the health sector is often confusing and does not equate with a consistent set of national standards. By formally setting competencies for advanced and specialist clinical practice, we will clarify roles for practitioners, their employers and importantly, the public. They will know that someone who says they are working at a higher level will be regulated and will have met competencies specific to that role.

A task and finish group was formed by NMC in 2003 to determine a new post-registration framework for the nursing part of the register, with the aim of protecting the title of some advanced and specialist practice roles through the setting of agreed competencies. This group has worked with different stakeholder groups, including the Department of Health, to review competencies and titles in nursing.

The NMC (2004) consultation document outlines the characteristics of a nurse working at a level beyond initial registration and they propose a definition for a nurse working at this level (Box 20.3). They clearly state they do not intend to develop standards and competencies for expert knowledge for each specific field of practice and that the standard they propose is generic (NMC 2004). To this end, they suggest seven broad domains which include a range of generic competencies (Box 20.4), and suggest that the characteristics of nurses working at a level beyond initial registration are that they work both independently and interdependently by:

- taking responsibility for case management;
- making differential diagnoses;
- planning and providing care and treatment, including prescribing medication, in collaboration with others as appropriate;
- providing health education, counselling and leadership.

CMHNs in dementia care, working as individual practitioners and as part of a wider team, are likely to demonstrate such characteristics and these will more than likely be fundamental to their role.

The NMC intends that nurses will be able to register on an additional sub-part of the nursing part of the register and will seek evidence from nurses that they meet the required standard. Nurses will need to demonstrate they have maintained their competence and will

Box 20.3 Definition of a nurse practising at an advanced level

A registered nurse who has command of an expert knowledge base and clinical competence, is able to make complex clinical decisions using expert clinical judgement, is an essential member of an interdependent health-care team and whose role is determined by the context in which s/he practises.

Box 20.4 Proposed seven domains for advanced nursing practice

- The nurse–patient relationship
- Respecting culture and diversity
- Management of patient health/illness status
- The education function
- Professional role
- Managing and negotiating health-care delivery systems
- Monitoring and ensuring the quality of health-care practice.

need to re-register every three years. The NMC have determined that the supporting expert knowledge that will inform practice should reflect a Masters degree level of thinking and when nurses are assessed, the NMC will require them to provide a rationale for their actions (NMC 2004). Education at Masters level is generally considered the level necessary for nurses to work towards practice at an advanced level (Manley and Garbett 2000; Chief Nursing Officer 2004).

The NMC proposals recognize that nurses' knowledge can be acquired in a number of ways including learning from academic courses, from practice and from others, and state that these arrangements are likely to include assessment in practice and the production of a portfolio of evidence demonstrating how the competencies have been met. The NMC also suggest that nurses who hold a specialist practice qualification, such as the Community Specialist Practitioner qualification mentioned earlier, will equally be eligible to make use of the arrangements.

In addition to the work carried out by the NMC, in 2003, an advisory group led by the Chief Nursing Officer made recommendations to the Department of Health Strategic Learning and Research Advisory Group to strengthen the approach to education of nurses and midwives beyond registration (CNO 2004). The report uses the phrase 'learning beyond registration' to include four main areas:

1   ad hoc training, e.g. learning opportunities that deliver organizational focused updating;

2   continuing professional development;

3   education and training associated with acquiring additional knowledge, skills and competencies intended to enable the nurse to move to more advanced activity (the main focus of the document);

4   education that is relevant to the nurses' professional practice, e.g. a leadership programme or Masters degree in dementia.

Among a number of recommendations, the report suggests that achievement of competencies associated with advanced forms of prescribing should become a normal expectation of nurses seeking recognition as advanced practitioners, and suggests that substantive learning beyond registration should both build towards recognition as an advanced practitioner as well as offer stand-alone modules for those who wish to enhance their role in primary practice. They recommend accredited learning pathways are constructed comprising different modules including both theoretical and practical learning that give weight to the acquisition of clinical competence and build towards recognized awards at Masters and Doctoral level (CNO 2004).

The report emphasizes the full spectrum of learning beyond registration as well as the need for portable credits that have currency throughout both academic and professional systems. It highlights issues similar to those raised in the NMC consultation such as the importance of portfolios as a means of demonstrating learning at an advanced level, along with an emphasis on developing competence in prescribing. The challenges and complexities of nurse prescribing in dementia care are discussed in depth in Chapter 9. Although advanced practice in nursing is clearly about more than being able to prescribe, developments in nurse prescribing could be viewed as an opportunity for CMHNs to develop their roles. For example, CMHNs could directly influence and improve dementia care through addressing polypharmacy or withdrawal from inappropriately prescribed sedation, as well as through more conventional prescribing.

Accrediting learning beyond registration is also being considered as part of current work by the University of Salford (Eyres 2005) on developing an inter-professional framework for all health professional learning beyond initial registration (commissioned by the Department of Health in 2003). The outcomes of this work (see web link in reference list) will impact on nurses' development following registration. One of the project aims is to identify a shared credit framework for learning and examine the relationship between academic accreditation and work-based learning. The importance of connecting all learning with the workplace is emphasized and the work will cover all health-care staff groups within the scope of statutory regulation.

Implications for CMHN practice

These developments give rise to some important challenges. CMHNs need to consider how they will use these opportunities to contribute to developing the evidence base for their practice in dementia. The need to establish an 'evidence base' to underpin practice is important for a number of reasons. With a move towards increasingly time-limited psychosocial interventions, and the introduction of roles such as nurse prescribing and different roles for nurses suggested in the Mental Health Act Bill (Hulatt 2004), it is important to be aware of the potential these changes offer, as well as be active in exploring and articulating the caring and compassionate nature of CMHN work, and what it is that helps both those with dementia and their carers and supporters with their experience of such a potentially life-changing condition. CMHNs in dementia care have a real opportunity to work inclusively to develop competence in promoting health and well-being for people with complex and enduring mental health needs and their families and carers (a key nursing area in both the NMC (2004), proposed competencies and the Knowledge and Skills Framework (Department of Health, (2004)), as well as to take a lead role in both developing and using existing health promotion techniques and approaches to this end.

Developing the skills to evaluate practice and disseminate the findings to the profession and practice community is key to developing the CMHN role (Keady and Adams 2001). It could be argued that the challenge in this area is greater than in many others, as nursing expertise is difficult to articulate and test because it is made up of many forms of knowledge (Clarke et al. 2003). Showing the evidence base for our practice is not just a matter of doing what research tells us to do, it is about making explicit how we integrate theory, practice and our personal knowledge, putting what we do under a magnifying glass, and being clear about how this can promote health and well-being.

CMHNs also need to consider the value of eventually registering as an advanced practitioner in community mental health nursing in dementia, raising the profile of this area and contributing towards developing the evidence base for practice. As already suggested, admission to such registers is likely to be based on a combination of standards of education and competence (RCN 2004a). CMHNs, therefore, need to become familiar with the NMC work on advanced practice and be prepared to be assessed for advanced practitioner status through a range of means such as portfolios of evidence, and for the challenges of rigorous practice-based assessments. It is important to note, however, at the time of writing, the mechanisms for regulation of advanced practice have not yet been decided although the NMC (2004) consultation document gives some indication.

The recent work on education for nurses emphasizes the importance of shared learning and from learning in and from the workplace. Keady and Adams (2001) argue for education and development for CMHNs in dementia to reflect practice reality and emphasize skill acquisition. Formal learning usually covers only a small part of the necessary learning for work, indeed, Eraut (1998) states that most learning that takes place is informal, arising from the process of work itself, and from communication and interactions within the workplace. Learning through the workplace and developing necessary knowledge and skills is about learning to reflect on learning, put it into practice and deal with the challenges and problems it generates. It involves new learning and learning new ways of learning! This can be challenging and it is important that CMHNs are able to access support and supervision to support and sustain their development.

There are also important messages for organizations employing CMHNs in dementia. In today's health-care climate, the emphasis is on demonstrating evidence to support future resource funding and on developing the knowledge and skills of the workforce to deliver evidence-based health care. It is important that CMHNs in dementia define their role and purpose clearly, develop the appropriate competencies at an advanced level, and locate their practice within some kind of evaluative framework. They also need to think about ways of disseminating their work and publicizing their achievements. Managers can support CMHNs by working with them to develop an agreed education and development strategy that supports this and links CMHN work in dementia with the organization's aims. It could provide criteria for CMHNs to use when selecting academic courses, and offer the supervision and support they need to integrate knowledge and practice, and register as advanced practitioners in dementia care.

Developing competency, integrating education and practice through portfolio development

The next section of the chapter outlines some of the ways CMHNs could use portfolios to demonstrate competency, and describes a portfolio example of developing CMHN practice in dementia.

Competency frameworks

The recent nursing literature contains examples of different competency frameworks, some specialized and some generic. Whatever framework CMHNs use as the basis for developing competency, they will need to spend some time thinking and teasing out the relevance of the competency statements for their own practice. The areas of competency will indicate areas for assessment and CMHNs will need to agree on these as being relevant to their practice.

One example of a specialized nursing competency framework is the Admiral Nurses Competency Framework (Traynor and Dewing 2003). This provides a nursing framework, including eight core competencies that capture the work that Admiral Nurses undertake with people with dementia and their carers (see Box 20.5). This can be used with generic

Box 20.5 Admiral Nurses' core competencies

- Therapeutic interventions
- Advanced assessment skills
- Sharing information about dementia and carer issues
- Prioritizing work
- Health promotion
- Ethical and person-centred care
- Balancing the needs of the carer and the person with dementia
- Promoting best practice.

competencies, such as those proposed by the NMC (2004) to represent advanced or higher level practice.

CMHNs could also consider the validity of other possible sources. The domains described below integrate the main areas of the CMHN role (derived from Keady 2003) and the NMC Code of Conduct and could prove a useful basis for a framework.

- working collaboratively with the person with dementia, their carers and supporters and the wider team;
- being person-centred and developing person-centred practice;
- developing caring relationships;
- being trustworthy and practising ethically with particular regard to confidentiality and consent;
- working to identify and minimize risk;
- developing evidence-based practice with particular reference to screening and assessment, therapeutic interventions and promoting health and well-being.

Dewing and Traynor (2003) suggest that CMHNs could integrate the themes from National Service Framework for Older People (Department of Health 2001) into a framework to gather evidence, thereby supporting the delivery of this strategy.

Links between more specialized competencies and the generic competencies suggested by the NMC for advanced practitioners will need to be clear, and consistency between these and the Knowledge and Skills outlines, currently being developed in the NHS as part of Agenda for Change Knowledge and Skills framework, will need to be established, with CMHNs being a key part of this process. These outlines define the core and specific dimensions of each role and the knowledge and skills required for the post to inform learning and development needs (Department of Health 2004). CMHNs will need to be sure the frameworks they use facilitate the development of evidence-based care in dementia for nurses and the teams they work with.

Creating a portfolio

Using standards and competencies to develop practice will more than likely require the creation of a portfolio of evidence that maps across the competency areas, with a written summary of learning throughout the process. It is important to be clear about the reasons for creating a portfolio of practice. We may have our own individual reasons; our employers may require us to undertake this work; also portfolios are likely to be a requirement to register as an advanced practitioner. One of the authors (SAS) created her own portfolio of Consultant Admiral Nurse practice in her second year in the role in order to develop the role along with her ability to articulate more clearly what she does and why. Some of her Admiral Nurse colleagues gave the following reasons for embarking on this process:

- for my own ongoing learning and reflection
- I want to develop as an advanced Admiral Nurse
- to use the learning from my Masters degree in practice
- to make the Knowledge and Skills framework relevant to what I do
- to improve what I do
- to keep a record of my work and development
- to learn from my practice
- to improve the evidence base in dementia nursing.

Portfolios can have different purposes and these will guide their development. See Box 20.6. It is difficult to give a timescale for portfolio development. Portfolios in the RCN Expertise in Practice Project (2004c) took approximately nine months to a year for a nurse to produce with the help of their companion (RCN 2004b). Susan Ashcroft-Simpson's own portfolio of Consultant Admiral nursing practice took a year to complete.

Collecting the evidence

The sorts of evidence a CMHN may use in a portfolio could include client records, critical incidents, accounts, presentations, published material, project plans, or meeting minutes, and should reflect the variety of a CMHN's day-to-day work. Traynor and Dewing (2003)

Box 20.6 Ways to use portfolios

Portfolios are safe places to keep a record of learning achievements in the workplace and what these mean to practice. A portfolio may be a collection of work that describes learning, progress and actions over a period of time. It should be more than a collection of certificates and should capture evidence of competency and learning to demonstrate personal and professional growth, and to direct future learning and development. Portfolios can be used as means to accredit prior learning and to gain credits for an academic award, for example, or as a basis for developing academic work for a course or for integrating academic work into practice. They may contribute to appraisal/review or developing advanced practice status. They could also be viewed as a way of developing as a practitioner researcher, that is, developing the skills to research directly into one's practice (Reed and Proctor 1995).

include an extensive list of type of evidence in the Admiral Nurse Competency Framework and an example of CMHN portfolio evidence is featured later in the chapter.

Nurses practising at an advanced level will need to show evidence of the development and application of their knowledge and skills in their area of practice. Purely descriptive accounts of applying knowledge in practice will not be enough, nurses will need to develop critical appraisal skills to be able to use learning from attendance on a course in a practice situation and generate further learning from their practice. Whatever course or education programme they access, they will need to demonstrate the outcomes for their patients and clients through the evidence they produce. Creating a portfolio is one means of achieving this and is increasingly recognized as a means of demonstrating and assessing competence to practice.

Structuring a portfolio

Portfolios can have different structures and CMHNs need to consider how they can devise or adapt a structure that is suitable to their practice, and use any guidance published by the NMC and other nursing bodies, particularly if they are considering developing and demonstrating practice at an advanced level.

The following is a template adapted from Traynor and Dewing (2003) and RCN (2004b):

- Introduction with content list. This says what the portfolio contains, briefly.
- The analysis and explanation of how the competencies have been achieved. That is, the reflective summary. This links theory and practice through detailing learning about and from practice. It is important here to consider the different perspectives on your work. The summary describes the effects of your work on yourself and others and summarizes your learning, including the gaps and any actions you are going to take as a result. It can be organized into sections such as:
  - Introduction and methods, i.e. how you tackled gathering, interpreting and analysing evidence; how you addressed ethical issues, the way you assessed how the evidence and reflective summary met the competency criteria and level.
  - Dissemination plan, i.e. how you are going to let others know about your work.
  - A curriculum vitae with an outline of role and responsibilities.
  - Contact details of those who have facilitated your development of the portfolio, this maybe your supervisor, buddy or mentor and a short testimony from them.
  - The broad range of evidence that shows you have met the competency areas and level you are aiming for. It is important to be selective here and include evidence that is cross-referenced across all the competency areas.
  - Your reflective summary.
  - Conclusion and references.

At first glance, this may seem like a lot of work. Creating a portfolio of learning is a challenge, particularly in terms of protecting time for this in a busy working day. However, there will be flexibility with any portfolio structure and an important part of the process of building a portfolio will be to decide on the purpose(s) of the work and then discuss and agree a structure with your supervisor or supporter, using any relevant guidelines in order to fit the purpose(s). It is important to keep a portfolio under control. Using a ring-binder with different sections may be a useful approach and nurses could use audio tape, video or other creative methods to reduce the amount of paper. The most important part of the portfolio is the evidence section. A common mistake is to include too much evidence which then makes the summary difficult and time-consuming to complete. A piece of evidence that cross-references across many competencies is preferable to one that covers one or two areas as the example later in the chapter shows. Developing a portfolio means beginning to stand back and think critically. It can also act as a means to developing linguistic and literacy skills. However, this all comes with experience. Discovering how to use a portfolio may well be an outcome of experience in its development and use.

Support to develop portfolios

Your portfolio facilitator may be your clinical supervisor, a colleague, or a client for example. Whoever they are, it is important they are able to do the following:

- offer a supportive relationship;
- help to apply competencies to your specific practice area or situation;
- be able to discuss portfolio structure and help you make decisions on this;
- discuss how to achieve outcomes and on the evidence required to demonstrate learning and competency;
- give feedback on whether evidence is at correct level;
- support you with writing and reconstructing experiences in the required format for the reflective summary;
- agree ways of giving and receiving feedback;
- be clear about their own ways of doing things, their own practice values and own views on learning.

(*Source*: for dementia 2003)

Extract from a reflective summary

The following extract from a CMHN portfolio is a reflective piece and relates to work with a family. The evidence the CMHN produced in her portfolio linked to this extract also comprised clinical notes and a testimony from the carer she was working with. The CMHN used a reflective framework (adapted from Johns 1995) to frame her reflection and included the main learning and action points in the summary in her portfolio.

What do I feel about the experience?

Maureen cared for her mother who had dementia and who had just moved into residential care. Her father had died four months before. She was particularly close to her father and her grief and distress was having a significant impact upon her life and her ability to cope with her mother's situation. Maureen had recently been diagnosed as having clinical depression and was trying to balance a full-time job with her grief and emotional turmoil. She described her situation as follows:

It is difficult for me to know what to focus on, my mum or dad. Dad's death was terrible and I just couldn't see the wood for the trees. I was having two bereavements at once as my mum went into a home soon after dad's death and it was like experiencing a loss as great as when dad died. I am also trying to do a demanding job and am worried about my performance.

Initially Maureen's experience made me feel confused. I faced a dilemma about my role. Maureen was referred to me for help and advice around her mother's diagnosis and move into full-time care. My role is to provide this support for family carers of people with dementia. However, I was hit initially by the gravity of loss and bereavement that Maureen was experiencing following her father's death. I felt that my initial interventions needed to focus on her feelings regarding her father's death before I could help her move on to the needs concerning her mother. I discussed the dilemma with colleagues and with Maureen. As my confusion cleared I felt more certain that my priority was to provide support around the death and loss of Maureen's father who had held a pivotal role in her life. From early on I could see there was a wide range of needs and interventions that Maureen and I could work on together. It was important to explain my role to her and negotiate a series of sessions together based on what we eventually agreed her needs and goals were. In all, this situation made me feel a little overwhelmed and this was one way of me gaining a focus, but I was aware that the sessions needed to be fluid and responsive to changing needs.

What are the key themes/issues I needed to pay attention to?

Initially, I needed to find out more about Maureen as a person by listening to her. She needed to be able to trust me as a nurse and feel she could talk openly to me. She was feeling out of control and was experiencing multiple losses and I needed to find out more about how this was impacting on her. I needed to pay attention to building a relationship with Maureen, one in which openness and honesty underpinned a working relationship where she was an equal partner, bringing her own expertise and understanding to the work. I needed to identify with Maureen how she would know if the work around her grief for her father and sense of loss for her mother had been successful so that we could move forward with other issues at an appropriate pace. There was so much potential work that we could do together that I formed some themes to organize my work, which I agreed with Maureen.

The main themes and focus of my work were around supporting her through the grieving process for her father; supporting Maureen to explore and adjust to the many senses of loss that she was experiencing following her mother's dementia; working to treat and support her through her depression; enhancing Maureen's understanding of Alzheimer's disease and dementia with Lewy Bodies; enhancing her understanding of appropriate responses and care for her mother; and empowering her to eventually be able to pass on her learning to her family and to the staff of the home. I identified through my work with Maureen a learning need of my own. I wanted to explore grief and bereavement in more depth. I had an understanding of the traditional model of grief processes but felt this was an opportunity to expand my knowledge.

How do I feel the situation was managed and what were the influencing factors (internal and external)?

Maureen needed to trust me and feel comfortable with me before she could openly talk about her father and mother. This trust doesn't come overnight. I had to make myself available to Maureen by demonstrating compassion, empathy, trust and an ability to join her and walk alongside her on her journey. Taking this time and clarifying our relationship helped me see more clearly into the maze of Maureen's emotions and helped me help her grasp clear threads from a clouded picture. I needed to listen to Maureen's story and forget any agenda I might have as she had many different needs and the picture was confusing.

My relationship with Maureen's mother and the care team working with her was forged through working with Maureen and helping her develop ways of supporting her mother. I feel I managed the sessions with Maureen well. I was focused, used a broad evidence base for my interventions, explained this to Maureen and we agreed the goals through discussion and negotiation. Maureen was good to work with because she would reflect upon what we had talked about in our previous session. She often demonstrated a clear understanding of what we had discussed by giving examples of how she had incorporated some new knowledge, advice or skill into her everyday caring role with her mother. Maureen was also prepared. She had always thought through the issues she wanted to bring before each meeting which was helpful, as she brought her own sense of clarity to the discussions in what had started out being a tangled picture.

What were the consequences for all the stakeholders?

Maureen listed the consequences of our eight sessions together as:

- Getting the emotions out of the cupboard.
- Help to grieve for her father.
- Developing emotional care of her mother through seeing into her world.
- Continuing to earn respect of colleagues at work.
- Improved self-esteem.

The consequences for me were:

- Explaining and using theory to develop my work with Maureen.
- Real partnership working, encouraging Maureen to ask me difficult questions and to support me when I struggled to explain to her what I was doing and why.
- A sense of achievement as Maureen's depression began to lift, she regained control over her life and had purpose and direction.
- Influencing her mother's care in the nursing home positively.
- Helping Maureen to regain a sense of well-being.
- Developing my own knowledge and skills working with grief and bereavement.

The consequence for Maureen's mother was:

- Improved emotional care by the staff and her family.

Could the situation have been dealt with differently and what would the consequences have been?

I did consider working directly with the home staff to help increase their understanding of her mother's emotional needs and thus enhance her care. This would have achieved more speedy but perhaps limited results. The consequences of this would have been that Maureen might not have developed the close supportive relationship that she has since done with the home staff, and she might not have developed the strong sense of empowerment that she has today. Instead of this approach, I worked with Maureen when she was emotionally able, she then supported the staff by passing on her new learning to them in her own words. This helped her to gain a stronger sense of self-esteem and a stronger understanding of her mother's needs and her mother's experience.

What sources of knowledge could have influenced the situation and how can I make sense of this in terms of my practice?

Rogers' (1967) humanistic approach influenced my work, as did the National Institute of Clinical Excellence (NICE 2004) guidelines on depression. I felt Maureen was experiencing a grief reaction, and my experience that counselling and problem-solving style approaches do help within a holistic approach to care, informed my care plan. I have developed my understanding of bereavement and attachment and loss through doing this work with Maureen. Working with the whole system, i.e. Maureen, her mother, her colleagues and her mother's care team, has influenced my interest in systemic family work.

What are my action points?

The next step is to think about publishing this work with Maureen in a nursing or dementia journal as my supervisor feels this would be a useful practice piece for others to read. She has offered to help me with this and I've set myself the target of six months.

Summary of portfolio example

This portfolio extract starts to illustrate the evidence base and outcomes of CMHN work with clients and teams. It maps across the eight care competencies of the Admiral Nurse Competency Framework and the seven proposed domains for advanced nursing practice (NMC 2004). This reflective work demonstrates the CMHN's clinical and developmental skills and experience and her ability to think creatively from different perspectives. The example demonstrates integration of theory and practice and the use of critical thinking skills in a practice context. It is one example from a portfolio that is currently 'work in progress'.

Developing a portfolio is an ongoing process, as this reflects the nature of learning through the workplace. Once a portfolio has been created, it will need review and development over time to capture the learning through carrying out action plans and to continue to develop the evidence base for practice.

| Discussion

Traditionally, education in nursing has necessitated nurses leaving the practice area to study elsewhere. However, there is now growing emphasis and evidence to support the value of integrating education and practice in different ways. The move in post-registration nursing education and development from a predominantly classroom-based learning approach, to a focus on learning from and in practice is apparent in current review proposals (NMC 2004; CNO 2004). For CMHNs in dementia care, this provides the context for nursing practice to develop in a way that is responsive to the needs of people with dementia and their carers. There is also a growing move towards encouraging learning opportunities shared between different professions along with recognition of the need to recognize and accredit learning that is achieved through learning in the workplace (Eyres 2005). Nursing is moving towards becoming a competency-based profession and the work by the NMC (2004) with key nursing stakeholders, to create an agreed group of nursing domains and associated competencies at an Advanced Practice level supports this. CMHNs in dementia care should be encouraged and motivated to prepare themselves to register at this level, generating and making use of organizational and peer support for their learning and development. Registering as advanced practitioners will contribute towards the evidence base for nursing practice in dementia care and raise the profile of nursing in a field that is often believed to be of little import. These developments in nursing education undoubtedly bring challenges for CMHNs practising in this area. However, development and demonstration of competency to practise at an advanced level in this field can only contribute to improving the experience of care for people with dementia and their carers and families.

Summary

This chapter has focused on education and development for CMHNs working in dementia. The drivers for education review in nursing have been discussed and the emphasis has been on possibilities for CMHN development as advanced practitioners. The chapter has suggested ways for nurses to record and structure their work, showing the outcomes of their practice through creating a portfolio of evidence. Demonstrating ability to practise is particularly important in terms of accountability to the public; to support lifelong learning and career progression in nursing; and for the ongoing development of dementia practice and services.

Lessons for CMHN practice

- Integration of education into practice and the demonstration of resulting improvements, are fundamental to the cycle of learning, development and practice change in this field of nursing.

- Developing practice in a systematic and sustained way and integrating the 'best knowledge' into nursing practice are key to developing CMHN practice in dementia care.

- CMHNs in dementia care are encouraged to register as advanced practitioners when processes and mechanisms are agreed, emphasizing the need for and raising the profile of skilled nursing in this area.

- Underpinning role preparation and development for CMHNs in dementia care, with clinical supervision and a commitment to developing reflective practice, are recommended.

- In order to facilitate the development of advanced practitioners in dementia care, specialist competencies for community nursing in dementia need to relate to the Agenda for Change Knowledge and Skills Framework (Department of Health 2004) and to the NMC (2004) Advanced Practitioner domains and competencies, when agreed.

References

Chief Nursing Officer (2004) *Post Registration Development: A Framework for Planning, Commissioning and Delivering Learning Beyond Registration for Nurses and Midwives. A consultation.* London: CNO.

Clarke, C.L., Keady, J. and Adams, T. (2003) Integrating practice and knowledge in a clinical context, in J. Keady, C. Clarke and T. Adams (eds) *Community Mental Health Nursing and Dementia Care.* Maidenhead: Open University Press.

Coffey, M. and Hannigan, B. (2003) Education and training for community mental health nurses, in B. Hannigan and M. Coffey (eds) *The Handbook of Community Mental Health Nursing.* London: Routledge.

Department of Health (2001) *National Service Framework for Older People: Modern Standards and Service Models.* London: Department of Health.

Department of Health (2004) *The NHS Knowledge and Skills Framework (NHS KSF) and the Development Review Process.* London: Department of Health.

Dewing, J., Hancock, S., Brooks, J., Pedder, L., Adams, L., Riddaway, L., Uglow, J. and O'Connor, P. (2004) An account of 360° review as part of a practice development strategy. *Practice Development in Health Care*, 3(4): 193–209.

Dewing, J. and Traynor, V. (2003) Higher-level practice: addressing the learning needs for community mental health nursing practice in dementia care, in J. Keady, C. Clarke and T. Adams (eds) *Community Mental Health Nursing and Dementia Care.* Maidenhead: Open University Press.

Eraut, M. (1998) Concepts of competence, *Journal of Interprofessional Care*, 12(2): 127–39.

Eyres, R. (2005) *Health Professional Learning Beyond Registration.* Manchester: University of Salford. Web page: http://www.hplbr.org.uk/index.htm.

for dementia (2003) *Becoming a Competency Companion.* London: for dementia.

for dementia (2004) *Core Job Description Admiral Nurse.* London: for dementia.

Hulatt, I. (2004) The Mental Health Bill: united we stand, *Mental Health Practice*, 8(3): 17.

Johns, C.C. (1995) Framing learning through reflection within Carper's fundamental ways of knowing in nursing, *Journal of Advanced Nursing*, 22: 226–34.

Keady, J. (2003) People with dementia and their carers, in B. Hannigan and M. Coffey (eds) *The Handbook of Community Mental Health Nursing.* London: Routledge.

Keady, J. and Adams, T. (2001) Community mental health nurses in dementia care: their role and future. *Journal of Dementia Care*, March/April: 33–7.

Lintern, T., Woods, B. and Phair, L. (2000) Training is not enough to change care practice, *Journal of Dementia Care*, 8(2): 15–17.

Manley, K. (1996) *Consultancy: Masters in Nursing Distance Learning Module.* London: RCN.

Manley, K. and Garbett, R. (2000) Paying Peter and Paul: reconciling concepts of expertise with competency for a clinical career structure, *Journal of Clinical Nursing*, 9: 347–59.

Morrissey, M. (1999) Current issues in care, in M. Morrissey and A.L. Cookley (eds) *Alzheimer's Disease: Beyond the Medical Model.* Salisbury: Quay Books, Mark Allen Publishing Ltd.

National Institute of Clinical Excellence (2004) *Quick Reference Guide: Depression: Management of Depression in Primary and Secondary Care.* Clinical Guideline 23. London: National Institute of Clinical Excellence.

Nursing and Midwifery Council (2004) *Consultation on a Framework for the Standard for Post-registration Nursing.* London: NMC.

Pulsford, D. et al. (2003) The contribution of higher education to dementia care, *Journal of Dementia Care*, 11(4): 27–9.

Reed, J. and Proctor, S. (1995) *Practitioner Research in Health Care: The Inside Story.* London: Chapman and Hall.

Rogers, C. (1967) *On Becoming a Person.* London: Constable.

Royal College of Nursing (2004a) *The Future Nurse: The Future for Nurse Education.* London: RCN.

Royal College of Nursing (2004b) *Becoming an RCN Accredited Facilitator. Part 3: Developing Your Portfolio – Methods for Gathering and Analysing Evidence.* London: Royal College of Nursing Institute.

Royal College of Nursing (2004c) *Expertise in Practice Project: Exploring Expertise.* London: Royal College of Nursing Institute.

Soliman, A. (2003) Admiral Nurses: a model of family assessment and intervention, in J. Keady, C. Clarke and T. Adams (eds) *Community Mental Health Nursing and Dementia Care.* Maidenhead: Open University Press.

Traynor, V. and Dewing, J. (2003) *The Admiral Nurses Competency Framework.* London: for dementia.

United Kingdom Central Council for Nursing Midwifery and Health Visiting (1994) *The Future of Professional Practice: The Council's Standards for Education and Practice Following Registration.* London: UKCC.

United Kingdom Central Council for Nursing Midwifery and Health Visiting (1995) *PREP and You.* London: UKCC.

United Kingdom Central Council for Nursing Midwifery and Health Visiting (1999) *A Higher Level of Practice: Report on the Consultation on the UKCC's Proposals for a Revised Regulatory Framework for Post-Registration.* London: UKCC.

United Kingdom Central Council for Nursing Midwifery and Health Visiting (2002) *Report of the Higher Level of Practice Pilot and Project.* London: UKCC.

Wallis, L. (2004) Personal life experiences can count in portfolios, *Nursing Standard*, 18(36): 11.

|21

Out of our history and into our future
Reflections on developing CMHN practice

Charlotte L. Clarke

Introduction

In this chapter I would like to analyse the relationship between what we actually practise, what we believe ourselves to be achieving through practising in this way, and the social and political forces that shape the way in which services are provided and care delivered. It is only through an analysis of this kind that we can appreciate the relationship between ourselves and our actions and the needs of those who are to benefit from our intervention. And it is this relationship that is fundamental to creating the energy to develop practice.

In this analysis I will draw together a number of research studies that form a programme of research into the processes of developing practice in health care, synthesizing some of the developing knowledge from these alongside the work of many eminent writers and researchers in the field. We will start off by examining health needs, moving on to explore health-care needs, and the needs of health-care organizations. As we move through these areas I would like also to throw down a few challenges to us personally, professionally and organizationally in order to shine a light on where perhaps we may want to move to. I don't mean to make assumptions about wanting to move anywhere, but if we are all totally satisfied with where we are now then I wonder why we are writing books such as this (and you are reading them!). We have an inherent curiosity to learn and to try to do things differently – those who receive our care, on the other hand, live every day with the frustrations, the destruction and the rewards of dementia. Curiosity and learning and improving are not a luxury, they are imperative if we are to fulfil our responsibility and duty of care to those who access our services. The first step is to be dissatisfied with where you are now.

Health needs

Health need is a surprisingly complex issue and we need to step back from the individual client in order to understand the dynamics at play and the way in which they shape what we understand an individual's health needs to be. Here are a few stark messages from others who have felt uncomfortable with where they are or see others being.

Processes of care within a psychiatric medical model result 'in a contrived and sanctioned dehumanisation of the person' (Hall 1996), and in illuminative accounts such as: 'I felt as though I was a heartless magician, demonstrating to these people the growing insubstantiality of their memory, providing them with an explicit display of the shrinking limits of their minds' (McKee 1999).

Society defines and redefines the dividing line that determines diagnosis and differentiates normal from abnormal – this is not an objective diagnosis but a position of 'moral rectitude' (Harding and Palfrey 1997) with value judgements placed on diagnostic indicators.

As long as there is a grain of truth in these statements, then it is important that we reflect on what these points mean for our practice and where they have come from, and how they shape the way in which we understand the health needs of our clients. There are many historical and cultural influences on what we think health need is. Previously, I have argued that dementia care practices, and the care of family carers, are underpinned by discrimination and reductionalism (Clarke 1999a). There are many dimensions to this:

- *Mental health status*. For a long time someone's mental (ill) health has been deployed as a reason for excluding them from participating in decision making and from articulating their own view of their needs (Barnett 1997). There are encouraging indications that this position is being challenged (e.g. Killick 1997; Crisp 1999) and methods are being developed to allow us to better engage with people in practice and in research (e.g. Wilkinson 2002). However, Sweeting and Gilhooly's (1997) articulation of the 'social death' of someone with dementia who is no longer regarded as a whole and valued person still has an uncomfortable resonance and we are in a very early stage of moving beyond that.

- *Dependency*. Hill (1999) argues that the binary division of dependent/independent is too simplistic and he calls for the interdependency between people to be more fully recognized. Such approaches to the complexity of dependency and independence have informed in part the emergence of relationship-centred care in the nursing of people with dementia (e.g. Clarke 1997; Nolan et al. 2004). Swain et al. (2003) also seek to disentangle what is meant by the concept of dependency, identifying the word 'independence' as having two meanings: (1) to need other people's help; (2) to be free from control in judgement, action, etc. This latter meaning is perhaps of particular concern to us in dementia care and is integrated with our developing an understanding of what it means to have insight and competence alongside the presence of dementia. If we are to support independence for people with dementia, then it is necessary for us to understand that this means freedom from control over their decisions and action. It does not just mean ability to manage without the help of others. Indeed, the help of others may allow the person with dementia to have control over their decisions and actions. Contrast this with a study that interviewed 20 nurses and found that 'for patients, dependency on care is a miserable loss of self-determination and self-worth' (Strandberg and Jansson 2003: 84).

- *Age*. Dementia has been seen to be a disease of largely an older sector of the population and has experienced therefore the age discrimination of resource allocation (Reed et al. 2004). This has fuelled and been fed by the therapeutic pessimism associated with dementia care and underdeveloped expertise and specialist practice (Brooker 2001). Recently this has been partially reversed due to emergence of pharmaceutical interventions for dementia and memory clinics, which need a workforce with high level of assessment skills. Luce et al. (2001) found that when compared with the memory clinic model, the traditional old age psychiatry route has patients referred who are both older and more advanced in the course of the dementia. That nursing people with dementia and their families demands a high level of expertise and skills has been promoted by *for dementia*, a London-based charity that has in the past decade developed a national network of Admiral Nurses, CMHNs who specialize in caring for families of people with dementia (see Chapter 20 in this book).

- *Gender*. Carter (1999) links care *in* the community to care *by* the community to care *by* women in the home. Likewise, Dalley argues that 'community care, then, is based on an ideology of familism which in turn rests on a gendered division of labour within the domestic sphere' (1993: 18). It requires a societal movement of gender perceptions for this position to have changed within the past few years.

- *Culture*. Arber and Ginn (1997) argue that culture impacts in families through their capacity to lever additional resources to manage an enduring health-care need such as dementia. In particular, this is bound up with class and the stratification of income. Cloutterbuck and Mahoney found that there was cultural differentiation in levels of respect and disrespect, writing that 'many African Americans view accessing and receiving healthcare as a potentially degrading, demeaning or humiliating experience. They fear racism or segregation of feelings of powerlessness and alienation in the system' (2003: 234). Ethnicity in dementia care has only recently received attention, with valuable work undertaken by Stuckey (2003), Farran et al. (2003), Nightingale (2003) and in this book, by Jenny Mackenzie in Chapter 6.

- *Biography*. The need for an intimate knowledge of the person's life story is being increasingly recognized as necessary to providing effective dementia care (Crisp 1995, 1999; Keady 1997; Keady and Gilleard 1999). This is the personal knowledge known of by family carers and people with dementia but of limited availability to professional carers (Clarke and Heyman 1998). Without access to this knowledge, our awareness of the person who has dementia is restricted and our ability to allow their biography to inform present intervention and future planning is consequently limited.

- *Focus of care*. There is a long history of being focused on the needs of the family carer and relieving them of the 'burden' of care but this dismisses the relationship between the family carer and the person with dementia (Kitson 1987; Orona 1990; Clarke 1997). For example, Adams (1999) describes how the person with dementia was not regarded by CMHNs as a legitimate target for therapeutic intervention and care was diverted into supporting the carer. This has changed considerably with the emergence of person-centred care practices (Brooker 2001) and the advent of assessment for dementia at earlier stages of memory loss and the introduction of memory clinics, with early intervention advocated with the person with dementia (e.g. Alzheimer Scotland Action on Dementia 1994, 2003; Gilliard and Gwilliam 1996; Moniz-Cook and Woods 1997). There is a need, currently unfulfilled, for interventions that focus on, and respect, relationships within families (Clarke 1997; Carter 1999).

- *Health status*. The past decade has seen a notable shift to understanding and engaging with some of the diversity of need in dementia. This is in part reflected by the growth of activity in areas of care for people with dementia that have been previously neglected, such as sexual health (Archibald 1995, 1997) and spiritual health (Barnett 1995; Froggatt and Moffitt 1997; Katsuno 2003; Snyder 2003). These reflect the need to focus on well-being rather than the eradication of disease that was promoted by Kitwood and Bredin (1992).

These historical and cultural influences on the way that the needs of someone with dementia are understood reflect changes to the underlying social position about the role of cognition in society and in being a person. Reed et al. (2004) make the distinction between self as a cognitive entity and self as a product of relationships. The latter (interactionist) position is supported by Kitwood and Bredin (1992) who suggest that as cognitive ability changes, people become increasingly reliant on others for a sense of self-identity (see also Orona 1990; Sabat and Harré 1992) leading us to value and nurture those relationships. The position of self as cognitive entity results in dementia being seen to be so pervasive that the person is substantially and irreversibly changed – socially dead – and allows distancing by those around them in order to define themselves as sane and normal (Hall 1996; Reed 1999). In the quote below, Friedell (2002: 361) reflects on the personal impact of this perceived fragmentation of what it is to be human:

> for me the horror of AD is summed up in a statement by Dempsey and Baago (1998 p. 84): 'while the physical being of an individual with a dementing illness remains intact, the very essence of a person – the psycho-social self – slowly disintegrates'. It can be questioned how true this is. Nevertheless, their statement well expresses the horror, with its uncanniness of the slow disintegration of a self whose essence, presumably, is to integrate. Just how could one even conceive of a self slowly disintegrating?

While Friedell, as a person with dementia, finds it hard to conceive of the self disintegrating, it was clearly not beyond J.K. Rowling to do so. In *The Prisoner of Azkaban* (1999), she describes creatures that suck out your soul. These creatures are called dementors and are portrayed as a source of terror for others.

In a cognitively defined and dependent society, the society itself plays a part in disabling people with dementia: 'it is the complexity of society that contributes to reducing the functional ability of people with memory problems' (Reed et al. 2004: 81). For example, Friedell found himself after diagnosis with dementia 'transmogrified into a woman. He was supposed to be weak at sustained attention ("flighty"), poor at logic and long-range planning, but great at living in the moment, at smelling the flowers and at appreciating the warmth of touch' (Friedell and Bryden 2002: 131). This was an expectation that was rejected!: 'Living in the here and now is not sufficient; one must be capable of cherishing memories and envisioning the future' (Friedell 2002).

There are undoubtedly culturally diverse ways of understanding and responding to dementia. For example, Cloutterbuck and Mahoney (2003) found that the 'toleration of cognitive and behavioural changes' and respect for dignity and independence for as long as possible in African American families was a strength, although it also tended to result in delays in seeking assessment and diagnosis. However, the role of our society and the impact of globalization cannot be underestimated, influencing as it does the social and financial infrastructure that is in place for older and disabled people as well as our understanding of what dementia is and therefore what the needs of someone with dementia might be. For instance, Bond and Corner (2004) describe the politicization of Alzheimer's disease, it being important that it is seen as pathological to allow access to research funds. In particular, they highlight the way in which 'mild cognitive impairment' has emerged as a new diagnostic label and the significance of that for research and clinical funding, the experience of people and professional intervention.

There are, then, processes that promote a cognitive understanding of dementia as a pathology and with, therefore, a set of assumptions about the need for assessment and intervention. There are also processes that contend that this is an inadequate understanding of dementia and of health need. Indeed, Berrios writes, 'during the last few years, the cognitive paradigm has become an obstacle, and a gradual re-expansion of the symptomatology of dementia is fortunately taking place' (2000: 10). It is in this context that a range of frameworks of assessment and intervention are now emerging, such as relationship-centred care (Nolan et al. 2002; Nolan et al. 2004). Likewise, Coleman and Mills (2001) argue that 'contemporary societies need to develop new cultures of dementia care drawing on insights from the world's faiths and traditions'. In the theory of normalization, developed through a grounded theory study of family carers of people with dementia, we can see that families focus on their continuing relationship with a person with dementia; that professionals often focus on the pathology and deficits of the individual and carer burden; and that there is a need to focus on the interpersonal dimensions of families and care (Clarke 1997). These are approaches to understanding the health need of people with dementia and their families that are 'clearly contradictory to the story of deviance, difficulty, and despair' (Robinson 1993).

Here then is our first set of challenges:

- to adjust our lens of focus and *reframe* health need;
- to come out of our *cognitively bound* way of thinking;
- to recognize *enduring ability*.

Health-care need

There is also a set of historical and cultural influences on health-care 'need'. Some of these are bound with the legacy of health-care delivery models and infrastructure, and the repeated efforts of policy to adjust the way in which health care is delivered bears testimony to the intractable nature of these patterns of service delivery (e.g. Iles and Sutherland 2001; Newman and Maylor 2002). These include issues such as the promoted shift from secondary to primary care (Iliffe 1997; Kavanagh and Knapp 1998; Iliffe et al. 2000) and although people with dementia and their families are undoubtedly now better supported to remain in their own homes and communities (e.g. Fortinsky et al. 2002), there are still an enormous number of people with dementia in long-term residential or inpatient care. The danger of having to work with inflexible delivery models and infrastructure is that they come to determine perceived health need. For example, very few people with dementia actually need respite care but it is one of few interventions available to allow the family carer to relinquish day-to-day care activity for a short period of time. Indeed, it is a reflection of the medicalization and associated assumed pathology of caring activity that allows us to even frame respite as a health-care rather than social care activity.

Another key influence on health-care need is the process by which professionals and services define need. In dementia care, as with other areas of enduring health care and social care need, there are marked differences between the dominant knowledge of professional and lay carers (e.g. Clarke and Heyman 1998). The family carer of a person with dementia has a knowledge of that person that is normally denied to practitioners and that is inevitably drawn from a domain of personal values and meanings (Nolan and Keady 2001). Practitioners have a knowledge base that arises from their past knowledge and experiences of caring for people with dementia. The care provided by practitioners is determined by a knowledge of the 'right' way of caring. This is potentially assumptive of a single evidence base and may lack acknowledgement of the values and meanings associated with the knowledge domains of the family carer or person with dementia. There are three linked dimensions to this apparent mismatch between health need and service provision to meet that need (Clarke 1999b):

1   There are considerable differences between lay and professional conceptions of health and pathology.

2   There is philosophical diversity in professional practice ranging from pathophysiological models through to interactionalist, social constructionist and socio-critical models, each bringing its own set of assumptions about dementia causality, assessment, intervention, role of the family and relationship between professionals and client.

3   These conflicting knowledge domains generate ethical dilemmas in clinical decision-making.

For example, in a study into the construction and management of risk in dementia care, Clarke et al. (2004a) were concerned that risk assessment and management are processes that have the potential to marginalize and exclude people from social participation and that power can be exerted through the status of knowledge and the ability to effect action (people with dementia being quite powerless). The ethical issues around risk management demand that practice that is defensible is promoted rather than defensive practice dominating. In particular, professionals, families and people with dementia need to recognize the context of meaning in which their expertise is embedded and make these meanings accessible to each other. Bond et al. (2002) argue that a diagnosis of dementia can lead to professional judgements about lack of insight that result in depersonalization and loss of independence, and in this way removal from the probabilities of risk.

Here then is our second set of challenges:

*   to know of our *differences*;
*   to value our *diversity*;
*   to work in *partnership* with service users.

The knowledge needs of health care

Health care itself has a set of needs that are influenced by its own organizational biography, and often it is these needs that preside over the needs of individual clients and families. In the UK, some of these issues concern the evolution of the National Health Service (NHS) – that it is actually multiple NHS organisations and so tensions ripple through the system between developing local services to meet local need and national-driven policy and services; and that the internal marketplace approach to providing services impacts still on the way in which these NHS organizations work together.

The very notion of the NHS is of course laden with a set of boundaries and borders, including the boundaries of health and social care and of primary and secondary care (Manthorpe et al. 2003). These are reinforced by inter-professional guardedness, the overlaying of policies such that tensions and conflicts of purpose are created and by the essence of the NHS as a service attending to the well-being of those who are unwell. It is therefore an 'ill-health' service (or 'disease-ridden' as described by one study participant in the following study!). This soft systems methodology evaluation of partnership working and community development described the dynamics of engagement and entrenchment that shape the needs of any health provider organization. Patterns of entrenchment are those in which decisions and actions reinforce historical patterns of service delivery, health is clinically (ill-health) defined, power continues to be distributed according to traditional hierarchies, change upholds disease-orientated individualistic definitions of health and the historical distribution of power. One the other hand, patterns of engagement are those in which decisions and actions focus on meeting population health need, regardless of traditional boundaries of service delivery. Health is defined as a universal attribute possessed by all, available to all, and the responsibility of all. Change challenges traditional power hierarchies and promotes partnership working across professions, organizations and statutory and voluntary care sectors.

Underpinning several issues here is the way in which knowledge is created, communicated and used in services and in a way that seeks to minimize the loss of knowledge to the system. In a study of adult mental health services that developed a new pattern of service delivery (involving a higher proportion of non-professionally qualified staff; shared health and social care staff offices and high level of joint-disciplinary activity between CMHNs and social workers) (Gibb et al. 2002), it was possible to identify ways in which the service had developed so positively. These included: feeding service user knowledge into the care system; minimizing information transaction time (especially between the social workers and the CMHN); creating an early warning system; interdisciplinary knowledge exchange; and an increased capacity for receptivity and critical analysis of knowledge. Similarly, Garvin (1993) emphasizes the importance of quick and efficient transmission of knowledge through an organization in order to enhance decision-making, inform new policy and practice and provide the capacity for effective action (Senge 1990).

Here then is our third set of challenges:

- to develop practices and services across *boundaries*;
- to conceptualize *health* and the role of the NHS;
- to *capture knowledge* and orientate services to service users;
- to put knowledge to *work*;
- to prevent the *haemorrhaging* of knowledge.

Needs of health-care organizations

There are a number of ways in which the whole industry of health care needs to be able to perpetuate itself, and these are manifest in the following ways: emergence of self-sustaining organizations; transfer from non-human to human capital resource base; recognition of the need for lifelong learning of the workforce.

In relation to self-sustenance, health-care organizations need to be attentive to their own organizational needs if they are to be sustainable and continue to be able to deliver health care (Good 2001). This means that they need to attend to the accountability and reporting mechanisms placed upon them to a wide variety of stakeholders, but not least those that fund the organization's activities. At times this results in organizational needs appearing to drive and even supersede the needs of the service user but this only happens when the performance management criteria do not accord with service user need and it is important to examine the value base of the criteria. The NHS Modernisation Agency and National Health Service University (NHSU) have developed and promoted mechanisms for developing practice and services, and increasingly connect these to the discipline of improvement (see Clarke et al. 2004b) which rests on the belief that:

- All work is process.
- All processes should meet the needs of users and carers.
- All processes can be redesigned and improved.
- Everyone should be involved in improving services.

The discipline of improvement has evolved from notions of technical-rationality (services being seen to develop through logically deduced alterations to processes and structures) to embracing more post-modern notions of learning, participation, process and context specificity. It supports the generation of local solutions to local problems yet retains the promotion of universal principles.

In any change to practices it is essential to connect up the needs of the service user, the practitioners and the organization. There is ample evidence to suggest that ad hoc unplanned implementation of change does not result in the desired outcomes (e.g Taylor and Hirst 2001; Good 2001). Heller and Arozullah (2001) identified four factors for successful implementation of practice change: (1) aligning the practice with the strategic goals of the organization; (2) obtaining active senior leadership commitment, including allocation of resources; (3) securing the appropriate infrastructure to facilitate integration of recommended actions into daily practice; and (4) setting up systematic communications with all stakeholders.

Traditionally, the power of organizations has been exerted and sustained through their infrastructure and buildings, their non-human capital resource base. Now it is much more acknowledged that it is people, the human capital of an organization, that are its power base (Good 2001). In particular, the human capital is important because of its role in developing, communicating and using knowledge. To this end, the vast investment in professional development of nursing staff in the UK in recent decades has now created the critical mass necessary for knowledge management to be a very valuable commodity for health-care organization. This is enhanced by those staff who have post-registration and postgraduate experiences now attaining senior management and leadership roles and in turn promoting a questioning approach in their staff. Indeed, the Institute for Healthcare Improvement (2000) urges us to consider professional subject matter as a core component of improvement in health care. It is this professional knowledge base that is essential to driving forward patient care. First, because it is the ethical base of practice that is essential to the adoption and sustaining of change (Berwick et al. 2001; Manthorpe 2001; Monaghan and Begley 2004); and, second, because for any service or practice change to take place, the staff must have or be able to acquire the expertise to deliver the new way of working.

There is a shift from nursing using a knowledge base learnt in pre-registration training with subsequent education regarded as unnecessary (and, yes, I have worked in that place too!), to nursing knowledge being regarded as constantly evolving and staff education of considerable priority. Lifelong learning is starting to replace the 'learned for life' beliefs of earlier decades and personal learning through reflection is instrumental in creating practitioners who can learn to change health and social care in ways that are 'more congruent with the values and theories they espouse' (Greenwood 1998). Garvin (1993) recognizes that beyond 'high philosophy and grand themes' lies the gritty detail of practice. Like Schön (1983), who reminds us of 'the swampy lowlands' of practice, Garvin (1993) advocates the notion of learning organizations where the prevailing philosophy is one of continuous improvement requiring a commitment to lifelong learning, both for the individual and for the organization. We are reminded of the danger of failing to fully acknowledged workforce learning needs by Manthorpe et al. (2003) who relate that generalist staff reported a lack of confidence in managing dementia within primary care and referred people on to secondary care providers.

Brechin (2000) describes contemporary health-care working as:

> one of fire-fighting; managing time constraints; dealing with conflicting demands; setting difficult priorities; managing tricky relationships; finding short cuts; dealing with stress and frustration (both internal and external); and struggling to hang onto simply doing the job. It is about operating within organisational and social constraints as an individual, feeling accountable and responsible, yet often powerless and lacking any real autonomy.

> (Brechin 2000: 15)

Brechin goes on to describe a model of critical practice that is fundamental to developing practice and that encapsulates many of the things we have discussed in this chapter and has the following domains:

- critical reflexivity;
- engaged self;
- negotiated understanding and interventions;
- questioning personal assumptions and values;
- critical analysis;
- evaluation of knowledge, theories, policies and practice;
- recognition of multiple perspectives;
- different levels of analysis;
- ongoing enquiry;
- critical action;
- sound skill base used with awareness of context;
- operating to challenge structural disadvantage;
- working with difference towards empowerment.

Here then is our last set of challenges:

- to provide *sustainable whole-system* development;
- to realize that *people* are the resource;
- to ensure *lifelong learning* in a volatile policy environment.

Summary

If dissatisfaction is our starting point, then we need to be able to do something with that feeling! It needs to be supported to develop into a curiosity about other ways of doing things and we need to be provided with the wherewithal to satisfy that curiosity and find a more fulfilling and rewarding way of practising and meeting the health needs of people with dementia and their families,

One way of achieving this is to create learning communities – communities to which we belong and which are characterized by qualities that provide an environment of sustainable and sustained critical enquiry. We need to create communities that have the capacity to learn how to do the following:

- to *integrate* closely learning, practice and knowledge development;
- to respect the interdependence of professional and organizational *learning*;
- to realize that the *power and energy* of practitioners to move forward patient care is one of the biggest opportunities facing health and social care as it moves towards being knowledge-orientated;
- to tap into the *knowledge creation* potential of practitioners;
- to work with the *contexts* of organizational care delivery;
- to learn how to *reconceptualize* health need, health care and organizational development.

In short, we need to create communities that create the future for people with dementia, their families, the staff who work with them and the organizations in which they are employed. This is a set of components that constitute developing dementia care, and is something that every single one us has some influence over, an influence that we are obliged to exert in order to provide optimal services and practices for people with dementia.

References

Adams, T. (1999) Developing partnership in the work of community psychiatric nurses with older people with dementia, in T. Adams and C.L. Clarke (eds) *Dementia Care: Developing Partnerships in Practice*. London: Baillière Tindall.

Alzheimer Scotland Action on Dementia (1994) *Agenda for Dementia: Improving the Care of People with Dementia and Their Carers in Scotland*. Edinburgh: Alzheimer Scotland Action on Dementia.

Alzheimer Scotland Action on Dementia (2003) *Making the Journey Brighter: Early Diagnosis and Support Services for People with Dementia and their Carers*. Edinburgh: Alzheimer Scotland Action on Dementia.

Arber, S. and Ginn, J. (1997) Class, caring and the life course, in S. Arber and M. Evandrou (eds) *Ageing, Independence and the Life Course*, 2nd edn. London: Jessica Kingsley.

Archibald, C. (1995) Sexuality and the sexual needs of the person with dementia, in T. Kitwood and S. Benson (eds) *The New Culture of Dementia Care*. London: Hawker.

Archibald, C. (1997) Sexuality and dementia? in M. Marshall (ed.) *The State of the Art in Dementia Care*. London: Centre for Policy on Ageing.

Barnett, E. (1995) Broadening our approach to spirituality, in T. Kitwood and S. Benson (eds) *The New Culture of Dementia Care*. London: Hawker.

Barnett, E. (1997) Collaboration and interdependence: care as a two-way street, in M. Marshall (ed.) *The State of the Art in Dementia Care*. London: Centre for Policy on Ageing.

Berrios, G. (2000) Dementia: historical overview, in J. O'Brien, D. Ames and A. Burn (eds) *Dementia*, 2nd edn. London: Arnold.

Berwick, D., Davidoff, F., Hiatt, H. and Smith, R. (2001) Refining and implementing the Tavistock principles for everyone in health care, *BMJ*, 232(7313): 616–20.

Bond, J. and Corner, L. (2004) *Quality of Life and Older People*. Maidenhead: Open University Press.

Bond, J., Corner, L., Lilley, A. and Ellwood, C. (2002) Medicalization of insight and care-givers' responses to risk in dementia, *Dementia*, 1(3): 313–28.

Brechin, A. (2000) Introducing critical practice, in A. Brechin, H. Brown and M.A. Eby (eds) *Critical Practice in Health and Social Care*. London: Sage Publications.

Brooker, D. (2001) Therapeutic activity, in C. Cantley (ed.) *A Handbook of Dementia Care*. Buckingham: Open University Press.

Carter, C.E. (1999) The family caring experiences of married women in dementia care, in T. Adams and C.L. Clarke (eds) *Dementia Care: Developing Partnerships in Practice*. London: Baillière Tindall.

Clarke, C.L. (1997) In sickness and in health: remembering the relationship in family caregiving for people with dementia, in M. Marshall (ed.) *The State of the Art in Dementia Care*. London: Centre for Policy on Ageing.

Clarke, C.L. (1999a) Taking partnership in dementia care forward, in T. Adams and C.L. Clarke (eds) *Dementia Care: Developing Partnerships in Practice*. London: Baillière Tindall.

Clarke, C.L. (1999b) Dementia care partnerships: knowledge and ownership, in T. Adams and C.L. Clarke (eds) *Dementia Care: Developing Partnerships in Practice*. London: Baillière Tindall.

Clarke, C.L. and Heyman, B. (1998) Risk management for people with dementia, in B. Heyman (ed.) *Risk, Health and Healthcare: A Qualitative Approach*. London: Chapman and Hall.

Clarke, C., Luce, A., Gibb, C., Williams, L., Keady, J., Cook, A. and Wilkinson, H. (2004a) Contemporary risk management in dementia: an organisational survey of practices and inclusion of people with dementia, *Signpost*, 9(1): 27–31.

Clarke, C.L., Reed, J., Wainwright, D., McClelland, S., Swallow, V., Harden, J., Walton, G. and Walsh, A. (2004b) The discipline of improvement: something old, something new? *Journal of Nursing Management*, 12: 85–96.

Cloutterbuck, J. and Mahoney, D.F. (2003) African American dementia caregivers: the duality of respect, *Dementia*, 2(2): 221–43.

Coleman, P.G. and Mills, M.A. (2001) Philosophical and spiritual perspectives, in C. Cantley (ed.) *A Handbook of Dementia Care*. Buckingham: Open University Press.

Crisp, J. (1995) Making sense of the stories that people with Alzheimer's tell: a journey with my mother, *Nursing Inquiry*, 2: 133–40.

Crisp, J. (1999) Towards a partnership in maintaining personhood, in T. Adams and C.L. Clarke (eds) *Dementia Care*. London: Baillière Tindall.

Dalley, G. (1993) The ideological foundations of informal care, in A. Kitson (ed.) *Nursing: Art and Science*. London: Chapman and Hall.

Dempsey, M. and Baago, S. (1998) Latent grief: the unique and hidden grief of carers of loved ones with dementia, *American Journal of Alzheimer's Disease*, 13(2): 84–91.

Farran, C.J., Paun, O. and Elliott, M.H. (2003) Spirituality in multicultural caregivers of persons with dementia, *Dementia*, 2(3): 353–77.

Fish, D. and Coles, C. (1998) *Developing Professional Judgement in Health Care*. Oxford: Butterworths Heinemann.

Fortinsky, R.H., Unson, C.G. and Garcia, R.I. (2002) Helping family caregivers by linking primary care physicians with community-based dementia care services, *Dementia*, 1(2): 227–40.

Friedell, M. (2002) Awareness: a personal memoir on the declining quality of life in Alzheimer's, *Dementia*, 1(3): 359–66.

Friedell, M. and Bryden, C. (2002) Editorial, *Dementia*, 1(2): 131–3.

Froggatt, A. and Moffitt, L. (1997) Spiritual needs and religious practice in dementia care, in M. Marshall (ed.) *The State of the Art in Dementia Care*. London: Centre for Policy on Ageing.

Garvin, D.A. (1993) Building a learning organisation, *Harvard Business Review*, 71(4): 78–92.

Gibb, C.E., Morrow, M., Clarke, C.L., Cook, G., Gertig, P. and Ramprogus, V. (2002) Transdisciplinary working: evaluating the development of health and social care provision in mental health, *Journal of Mental Health*, 11(3): 339–50.

Gilliard, J. and Gwilliam, C. (1996) Sharing the diagnosis: a survey of memory clinics, their policies on informing people with dementia and their families, and the support they offer, *International Journal of Geriatric Psychiatry*, 11: 1001–4.

Good, V. (2001) Developing service organizations, in C. Cantley (ed.) *A Handbook of Dementia Care*. Buckingham: Open University Press.

Greenwood, J. (1998) The role of reflection in single and double loop learning, *Journal of Advanced Nursing*, 27: 1048–53.

Hall, B.A. (1996) The psychiatric model: a critical analysis of its undermining effects on nursing in chronic mental health, *Advances in Nursing Science*, 18: 16–26.

Harding, N. and Palfrey, C. (1997) *The Social Construction of Dementia: Confused Professions?* London: Jessica Kingsley.

Heller, C. and Arozullah, A. (2001) Implementing change: it's as hard as it looks, *Disease Management and Health Outcomes*, 9(10): 551–63.

Hill, T.M. (1999) Western medicine and dementia: a deconstruction, in T. Adams and C.L. Clarke (eds) *Dementia Care: Developing Partnerships in Practice*. London: Baillière Tindall.

Iles, V. and Sutherland, K. (2001) *Organisational Change*. London: NCCSDO.

Iliffe, S. (1997) Can delays in the recognition of dementia in primary care be avoided? *Aging and Mental Health*, 1(1): 7–10.

Iliffe, S., Walters, K. and Rait, G. (2000) Shortcomings in the diagnosis and management of dementia in primary care: towards an educational strategy, *Aging and Mental Health*, 4(4): 286–91.

Institute for Healthcare Improvement (2000) *Health Professional Learning about the Improvement of Health Care*. London: Institute for Healthcare Improvement.

Katsuno, T. (2003) Personal spirituality of persons with early-stage dementia: is it related to perceived quality of life? *Dementia*, 2(3): 315–35.

Kavanagh, S. and Knapp, M. (1998) The impact on general practitioners of the changing balance of care for elderly people living in institutions, *British Medical Journal*, 317: 322–7.

Keady, J. (1997) Maintaining involvement: a meta concept to describe the dynamics of dementia, in M. Marshall (ed.) *The State of the Art in Dementia Care*. London: Centre for Policy on Ageing.

Keady, J. and Gilleard, J. (1999) The early experience of Alzheimer's disease: implications for partnership and practice, in T. Adams and C.L. Clarke (eds) *Dementia Care: Developing Partnerships in Practice*. London: Baillière Tindall.

Killick, J. (1997) Confidences: the experience of writing with people with dementia, in M. Marshall (ed.) *The State of the Art in Dementia Care*. London: Centre for Policy on Ageing.

Kitson, A.L. (1987) A comparative analysis of lay-caring and professional (nursing) caring relationships, *International Journal of Nursing Studies*, 24: 155–65.

Kitwood, T. and Bredin, K. (1992) Towards a theory of dementia care: personhood and well-being, *Ageing and Society*, 12: 269–87.

McKee, K.J. (1999) This is your life: research paradigms in dementia care, in T. Adams and C.L. Clarke (eds) *Dementia Care: Developing Partnerships in Practice*. London: Baillière Tindall.

Luce, A., McKeith, I., Daniel, S. and O'Brien, J. (2001) How do memory clinics compare with traditional old age psychiatry services? *International Journal of Geriatric Psychiatry*, 16: 837–45.

Manthorpe, J. (2001) Ethical ideals and practice, in C. Cantley (ed.) *A Handbook of Dementia Care*. Buckingham: Open University Press.

Manthorpe, J., Iliffe, S. and Eden, A. (2003) The implications of the early recognition of dementia for multiprofessional teamworking: conflicts and contradictions in practitioner perspectives, *Dementia*, 2(2): 163–79.

Monaghan, C. and Begley, A. (2004) Dementia diagnosis and disclosure: a dilemma in practice, *International Journal of Older People Nursing*, 13(3a): 22–9.

Moniz-Cook, E. and Woods, R.T. (1997) The role of memory clinics and psychosocial intervention in the early stages of dementia, *International Journal of Geriatric Psychiatry*, 12: 1143–5.

Newman, K. and Maylor, U. (2002) The NHS Plan: nurse satisfaction, commitment and retention strategies, *Health Services Management Research*, 15(2): 93–105.

Nightingale, M.C. (2003) Religion, spirituality, and ethnicity: what it means for caregivers of persons with Alzheimer's disease and related disorders, *Dementia*, 2(3): 379–91.

Nolan, M., Davies, S., Brown, J., Keady, J. and Nolan, J. (2004) Beyond 'person-centred' care: a new vision for gerontological nursing, *International Journal of Older People Nursing*, 13(3a): 45–53.

Nolan, M. and Keady, J. (2001) Working with carers, in C. Cantley (ed.) *A Handbook of Dementia Care*. Maidenhead: Open University Press.

Nolan, M., Ryan, T., Enderby, P. and Reid, D. (2002) Towards a more inclusive vision of dementia care practice and research, *Dementia*, 1(2): 193–211.

Orona, C.J. (1990) Temporality and identity loss due to Alzheimer's disease, *Social Science in Medicine*, 30: 1247–56.

Reed, J. (1999) Keeping a distance: the reactions of older people in care homes to confused fellow residents, in T. Adams and C.L. Clarke (eds) *Dementia Care: Developing Partnerships in Practice*. London: Baillière Tindall.

Reed, J., Stanley, D. and Clarke, C. (2004) *Health, Well-being and Older People*. Bristol: The Policy Press.

Robinson, C.A. (1993) Managing life with a chronic condition: the story of normalisation, *Qualitative Health Research*, 3: 6–28.

Rowling, J.K. (1999) *The Prisoner of Azkaban*. New York: Scholastic Inc.

Sabat, S. and Harré, R. (1992) The construction and deconstruction of self in Alzheimer's disease, *Ageing and Society*, 12: 443–61.

Schön, D. (1983) *The Reflective Practitioner: How Professionals Learn in Action*. New York: Basic Books.

Senge, P. (1990) *The Fifth Discipline: the Art and Practice of the Learning Organisation*. London: Doubleday/Century Business.

Snyder, L. (2003) Satisfactions and challenges in spiritual faith and practice for persons with dementia, *Dementia*, 2(3): 299–313.

Strandberg, G. and Jansson, L. (2003) Meaning of dependency on care as narrated by nurses, *Scandinavian Journal of Caring Sciences*, 17(1): 84–91.

Stuckey, J.C. (2003) Faith, aging and dementia: experiences of Christian, Jewish, and non-religious spousal caregivers and older adults, *Dementia*, 2(3): 337–52.

Swain, J., French, S. and Cameron, C. (2003) *Controversial Issues in a Disabling Society*. Buckingham: Open University Press.

Sweeting, H. and Gilhooly, M. (1997) Dementia and the social phenomenon of social death, *Sociology of Health and Illness*, 19: 93–117.

Taylor, P. and Hirst, J. (2001) Facilitating effective change and continuous improvement, *Journal of Change Management*, 2(1): 67–71.

Wilkinson, H. (ed.) (2002) *The Perspectives of People with Dementia: Research Methods and Motivations*. London: Jessica Kingsley.

22

Signposts to the future
Some personal reflections and messages for CMHN practice

John Keady, Charlotte L. Clarke, Sean Page and Trevor Adams

Introduction

In the Foreword to this book, Professor Mike Nolan outlined the importance of community mental health nursing to dementia care and generously stated that the text had messages that could transcend this specific professional grouping. We certainly hope this proves to be the case as there is much to learn and share within the field of dementia care practice, and from other disciplines and stakeholder groups more generally. However, in this final, brief, concluding chapter, we would like to return to the primary purpose of the text and focus upon the work of the community mental health nurse (CMHN) in dementia care by documenting some reflections and messages for the profession. This could be considered a rather self-indulgent and self-important exercise, but in our opinion it is all the more pressing as, nationally, dementia care services seek to establish themselves as either medical or social care services. Arguably, this leaves the CMHN standing at a crossroads where the path to follow is far from clear.

Moreover, given the absence, to date, of a (UK) funded national study on the work and evidence-base of the CMHN in dementia care – something that we have been advocating for some time now (Keady 1996) – coupled with a void in the national leadership and steering of the profession, the potential for CMHNs to be vulnerable to change and the re-ordered priorities of employing organizations is considerable. Indeed, the more (mental) health policy and social structures dilute the discourse around the place of nursing in dementia care, the greater the likelihood of dementia being removed from a national agenda on what constitutes a meaningful, efficient and effective mental health nursing workforce. Without strong leadership, political will and commitment to inclusion, such a scenario, as negative and unwelcome as it may appear, may become a self-fulfilling prophecy.

As Editors (collectively) of the two volumes of *Community Mental Health Nursing and Dementia Care*, we have approached this final chapter by pooling our thoughts and developing a bullet-pointed list – some of which are rambling and lengthy, others short and concise – on what we see as a range of challenges and opportunities facing CMHNs who work with people with dementia and their families. These messages are drawn from a number of sources. Some have been based upon the overarching threads and contributions found in the two volumes, while others are simply the result of a wish-list, exposure/sensitivity to practice/policy and clear blue sky thinking. They are intended neither to be hierarchical nor definitive, simply a pathway to illuminate our own understandings and priorities. However, readers are invited to act on, debate, remove and add to the list as they see fit.

Thoughts and messages

On CMHN practice and research

- While our two edited volumes provide, we hope, a context for a deeper and more appreciative understanding of CMHN practice in dementia care, it can be no more than an introduction to the field. There remains a significant need to find consensus and agreement about CMHN practice in dementia care in order to define its field of contribution, describe, develop and test its evidence-base and unify approaches to assessment, intervention and reporting.

- CMHNs in dementia care meet and interact with potential participants for research endeavour just about every day of their working lives, namely their case-loads. The use of practitioner-research methods (Reed and Procter 1995), and the production of imaginative and practice-relevant research questions, could turn everyday encounters into evidence for peer dissemination. Naturally, this approach is subject to consent and NHS research and governance procedures, but the implications of adopting such a methodology could pay dividends. For instance, separate CMHN practitioner-research studies in North Wales and Manchester have combined a longitudinal, in-depth case study design with an underpinning narrative/constructivist approach in order to develop:

  - a life review procedure to enrich and inform cognitive assessment within a memory clinic setting (Keady *et al.* 2005);

  - the use of ecomaps and genograms as foundations for early-stage intervention, decision-making and support (Keady *et al.* 2004); and

  - a negotiated sessional plan for the family support of a parent with dementia using a relationship-centred approach (Keady *et al.* in press).

  The field is ripe for additional studies and the compilation and dissemination of evidence from everyday experience.

- The role of the CMHN in health promotion work is an under-developed, reported and evaluated aspect of dementia care practice.

- The 'cure v. care' model has not been applicable to mental health where the doctor may have problems in understanding, let alone curing, severe, chronic or enduring mental health problems, and where nurses have generally preferred to care about people rather than take care of them. This view is recognized by the Chief Nursing Officer in her recent review of mental health nursing (DOH 2006a) where the value of positive therapeutic relations is highlighted and where the recovery model (Anthony 1993) is recommended as the basis for nursing practice. Around these views is a broader change agenda from which recurrent themes, such as the importance of holistic and evidence-based care, can emerge. For CMHNs in dementia care, the challenge is to mine and exploit such opportunities.

- In the future, CMHNs roles and relationships, especially with psychiatrists, will continue to change and develop. The Department of Health are of the opinion that the cultural change within health care alongside demographic pressures means that there is a need for a new and changing role for the psychiatrist; this is articulated through the *New Ways of Working* document (DH 2006b). The proposal is that a consultant psychiatrist may be used to best effect by concentrating on those people with the greatest needs and that other responsibilities should be redistributed throughout the multi-disciplinary team. With a continuing emphasis being placed upon the early detection, diagnosis and treatment of mental health problems, it seems likely that, in the future, CMHNs are going to be asked to 'step up to the mark' and assume responsibility for the management of those with early dementia.

- The specialization of nursing into dementia care has been fuelled by the belief that people with dementia can benefit from interventions delivered by a highly skilled workforce. The opportunity for this has to be seized, in part through changing service models such as memory clinics which have provided CMHNs with access to people with increasingly early stages of cognitive loss, and in part through developing a greater awareness of the needs of those beyond the person with dementia, as is the case with Admiral Nursing. As an illustration, Page et al. (in press) have shown that specialist memory clinic nurses can diagnose dementia with 94 per cent accuracy, achieving a kappa of 0.88, which represents an almost perfect degree of agreement with later 'psychiatrist made' diagnosis (Macclure and Willett 1987). Additional randomized controlled studies are required to demonstrate CMHN competencies at assessment, diagnosis, disclosing diagnosis, prescribing, delivering an array of psychosocial interventions and crisis management.

- CMHN practice in dementia care is predominantly constructed from a relational and family-centred context with its efficacy demonstrated through the interpersonal skills, practice experience and knowledge of the CMHN. To date, the role has been defined through sustained and prolonged engagement where the CMHN has entered into the daily life and fabric of the family. In the future, the sustainability of such long-term relationships is likely to come under increasing scrutiny and threat (from the health service's drive for efficiency and cost savings if nothing else), and therefore CMHNs will need to embrace more targeted and time-limited interventions with those with the most complex needs. The training and case supervision of non-professionally qualified staff, e.g. NVQ level care staff, are likely to replace the previously held 'lengthy relationships' of old, bringing new skills of negotiation, sharing core skills, staff empowerment and supervision to the fore, as has recently been demonstrated in a pilot project in the north of England (Ryan et al. 2004).

- The role, training and team location of CMHNs involved in palliative and end-stage dementia are yet to be fully reported, despite their (potential) presence in such services being broadly welcomed (Robinson et al. 2005). Additional practice reporting, research commentary and pilot projects are required to further define this role.

- It is imperative that CMHNs publish more widely in a variety of outlets and sources, from *Newsletters* through to book chapters, practice journals and peer reviewed articles. The profession needs a body of evidence to show to service users (not simply NHS managers) that their role is part of a specialist area of practice with a unifying theme. On this latter point, we would recommend the adoption of a rehabilitative approach to dementia care practice and nursing, not a focus on deficits or recovery.

On mental health policy and education

- Recent reviews into mental health nursing in England (DOH 2006a) and Scotland (Scottish Executive 2006) contain similar shortcomings with respect to dementia care nursing. Underpinning each Review is the 'recovery approach'. This approach, as intimated in our previous bullet point, does not fit in very well with nursing people who have a progressive and degenerative condition. While the idea of recovery has been developed with respect to younger people with mental health conditions, little work has shown the use and value of the approach when nursing people with dementia. The idea of recovery is largely an unexplored and untested idea with respect to dementia care nursing and seems to owe more to nursing other client-groups within mental health care.

- *From Values to Action* (DOH 2006a) is primarily a consultative document and comprises opinions of different people and bodies involved in the provision of mental health care. However, the Review gives little indication as to what extent the consultation specifically addressed people with dementia and dementia care nursing. Indeed, the focus on the recovery approach confirms suspicions that the consultation period was primarily concerned with younger people with mental health conditions rather people with dementia. The recommendations of the Review seem to be about another area of nursing rather than dementia care nursing. This begs the question as to why CMHN practice, and dementia care nursing more broadly, has not received a review of its own. Commissioning such a study would help to allay some of the underlying suspicions and concerns about the place of dementia care nursing within mental health nursing more broadly.

- A set of capabilities and competencies for mental health nurses accompanied the publication of *From Values to Action* (DH 2006a). While they do not specifically relate to mental health nursing to people with dementia, and thus raise the question of whether they are applicable to nursing people with dementia, a further shortcoming may be identified. This shortcoming relates to the atheoretical nature of capabilities and competencies in which nurses are not offered a framework that allows them to understand the relationship between different social phenomena within specific clinical situations. Thus a particular capability or competence may advocate that mental health nurses should work with the person who has dementia and their family, but give no indication about psychological or sociological theories and how they may interact with each other. The Review's emphasis on capabilities and competencies allows mental health nursing to be constructed in the same way and does not link the essential relationship between capabilities and competences with wider theoretical, explanatory frameworks. Failing to highlight this link:

  o reduces the ability of nurses to contribute towards sound and evidence-based decision-making;

  o creates a low level version of mental health nursing that seriously affects their standing within multi-disciplinary mental health teams; and

○   brings about situations in which nurses may put clients at risk as a result of their
limited and superficial training and educational background.

- There is an urgent need to make explicit the content of, and exposure to, dementia
care education across all specialisms in pre-registration nurse education. Working with
people with dementia and their families is not the sole preserve of CMHNs, or any
other mental health-trained staff but, arguably, it is the responsibility of CMHNs to
disseminate their knowledge and practice to the nursing profession as a whole.
Providing educational consultancy would appear an important future role, as is the
training and consultancy role to primary care staff as recommended a few years ago
by the Audit Commission's (2000) *Forget Me Not* report. Recent research has
highlighted the importance of training primary care staff about dementia through a
structured and time-limited educational programme (Downs et al. 2006). Indeed,
these authors demonstrated through a randomized controlled trial that the delivery of
such programmes helped to improve earlier detection rates, raised the quality and
quantity of case note entries and facilitated the use of more case-sensitive screening
and assessment tools in primary care practice (Wilcock et al. 2003; Downs et al. 2006).
This evidence-base could be used by CMHNs within their own practice locality to
further develop and influence care practice.

- People with dementia and their families need to be involved in setting the agenda
for CMHN practice and in articulating the educational, research and practice
programmes that underpin mental health nursing values and discourse. This needs to
be lifted beyond the rhetorical and woven into the fabric of everyday life and practice.
People with dementia, their families and social networks/communities are the greatest
strength and asset that the profession has.

A final word

The opportunity to edit the two *Community Mental Health Nursing and Dementia Care*
books has been a real privilege and has opened our eyes to the complexity, diversity and
sheer dedication of CMHNs in the United Kingdom, Ireland and other parts of the world
to providing high quality, person-centred nursing care to people with dementia and their
families, often in difficult and demanding situations. People with dementia and their
families need the services of CMHNs and CMHNs need access to people with dementia
and their families. It is a tautology that has been evident for the past 50 years. The next
50 years will pose many challenges, but whoever, at this time, is editing texts on the practice
of mental health nursing, it is crucial that the voice and experience of people with dementia
and their families are centre stage and integral to its contents. Any other outcome would be
hard to contemplate.

References

Anthony, W.A. (1993) Recovery from mental illness: the guiding vision of the mental health service
system in the 1990's, *Psychosocial Rehabilitation Journal*, 16: 11–23.
Audit Commission (2000) *Forget Me Not: Mental Health Services for Older People*. London: Audit
Commission.

Department of Health (2006a) *From Values to Action: The Chief Nursing Officer's Review of Mental Health Nursing*. London: Department of Health.

Department of Health (2006b) *New Ways of Working for Psychiatrists: Enhancing Effective, Person-centred Services through New Ways of Working in Multidisciplinary and Multi-agency Contexts. Final Report 'But Not the End of the Story'*. London: Department of Health.

Downs, M., Turner, S., Bryans, M., Wilcock, J., Keady, J., Levin, E., O'Carroll, R., Howie, K. and Iliffe, S. (2006) Effectiveness of educational interventions in improving detection and management of dementia in primary care: cluster randomised controlled study, *British Medical Journal*, 332: 692–6.

Keady, J. (1996) The experience of dementia: a review of the literature and implications for nursing practice, *Journal of Clinical Nursing*, 5(5): 275–88.

Keady, J., Ashcroft-Simpson, S., Halligan, K. and Williams, S. (in press) Admiral Nursing and the family care of a parent with dementia: using autobiographical narrative as grounding for negotiated clinical practice and decision-making, *Scandinavian Journal of Caring Sciences*.

Keady, J., Williams, S. and Hughes-Roberts, J. (2005) Emancipatory practice development through life-story work: changing care in a memory clinic in North Wales, *Practice Development in Health Care*, 4(4): 203–12.

Keady, J., Woods, B., Hahn, S. and Hill, J. (2004) Community mental health nursing and early intervention in dementia: developing practice through a single case history, *International Journal of Older People Nursing*, 13(6b): 57–67.

Maclure, M. and Willett, W.C. (1987) Misinterpretation and misuse of the kappa statistic, *American Journal of Epidemiology*, 126: 161–9.

Ryan, T., Nolan, M., Enderby, P. and Reid, D. (2004) 'Part of the family': sources of job satisfaction among a group of community-based dementia care workers, *Health and Social Care in the Community*, 12(2): 111–18.

Page, S., Hope, K., Bee, P. and Burns, A. (in press) Nurse diagnosis of Dementia: a potential change in practice, *International Journal of Geriatric Psychiatry*.

Reed, J. and Procter, S. (1995) *Practitioner Research in Health Care: The Inside Story*. London: Chapman and Hall.

Robinson, L., Hughes, J., Daley, S., Keady, J., Ballard, C. and Volicer, L. (2005) End-of-life care and dementia, *Reviews in Clinical Gerontology*, 15: 135–48.

Scottish Executive (2006) *Rights, Relationships and Recovery: The Report of the National Review of Mental Health Nursing in Scotland*. Edinburgh: Scottish Executive.

Wilcock, J., Iliffe, S., Walters, K., Rait, G., Austin, T., Turner, S., Bryans, M., Downs, M., O'Carroll, R.E. and Keady, J. (2003) The development of an evidence-based curriculum for dementia care training in general practice, *Education and Ageing*, 17(2/3): 217–36.

Index

COMMUNITY MENTAL HEALTH NURSING AND DEMENTIA CARE
PRACTICE PERSPECTIVES

John Keady, Charlotte L. Clarke and Trevor Adams

A rounded account of Community Mental Health Nurses' practice in dementia care has been long overdue. This is the first book to focus on the role of Community Mental Health Nurses in their highly valued work with both people with dementia and their families.

This book:

- explores the complexity and diversity of Community Mental Health Nurse work;
- captures perspectives from along the trajectory of dementia;
- identifies assessment and intervention approaches;
- discusses an emerging evidence base for implications in practice.

Contributions to this collection of essays and articles are drawn from Community Mental Health Nurse practitioners and researchers at the forefront of their fields.

It is key reading for practitioners, researchers, students, managers and policy makers in the field of community mental health nursing and/or dementia care.

Contributors
Trevor Adams, Peter Ashton, Gill Boardman, Angela Carradice, Chris Clark, Charlotte L. Clarke, Jan Dewing, Sue Hahn, Mark Holman, John Keady, Kath Lowery, Jill Manthorpe, Cathy Mawhinney, Anne Mason, Paul McCloskey, Anne McKinley, Linda Miller, Gordon Mitchell, Elinor Moore, Michelle Murray, Mike Nolan, Peter Nolan, Tracy Packer, Sean Page, Marilla Pugh, Helen Pusey, Assumpta Ryan, Alison Soliman, Vicki Traynor, Dot Weaks, Heather Wilkinson.

Contents
*Contributors – Acknowledgements – Editorial note – Foreword by Professor Mike Nolan – Introduction – **Part One: Setting the scene: the landscape of contemporary community mental health nursing practice in dementia care** – Voices from the past – Integrating practice and knowledge in a clinical context – Multidisciplinary teamworking – 'We put our heads together' – Risk and dementia – **Part Two: Dementia care nursing in the community: assessment and practice approaches** – Assessment and therapeutic approaches for community mental health nursing dementia care practice – Cognitive-behavioural interventions in dementia – Turning rhetoric into reality – From screening to intervention – The community mental health nurse role in sharing a diagnosis of dementia – Group therapy – Psychosocial interventions with family carers of people with dementia – Admiral nurses – Normalization as a philosophy of dementia care – Assessing and responding to challenging behaviour in dementia – **Part Three: Leading and developing community mental health nursing in dementia** – Clinical supervision and dementia care – Multi-agency and inter-agency working – Higher level practice – Index.*

320pp   0 335 21142 9 (Paperback)   0 335 21143 7 (Hardback)

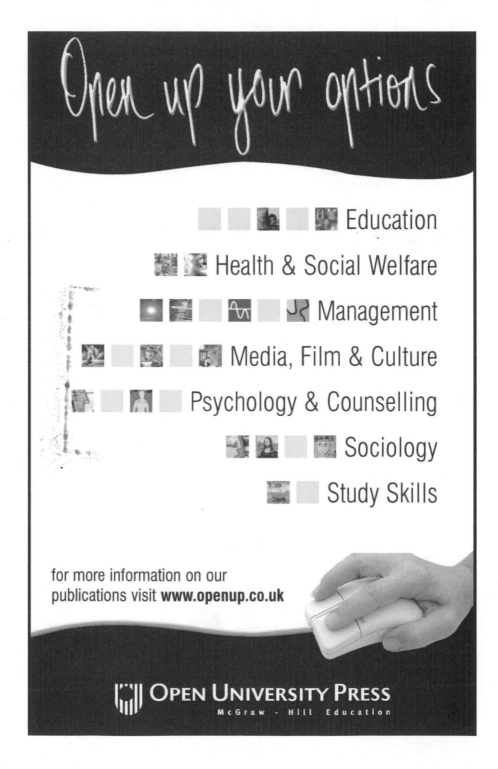